Health Care
in Nicaragua

HEALTH CARE IN NICARAGUA

Primary Care Under Changing Regimes

Richard Garfield

Glen Williams

New York   Oxford
OXFORD UNIVERSITY PRESS
1992

Oxford University Press

Oxford   New York   Toronto
Delhi   Bombay   Calcutta   Madras   Karachi
Kualu Lumpur   Singapore   Hong Kong   Tokyo
Nairobi   Dar es Salaam   Cape Town
Melbourne   Auckland

and associated companies in
Berlin   Ibadan

Published by Oxford University Press, Inc.,
200 Madison Avenue, New York, New York 10016

Oxford is a registered trademark of Oxford University Press

Library of Congress Cataloging-in-Publication Data
Garfield, R. M.
Health care in Nicaragua : primary care under changing regimes /
Richard Garfield, Glen Williams.
p. cm.   Includes bibliographical references and index.
ISBN 0-19-506753-3
1. Public health—Nicaragua.   I. Williams, Glen.
II. Title. [DNLM: 1. Delivery of Health Care—Nicaragua.
2. Health Planning—Nicaragua.   3. Health Policy—Nicaragua.
4. Primary Health Care.   W 84.6 G231h]
RA454.N5G37   1992
362.1′097285—dc20   DNLM/DLC
for Library of Congress   91-32069

9 8 7 6 5 4 3 2 1

Printed in the United States of America
on acid-free paper

Foreword

Nicaragua's long and beleaguered quest for self-determination shows that a popular revolution—unlike a coup—is not won definitively through armed struggle. Nor is democracy invariably assured by holding elections, no matter how fairly votes are counted. A people's revolution, like true democracy, entails progressive transformation of social structures. It is a process that necessarily continues long after the last shots are fired.

In this updated edition of their book, Richard Garfield and Glen Williams make it clear that the Nicaraguan revolution has neither been won nor lost; it is still underway. During eleven years as Nicaragua's government, the Sandinistas made enormous gains in health, education, and fairer distribution of land, wealth, and resources. They also made some serious miscalculations. Both successes and mistakes are objectively discussed by Garfield and Williams in this book.

As for mistakes, it is often said of the top Sandinista leaders that power went to their heads, that they became overly militant or increasingly authoritarian (their enemies say "totalitarian"), that they gradually distanced themselves from the will of the people and for this reason lost popular support.

There is little question, however, that toward the end of the eighties the main reasons for the diminishing popular support for the Sandinista government were the persistently worsening economic crisis and the relentless terrorism of the Contras. Both, of course, were a direct result of the U.S. government's strategy of "low-intensity conflict." Rather than aiming at a decisive military victory, this strategy was designed to gradually erode popular support for the revolutionary government. Relentless military hostilities and undermining of the economy unleashed a vicious cycle of growing public unrest and increasingly heavy-handed governmental control. Resultant abuses of authority were then blown out of proportion so as to bear out the U.S. charges of totalitarian rule. The final goal was to foment a popular uprising or, in lieu of that, to oust the Sandinistas by tampering with Nicaragua's national elections.

Although the Sandinista leadership did make some serious mistakes, it maintained a deep, consistent commitment to equity. Compared to most governments in the Americas (including the U.S. government), the Sandinistas were remarkably open and responsive to the will of farmworkers, laborers, low-income groups, women, organizations of disabled persons, and other sectors ignored or marginalized by most governments. The growing inability to meet people's most basic needs was less a measure of Sandinista mismanagement than of the brutal effectiveness of low-intensity conflict—a relentless war of attrition waged by the world's most powerful nation. Nowhere was the Sandinista government more responsive to the needs and wishes of the people than in the areas of health and education. Yet, when resources are limited, decisions about where to allocate them most effectively are often difficult.

Under Somoza—as in many countries where human rights are systematically denied—community-based health initiatives in Nicaragua became a springboard for critical analysis of health-related grievances, and provided a forum for strategic planning, group action, and cooperative self-defense. By encouraging people to diagnose the causes of their common ills, community health workers became increasingly politicized. In turn, they helped groups of people reflect upon their situation and plan organized action to cope with the underlying man-made causes of poor health. They became increasingly aware that health problems often had their roots unjust social structures. Thus health workers committed to people's overall well-being gradually assumed a central role as "agents of social change." As agents of change, community health workers were also branded as subversives by those set on preserving the inequities of the status quo. Selective targeting of health workers is, of course, not unique to Nicaragua. Community health workers have been brutally attacked in El Salvador, Guatemala, South Africa, the Philippines, and other places where ruling elites try to crush people's attempts at self-determination. By contrast, government health workers and health posts have been savagely targeted by mercenary rebels and guerrilla terrorists such as UNITA in Angola, RENAMO in Mozambique, the contras in post-Somoza Nicaragua, and most recently by vigilante "settlers" in the West Bank. All these mercenary groups were backed by regional superpowers (e.g. South Africa, the United States, and Israel) bent on crushing people-centered governments committed to self-determination and equity-oriented development.

By the late seventies, an extensive network of nongovernmental community health programs extended throughout Nicaragua, especially in rural areas and poverty-stricken urban *barrios*. When I visited in 1977, these grassroots health initiatives were playing a key role in mobilizing people in defense of their well-being and rights. Community health programs and workers were already under attack. In a vain attempt to co-opt these independent health programs or make them redundant. Somoza's health ministry—with help from USAID—launched a project to train local "health promoters." Beneath its pro-people façade, the government program was still topdown, and was weakened by endless restrictive, disempowering "norms." In sum, it was more limiting than liberating. Predictably, the government program failed to get off the ground, while the informal network of nongovernmental programs continued to expand.

The network of people-centered health initiatives was a key element in the awakening and mobilization of the people that finally led to liberation from the Somoza dictatorship. Likewise, in the Philippines, the massive, peaceful uprising of millions of people that resulted in the overthrow of the dictator Ferdinand Marcos did not just happen spontaneously. Years of awakening and grassroots mobilization had paved the way. The nationwide "community-based health care" movement, largely spearheaded by adherents of liberation theology, played a crucial role in this process. Facilitators of community discussion groups led participants through a process of "structural analysis" in which they traced the societal causes of poor health and then worked toward collective solutions. As a result, many progressive doctors, health workers, educators, and religious leaders were arrested, and some were tortured and killed. These abuses precipitated mass demonstrations and strengthened demands for a government more responsive to basic human needs.

In many parts of the world, progressive health movements play an important role in popular struggles against repressive regimes. This is true in El Salvador and Guatemala, where village health workers are playing a social role similar to that which they played in somocista Nicaragua. It is true in South Africa, where conscientious health professionals—outraged by the South African Medical Association's coverup of its members' implication in the torture and death of Black Consciousness leader Steve Biko—formed the alternative National Medical and Dental Association (NAMDA), which is committed to ending apartheid. And it is true of the Occupied Territories, where one third of Arab doctors have joined the Union of Palestinian Medical Relief Committees, which trains community health activists and stands up against the Israeli government's routine violations of Palestinians' health and rights.

Nicaragua and the Philippines have provided the world with two outstanding examples of how "people power" can topple oppressive dictators. Unfortunately, for both these nations, the real and potential social gains of liberation (including far-reaching improvements in health) were soon seriously compromised. In both cases, the U.S. government has helped a privileged, self-seeking minority to undermine the progress and popular support of the nations' new leaders.

In spite of setbacks, the people-centered struggle for health continues in both Nicaragua and the Philippines, as it does in El Salvador, Guatemala, the West Bank, South Africa, and other countries where unfair social structures make self-help imperative.

In the final two chapters of this book, which appear for the first time in this updated edition, the authors relate how, ironically, the overthrow of the Sandinistas and the consequent swing toward privatization of health care has in some ways pushed the Nicaraguan people toward a more decentralized, self-reliant approach. Less able to count on the government for equitable and affordable health services, community health workers and the public are turning to each other for mutual assistance and support.

Whether the remarkable improvements in health achieved during the eighties will be continued while the Sandinistas attempt to "rule from below" will depend on a number of factors, including international support for people-centered health and development initiatives begun by the Sandinistas. Some progressives, disillusioned by the Nicaraguan people's unwillingness to reelect the Sandinistas, have withdrawn their backing and assistance since the elections. But others have continued in solidarity with the troubled yet still viable revolution, lending a helping hand to the Nicaraguan people, who need it more than ever.

* * *

In 1980 representatives from the new Ministry of Health (MINSA) traveled to Project Piaxtla, the villager-run health care network in western Mexico with which I have been involved since 1965. By this time Project Piaxtla had become well known in much of Latin America, partly because of the villagers' health care handbook *Where There Is No Doctor,* which grew out of that experience.

The two visitors from MINSA, both Sandinistas and long-time community health activists, were committed to the idea that Nicaragua's revolutionary health policy should focus on community-based rather than hospital/doctor-oriented promotion of health. Their purpose in visiting the Mexican villager-run program was to explore participatory learning methods and to sharpen their perspectives for a "people-centered" approach, as well as to ask the help of the village team in drafting a community-oriented national health plan.

The debate in Nicaragua between community-based and hospital/doctor-oriented health care was subsequently resolved through a compromise. Large numbers of doctors and nurses and much larger numbers of community health workers (called *brigadistas*) were trained. However, the skills taught to the *brigadistas* were more restricted, especially in terms of curative care, than either we or the Sandinista advocates of a community-based approach would have liked. Even in revolutionary Nicaragua, many doctors were reluctant to let go of their monopoly on medical skills.

One outcome of the Sandinista health planners' visit to Mexico was a week-long workshop in which I participated in Ciudad Sandino, a sprawling, poor barrio lying on the outskirts of Managua. The workshop was organized by the local health committee and attended by health educators and local *brigadistas,* many of whom had become *multiplicadores* who were responsible for training and advising new *brigadistas.*

The workshop got off to a good start. Enthusiasm was high. Role plays, puppet shows, and the involvement of mothers, school teachers, and school children helped bring learning to life. Everyone was eager to continue. But after the first few days, a message arrived from the health ministry (MINSA) ordering that the workshop be suspended so that the *brigadistas* could take part in a national campaign against measles. A vaccination campaign of all the country's children had been scheduled for the coming weekend, and *brigadistas* were to give top priority to preparing the community for the campaign.

The workshop participants were distraught. They felt that they were learning exciting, valuable techniques for more effective health education, and were upset at the prospect of terminating the workshop. An emergency meeting was held with the town's health committee and community leaders. The community group drafted a message back to the health ministry, reminding it that the ministry's responsibility was to advise and provide backup to the *brigadistas* and community health committees, not to tell them what to do. The *brigadistas* pointed out that they were accountable to, and took their directives from, the community. The community committee had decided that the workshop was important and should continue. However, they explained, they agreed that the national measles campaign was also very important. Therefore they would continue the workshop, but with a strong emphasis on community activities designed to inform residents and make possible the fullest participation in the campaign.

I was astounded by the audacity of the *brigadistas* and town committee in challenging the authority of the health ministry! I think the fact that many of the *brigadistas* and *multiplicadores* were seasoned Sandinistas, who had first become health activists during the people's struggle to end tyrannical rule, had given them the strength and solidarity to stand up to abuse of authority, even when it came from their revolutionary government.

I was even more astounded when later that afternoon a reply came back from the health ministry, apologizing for having given such paternalistic orders. It praised the community for keeping the ministry in line and endorsed the *brigadistas'* plan to continue the workshop with a focus on preparing people for the measles campaign.

This confrontation between the ministry of health and the people of Ciudad Sandino, in which the ministry yielded to and respected the community's decision, did more than anything else I witnessed to convince me that the Nicaraguan revolution was not only people-supportive, but to a large extent people-directed. MINSA's respect for the community's judgement paid off. On the days leading up to the measles campaign, the workshop participants developed a wide range of activities engaging the community in learning about the importance of immunization. They conducted skits, told stories, and invited school children to take part in puppet shows.

One of the biggest successes of the workshop was a street theater production titled "The Measles Monster." In this skit the "monster"—an actor with a sweeping red cloak, a huge devil's mask, and giant, clawed hands—chases after children in the street, trying to catch those who have not been vaccinated against measles. After a wild chase, the monster catches a child (one of the actors) wearing a white happy-faced mask. The monster envelopes the boy in its cloak, and when the child reappears he is wearing another mask, covered with the red spots of measles. The boy becomes very sick and nearly dies. His distressed parents now realize that their fears had been misdirected and vow never to miss a vaccination date for their children in the future. At the end of the skit a loud-speaker calls out to the audience, "Why did the little boy get measles?" The question is repeatedly broadcast until everyone present shouts back, "Because he wasn't vaccinated!" Then the loud-speaker calls out, "And how did the community finally defeat the Measles Monster?" The audience shouts back, "They vaccinated all the children!" "Then what are you going to do this Saturday?" challenges the loud-speaker. And the audience trumpets back, "Vaccinate every child!"

It is anybody's guess how many children's lives this simple skit has helped to save. It has been reenacted in many parts of Nicaragua, modified and acted out in many parts of the world, and reproduced in Spanish and Portuguese editions of *Helping Health Workers Learn*.

On reflection, this street theater production of the Measles Monster—first created and performed by the *brigadistas* and children of Ciudad Sandino—communicates more than a message about how to prevent measles. Like the Nicaraguan revolution itself, it offers a vivid example of how ordinary people can triumph when they unite to overcome forces that threaten to destroy their health.

* * *

Why were the Reagan and Bush administrations so determined to "neutralize" the Sandinista government that they were willing to violate international law, make secret arms deals with Iran, lie to Congress and the public, and even finance illegal arms shipments to the Contras through trafficking of cocaine and heroin into the United States? What did the world's most powerful nation have to fear from a tiny, struggling nation like Nicaragua?

The answer is obvious but disturbing. The success of the Nicaragua revolution posed a threat to the national security of the world's power brokers (including the U.S. government, multinational big business, and the military-industrial complex), who put economic growth before equity and profit before people. For all its imperfections, Nicaragua under the Sandinistas served as a living prototype of an intrinsically nonviolent social order: a truly popular approach to government based on equity-oriented development rather than on growth-oriented development, on sharing rather than greed. The White House did not try to crush the Sandinista government because it was "undemocratic," but because the Sandinista government—with or without elections—was more responsive to the needs of all its citizens (hence, more truly democratic) than our own.

Much can be learned from the Nicaraguan experience. In this book, Richard Garfield and Glen Williams help show how the Nicaraguan revolution opened the way for a more participatory approach to health care and to remarkable improvements in the health in the face of formidable obstacles. Although the Sandinistas were defeated at the polls in 1990, the slogan "Sandino lives" still rings true in the hearts of millions of Nicaraguans. The Nicaraguan revolution—and the people-centered approach to health and development it engendered—remains a deep-seated force in Nicaraguan society. It deserves our comprehension and merits our support.

Together with the authors of this book, I believe that we must help the people of Nicaragua to achieve well-being and self-determination, and to renew the participatory, equity-oriented approach which gave the world a role model and the vision of a fairer, healthier society.

Palo Alto, California   *David Werner*

Preface

I first visited Nicaragua in 1980 for what was supposed to be a brief visit. From the airport I was whisked off to an old seminary, where new leaders were formulating health policy late into the night. Their optimism and commitment were irresistible. Soon I found myself a part of the system described and analyzed in this book.

The text is based in part on my experience working in the offices of nursing, malaria, epidemiology, and the public health school during the early eighties. I worked as a data analyst, administrator, trainer, clinician, and health educator. After joining the faculty of Columbia University in 1986, I continued collaborating in Nicaragua for short periods each year with the Ministry of Health (MINSA) and/or the Pan American Health Organization (PAHO).

Although it attempts an objective analysis, this book is no doubt influenced by my personal perspective. Like many other North Americans who went to Nicaragua in the eighties, I considered myself the inheritor of a tradition begun in the "freedom summers" in the U.S. South. What the civil rights movement represented domestically in the sixties, the primary health care strategy of the eighties represents internationally. At a time when the gap between the "haves" and the "have-nots" was growing in much of the world, in Nicaragua it was shrinking. Like the students who gave up their summers to confront racism in the Deep South, we saw in Nicaragua an important opportunity to promote justice and development. Such grandiose aims offered little consolation when hot, hungry, and broke in Managua. Yet, except for many boring and a few terrifying moments, my work there has been enormously satisfying.

One of my most surprising experiences was meeting Justo Pastor Zamora, a vice-minister of health under Somoza. In 1980, he had returned to his private practice, working as an orthopedist. Despite his excessive defenses of Somoza, he clearly was a generous and caring practitioner. He recounted to me the story of an American physician who visited the polio ward of El Retiro Hospital: "Everyone had abandoned these poor creatures. Paralysis had so affected them that they could not even cough—some of them were drowning in their own secretions because no one helped." The

American doctor, who suctioned the polio patients' mucus manually, became a model for Dr. Zamora. I was moved by his story, but saw it as an eloquent testimony to the failure of the old regime. A few individuals, no matter how caring, would never save the children or prevent polio. His own defense of the former regime seemed to me a reflection of the necessity for radical change ushered in by the Sandinista revolution.

My first exposure to rural Nicaragua came through Ania, the twelve-year-old daughter of the family with whom I lived. Ania was gracious, simple, and had killed one of Somoza's soldiers in the revolution a year earlier. She was now in charge of literacy training in a hilly, dry rural community in the central region of the country. This was outside the town of Acoyapa, in the Chontales province, six hours by jeep and half an hour on horseback from Managua. The town of Acoyapa had 8,000 people; the rural area where Ania lived had 100. The household where Ania stayed was made of sticks and straw and housed eight people, a pig, and two goats. Everything got wet when it rained and there was no water when the rain barrel was empty. The staple food was tortillas, made by the women from the year's stock of corn stored in a bin on one side of the room. I imagined what it must be like to watch the coming year's food supply dwindle after a bad harvest.

The nearest neighbor lived ten minutes away. In this area, the peasants had felt little of Somoza's fury and were now enjoying the fruits of the revolution that they were tentatively coming to accept. Their crops brought a better price, they were able to buy a kerosene lamp, and they anticipated a steady supply of staples like cooking oil, soap, and salt. All around the country, one felt optimism for progress.

How different it might have appeared had we known that the Contra war was coming. Chontales was one of the areas repeatedly attacked by the Contras between 1984 and 1987. A group from Harvard University surveyed health conditions in Acoyapa in 1987.[1] In all, three clinics in the area had been destroyed, two others had been attacked, and fifteen were closed due to the war. Prenatal care was still a priority in the remaining health centers, and 70 percent of mothers received prenatal care. But immunizations required active community participation, which fell under Contra-led terror. Only 40 percent of the children had immunization cards that were up to date. More than half of the people had a friend or relative killed in the war, and a quarter had received death threats from the Contras. More than 20 percent of the people then living in the town of Acoyapa had moved there since the war started, many to escape the greater dangers in surrounding rural areas. The war eventually affected the entire country's social fabric. I found it hard to believe when the Sandinistas lost the 1990 election and the war ended.

Books about socialist countries are often predictable or worse. Such books often tell more about the leaders' intentions than the results of their policies. Nicaragua has become such an ideological touchstone.

During the Somoza regime, a minister of health was asked the infant mortality rate. "What is the rate for Costa Rica?" he shot back. "Forty per 1,000," an assistant replied. "Then ours is 38," he responded.[2] The actual rate at that time was about 110, but many Sandinista supporters have inflated this figure to 200 or greater for the Somoza period.[3] Not to be outdone, new-right apologists for the Reagan "holy war" against Nicaragua went so far as to report a smallpox epidemic, although this disease had been eradicated from the entire globe seven years earlier![4]

The electoral defeat of the Sandinistas has not, unfortunately, brought an end to the manipulation of health data for narrow political gain. In early 1990, one solidarity publication in the United States commented on the importance of "defending" the Sandinista "achievement" of a national average infant mortality rate of 63.4 per 1,000 live births. Later in the year, after the Chamorro government replaced the Sandinistas, they decried the alarming "rise" in infant mortality to the same 63.4 per 1,000! A rightist group claimed that although mortality had fallen to 65 per 1,000 live births, in the last years of the Sandinista regime it returned to 90 per 1,000.[5]

I wanted to present a more critical and useful analysis. The outcomes of Nicaragua's health programs have been full of twists and turns. While the country's economy fell into shambles, its health system at first succeeded in continuing to improve the general public's well-being and later maintained a partial safety net for those in greatest need. This was due, as we show, to high levels of community participation, the mix of public and private services, and large-scale international assistance. The new government appears committed to continuing many of the effective health policies developed by the Sandinistas.

Several specialized topics receive only scant mention in this book. These include occupational health, intensive curative care, rehabilitation, and mental health. This limitation is the result of our focus on the main programs and problems facing the country. As an epidemiologist, my emphasis is on analysis of data. My coauthor Glen Williams showed where personal experiences were needed to highlight the data. We hope our style brings to life the data that represent people, and makes clear the impact of the health system in their lives.

The primary care strategy, developed near the end of the seventies and implemented in the eighties, concentrated on simple, inexpensive health technologies.[6] UNICEF, for example, identified a basic "package" of services needed for child health to include growth monitoring, oral rehydration, breast-feeding, and immunization. Even without doctors and hospitals, the wide use of these four low-cost approaches would likely cut child deaths in half.

Perhaps the most important component of the primary care strategy outlined in Alma Ata in 1978 was "political will." The Sandinistas began with lofty goals and costly assumptions about what good health care would require. Dialogue among health professionals and demands from the population subsequently led to more modest approaches. Five years of economic strangulation and eight years of war dictated a low-cost, sustainable approach. This decision involved changes in the number and type of health professionals trained, the number and type of medicines distributed, the nature of health campaigns, the role of international assistance, and the type of medical care practiced. The post-Sandinista system is attempting to preserve this low-cost survival system while rebuilding the professional private health system.

We examine efforts by health leaders to involve communities in setting priorities and implementing health programs. We analyze the weaknesses, limitations, and failures of the health system, as well as its achievements. This is not a story of overnight miracles but of hard-won successes, daunting challenges, and painful failures.

The Nicaraguan experience should be useful to many other developing countries. Despite a decade of natural disasters, political upheaval, economic decline, and war, Nicaragua maintained a system of care that responds to the needs of most people. Other societies afflicted by economic decline and deteriorating health systems can develop similarly effective approaches.

This book was developed with the assistance of and published in an earlier version by OXFAM in the United Kingdom. The current text benefits from three more years of data, experience, and discussion. It is not merely an expanded version of the original text but one that is more explicitly analytical, makes more comparisons to other developing countries, and refers more extensively to international debates in health policy circles.

Chapters 1 through 6 chronicle the evolution of health services during the eighties. Chapters 7 through 12 analyze topics of particular interest in more detail. Changes in health policy during the first year of post-Sandinista administration are detailed in Chapter 13. Key topics are discussed in more depth in the concluding chapter. Pertinent data are presented in tables and graphs in the text. These and additional data, along with references to the sources of data, are detailed in the appendices.

New York   R. G.
June 1991

Acknowledgments

OXFAM-UK and NOVIB provided funds that helped make an early draft of this book possible. Other "internationalists" have helped by providing key material for this book. Most important among these are Glen Williams, who as cowriter and editor is single-handedly responsible for making this text readable. Other contributors include Peter Solis of England, who co-authored Chapter 12, Fritz Muller of Holland, who coauthored Chapter 10, and Sally McIntyre in Italy, who coauthored Chapter 7. Key material was also provided by Celine Woznica in Mexico on community participation in Ciudad Sandino (Chapter 3), Tim Takaro and Susan Cookson from the United States on the Contra war in Matagalpa (Chapter 5), Guiseppe Slater from California on hospital services (Chapter 6), Eugenio Taboada in Managua on the organization of health services (Chapter 2), Antonio Dajer in New York on ambulatory care (Chapter 6), Jeffrey Gates in New York on AIDS (Chapter 7), Ennio Cufino in Brazil on child health programs (Chapter 8), Nicky Low in England on post-Sandinista changes (Chapter 13), and Tom Frieden from New York on community participation and medical education (Chapters 4 and 9). Glen Williams and I take responsibility for the entire text, which was generated over numerous drafts developed between our homes in Oxford, Managua, and New York.

Ample support and encouragement for this project came from key Nicaraguan health leaders. These include, most importantly, Dora María Tellez, Leonel Arguello, Carolina Siu, Enrique Morales, Minister Ernesto Salmeron, Freddy Cardenas, Nubia Herrera, Carlos Lopez, José Ramon Cruz, Guillermo Gonzalez, Jorge Arostegui, and Ivan Tercero. Local representatives of UNICEF, including Ennio Cufino and Fernando Lezcano, and PAHO, including Carlos Linger, Miguel Marquez, Antonio Pages, Julio Caldera, and Isabel Turcios, played an important role. Much of the information in this book was collected during work on health projects; additional information was gathered from PAHO and MINSA offices in Managua and the outlying regions. Important editorial reviews were provided by Alan Meyers, Evelyn Mauss, William Bower, Harris Huberman, Paul Schneider, Tom Frieden, Sarah Jackson, Tim Takaro, Susan Cookson, Antonio Dajer, Jonathan Fox, Katheryn McGarrity, Claudia Garcia-Moreno, Victor Penchezadeh, Antonio Ugalde, Michael Zalkin, Eddy Coyle, Peter Sollis, and George Davey-Smith. Translations were made by Esperanza Soriano, editorial assistance was provided by Paul Schneider and Robert Gern, and graphic arts design was provided by David Kiam. We are also indebted to David Morely and Leonor Huper for their encouragement and assistance.

Contents

Abbreviations,   xxi

1. From Chaos to Crisis: Prior to 1979,   3
2. A Health Service for All: 1979–1983,   22
3. Community Participation,   35
4. Mass Mobilizations,   48
5. The War on Health,   67
6. From Expansion to Crisis Management: 1984–1990,   87
7. Women's Health,   112
8. Child Survival,   130
9. Health Professionals,   158
10. Medicines and Medical Equipment,   175
11. Stretching the Shrinking Cordoba,   190
12. Health in a Survival Economy,   201
13. After the Sandinistas,   218
14. The Nicaraguan Health Model,   231

Appendices,   243

A. General Health Data, 1974–1990,   244
B. Comparative Data on Health and Social Conditions in Central America,   261
C. Principal Causes of Death Among Hospitalized Patients, 1980–1987,   264
D. Demographic Variables, 1950–1990,   265
E. Hospital Admissions and Mortality Rates for Diarrheal Diseases, 1980–1987,   266

F. Recorded Deaths by Cause, 1983–1988,   267

G. Organizations That Coordinate Medical Assistance
    to Nicaragua,   268

Notes,   269
Additional Reading,   293
Index,   295

Abbreviations

ADN	Nicaraguan Demographic Association
AMNLAE	Louisa Amanda Espinosa Women's Association
APHA	American Public Health Association
ATC	Rural Workers Association
BCN	Banco Central de Nicaragua
CAHI	Central American Historical Institute
CAM	Center for Medical Supplies (MINSA)
CARE	Citizens Active in Relief Everywhere
CDS	Sandinista Defense Committees
CELADE	Latin American Demographic Center
CEPAD	Evangelical Committee for Aid and Development
CEPAL	Latin American Center for Population Studies
CEPS	Center for Popular Health Studies
CIAV	The International Verification and Support Commission
CIERA	Center for Information and Studies of the Agraria Reform
CIES	Center for Health Information and Studies
CPS	Popular Health Councils
DECOPS	Office for Popular Health Education and Communication (MINSA)
DINEI	National Division for Statistics and Information (MINSA)
ECLAC	Economic Commission for Latin America and the Caribbean
ENABAS	Nicaraguan Supply Company
FETSALUD	Federation of Health Workers
FSLN	Sandinista Front for the Liberation of Nicaragua
IADB	Inter-American Development Bank
INEC	National Institute for Studies and Censuses

INSS	National Institute for Social Security
INSSBI	National Institute for Social Security and Social Welfare
JGN	National Government of Reconstruction
MIDINRA	Ministry of Agrarian Reform
MIFIN	Ministry of Finance
MINSA	Ministry of Health
MIPLAN	Ministry of Planning
NCAHRN	National Central America Health Rights Network
OAS	Organization of American States
OMS	World Health Organization
OPS	Pan American Health Organization
OXFAM	Oxford Famine Relief
PAHO	Pan American Health Organization
PAN	National Food Program
UNAG	National Farmer's Union
UNAN	National Autonomous University
UNESCO	United Nations Education and Cultural Organization
UNICEF	United Nations Children's Fund
UNO	United Nicaragua—Opposition, political coalition headed by Violeta Chomorro
USAID	U.S. Agency for International Development
USHEW	U.S. Department of Health, Education, and Welfare
WHO	World Health Organization

Health Care
in Nicaragua

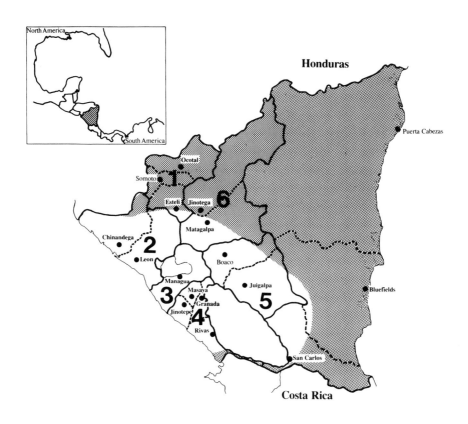

Region	Department	Population*	City
1	Nueva Segovia	144,700	Ocotal
	Madriz	90,300	Somoto
	Esteli	123,300	Esteli
2	Chinandega	298,700	Chinandega
	Leon	297,700	Leon
3	Managua	917,600	Managua
4	Masaya	207,000	Masaya
	Carazo	143,100	Jinotepe
	Grenada	132,900	Granada
	Rivas	115,700	Rivas
5	Chontales	87,400	Juigalpa
	Boaco	89,100	Boaco
6	Matagalpa	241,800	Matagalpa
	Jinotega	117,400	Jinotega
AZ#	North Zelaya	82,000	Puerta Cabezas
	South Zelaya	161,300	Bluefields
	Rio San Juan	35,600	San Carlos

War-Affected Areas

*Estimated Population in 1990 (Source: INEC)
#AZ is the Autonomous Zone

Map of Nicaragua. Inset shows area of detail.

1

From Chaos to Crisis:
Prior to 1979

> In Nicaragua, life is a slow death. I can't live it, nobody can.
> I'm going to fight for life in Nicaragua.
>
> DR. OSCAR DANILO ROSALES,
> killed in action, 27 August 1967)

At one minute past midnight on 23 December 1972, a devastating earthquake hit Managua. It killed 10,000 people, injured 20,000 more, and left three-quarters of the city's 400,000 residents homeless.[1,2] Panic reigned. Survivors rushed the injured to El Retiro—the city's central hospital—only to find it in ruins. Few doctors or nurses were on hand in any case. Many were busy caring for injured members of their own families or protecting the rubble of their homes from thieves. Others, fearing the deluge of patients at the hospital, simply stayed away.

The rule of the jungle quickly became the norm. Those who gained most were, as usual, President Anastasio Somoza-Debayle and his associates. They immediately went into action speculating in land and pocketing millions of dollars in aid, food, and supplies intended for earthquake victims.

Nicaragua has been visited by many natural and man-made disasters in this century. This book examines how health and health services have developed despite some of the greatest limitations found anywhere in the developing world.

The most visible aid from the government of the United States following the 1972 earthquake was barbed wire. It was used to cordon off the central city business district, supposedly to discourage looters. In fact, the barbed wire made looting easier for Somoza's armed forces. The U.S. government and voluntary agencies also sent large quantities of food and medical supplies, but little of it reached those in need.

A U.S. mobile military hospital, with a full contingent of surgical and support staff, arrived within forty-eight hours of the earthquake. The surgical team set up within the confines of the U.S. embassy, where patients with the "right" connections were admitted for treatment. So few were

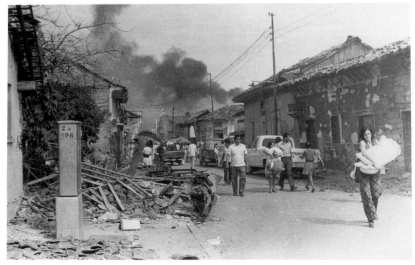

Residents flee as Managua burns following 1972 earthquake.

treated that doctors and nurses passed their time by playing volleyball in the embassy compound. Meanwhile, outside the embassy gate, thousands of people with serious injuries waited in vain for treatment. It was a scene that aptly symbolized Nicaraguan society: A poor majority were excluded by a tiny elite sustained by the United States.

One of the most dramatic economic links between the two countries was the infamous "Plasmaferesis" laboratory in Managua. Arnoldo Ramos was a Cuban expatriate who found safe haven in Nicaragua after the failed Bay of Pigs Invasion of Cuba in1961. He ran a profitable pharmaceutical company in partnership with the Somoza family. In an ingenious new scheme, Ramos and Somoza began exporting blood plasma to the United States in 1971. The "Plasmaferesis" laboratory quickly became one of Managua's major industries, employing 500 workers and producing 15 percent of the world's supply of blood plasma.

By 1975, thousands of people earned a living selling their blood for five dollars a pint to the laboratory. The plasma was then sold for about thirty dollars to dealers in the United States. Since blood donors also received a meal, "vampire Ramos" (as he was known) was never short of would-be donors. Many had recently come to the city from the rural north, where the Somozas had seized their lands for tobacco, sugar, and cotton plantations. The poor districts of Managua overflowed with thousands of ex-peasants who survived most of the year by selling blood, in addition to harvesting export crops on plantations for a few months each year.

The plasma business eventually contributed to the downfall of the Somoza regime. In 1977, the newspaper *La Prensa* reported horrific abuses

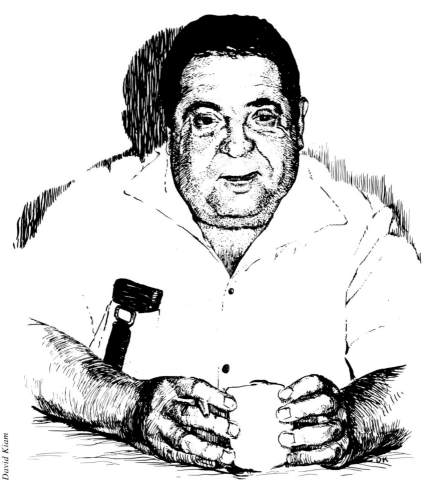

David Kiam

From a photo of Dr. Arnoldo Ramos, 'the vampire', published in the Somoza newspaper *Novedades* in 1977. The caption read, "Dr. Ramos is one of the most respected doctors in all Central America."

occurring in the "Plasmaferesis" laboratory. Front-page photos showing cadavers wholly drained of blood provoked a storm of public anger. Somoza's response was to have Pedro Juaquin Chamorro, editor of *La Prensa*, killed on 10 January 1978. A massive public reaction followed immediately. Angry crowds invaded the hospital where Chamorro's body was being held, and 40,000 people accompanied his coffin to the cemetery. Defying the much-feared National Guard, protesters put Somoza-owned businesses to the torch. Along with banks, factories, and finance houses, the infamous "Plasamferesis" laboratory went up in flames. Former *La Prensa* reporter Silvio Mora remembers: "The Guard watched with glazed eyes, lost and confused before a people which had lost its fear."

This burst of outrage was the spark from which the Sandinista Front for the Liberation of Nicaragua (FSLN) organized a general insurrection and, eighteen months later, overthrew the dictatorship. Somoza fought fiercely to maintain power. About 35,000 people died in the revolutionary war and much of the country's economic and social infrastructure was reduced to ruins.[3] When the Sandinistas finally took power on 19 July 1979, they inherited the highest per capital foreign debt in Latin America. The new government faced the immense task of reconstructing a bankrupt nation that for more than four decades had suffered under one of Latin America's most brutal, corrupt dictatorships. This chapter describes the country and social processes related to health that led to the establishment of the Sandinista government.

THE SANDINISTAS

Formed in 1961, the FSLN developed a mix of Marxism, Christian defense of the poor, and nationalism. It took its name from national hero Augusto Cesar Sandino, whose guerrilla army fought an occupying force of U.S. Marines to a standstill between 1927 and 1933. A thorn in the side of the U.S.-backed Nicaraguan government of the day, Sandino was murdered in 1934 on the orders of Anastasio Somoza García, then-head of the National Guard. In 1936, Somoza assumed the presidency, starting a dynasty that lasted forty-three years.[4,5]

In 1969, the FSLN proclaimed its intention to establish a state based on political pluralism, a mixed economy, and nonalignment in international affairs. They promised to form a government dedicated to pursuing "the logic of the majority" by promoting the interests of poor and marginalized—those who had suffered most under the Somoza regime.[6]

When their third general insurrection brought the Sandinistas to power in 1979, they transformed the executive into a multiparty junta of five persons while legislative power was held by a new National Assembly, dominated by Sandinista-related "mass" organizations. The most powerful group in the country was the nine-member dictatorate of the FSLN. This group had more authority than the executive over the many new governmental ministries established in 1979. Indeed, distinctions between the party and the state were difficult to discern during the first years of the Sandinista government.[7] In 1984, elections led to the first Sandinista president and vice-president and a constituent assembly made of the nine legal parties. Nonetheless, governmental powers gradually devolved to regional and municipal governments during the eighties.

This process took a radical new twist in 1990, when a coalition of center and rightist parties won the presidency through the election of Violeta Barrios de Chamorro, widow of newspaper editor Pedro Juaquin. In what was the first electoral transformation from socialism to capitalism in a developing country, the Sandinistas won control only of some towns and a department, along with the largest voting bloc in the National Assembly.

THE COUNTRY

Wedged between Honduras to the north and Costa Rica to the south, Nicaragua is the largest of the six countries of the Central American isthmus. The population is growing rapidly (see Figure 1–1).

The country has three main geographic regions. The western coast's fertile plains that are home to 60 percent of the people. Numerous volcanoes give the soil its fertility and formed the two great lakes, Lake Managua and Lake Nicaragua. The central uplands are a chain of rugged hills and mountains that run from the northern border almost down to Costa Rica in the south. This region has a temperate climate but little water, and is more sparsely populated. To the east is the so-called Atlantic coast—something of a misnomer for a region of rain forests, savannah, swamps, and lagoons. It occupies almost half the national territory but has only 10 percent of the population.

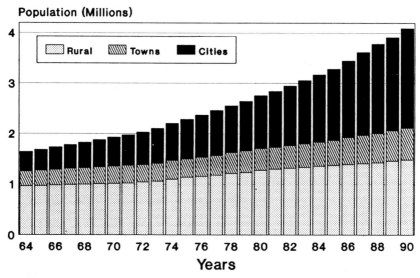

Figure 1–1 Estimated population, 1964–1990. From 1979 to 1990, the population increased by more than 50%. By 1991 it had doubled since the last national census in 1971. Most of this rise was in cities (more than 20,000 inhabitants), where population grew by 75% from 1979. In rural areas (less than 5,000 inhabitants), the population grew by about 25%. These figures assume a growth rate 6% higher than official estimates. The next national census is scheduled to begin in 1992.

The country is dotted with towns, villages, and dispersed rural dwell-
ings.[8] More than 5,000 communities are located in 135 municipalities. The
traditional geographical division is the department, of which there are sixteen. To encourage decentralization, the departments were organized in
1982 into six regions in the Pacific and upland territory and two "special
zones" on the Atlantic coast.[9] Since 1988 the Atlantic coast territories have
been redesignated the "autonomous zone" in recognition of a new measure
of self-governance in these indigenous areas.

The Pacific and upland regions, first colonized by Spain in the early
sixteenth century, are ethnically and culturally homogeneous. Almost all of
the people are Mestizo (of mixed Spanish and indigenous Indian ancestry),
Spanish-speaking, and Roman Catholic. The Atlantic coast, a sphere of
British influence for more than two centuries, is home to six different ethnic
groups. Half the population consists of Spanish-speaking Mestizos who
have migrated from the Pacific region. The largest ethnic minority is the
Miskito people, descendants of indigenous Indians and Afro-Caribbean
slaves or immigrants. The Miskitos still speak their own language and live
mainly in the north. The five non-Mestizo minorities of the Atlantic coast
belong mostly to the Moravian or other Protestant churches.

The economies of the three regions are quite distinct. The Pacific region

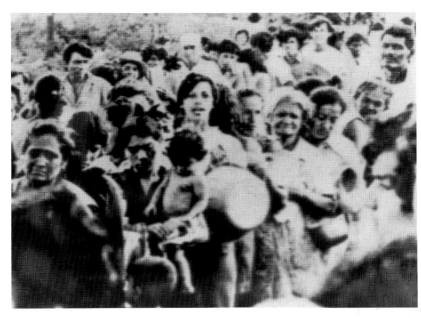

El Nuevo Diario

People made homeless in the 1972 earthquake wait for emergency food rations.
Much of the international aid was misappropriated by President Somoza and his
associates.

produces cotton and sugar for export, as well as maize, rice, and beans for domestic consumption. The central uplands are used primarily for cattle raising and coffee production. On the Atlantic coast, where communications are poorly developed and transport is conducted mainly by river, the main economic activities are lumbering, gold mining, fishing, and subsistence agriculture.

Subsistence agriculture was the main economic activity throughout the country prior to World War II. In the forties, export agriculture began to grow rapidly. The country generated the highest yields per acre and the highest level of capital inputs for agriculture in any Latin American country in the sixties.

A small group of landowners and entrepreneurs, headed by the Somoza family, controlled the economy of the Pacific region. By the seventies, thousands of small-scale farmers, forced off their land on the coastal plain to make way for export crops, worked as itinerant seasonal laborers on large estates. Wealth and income were highly skewed. Average per capita income of the richest 5 percent of the population was $5,409.[10] This was twenty-five times that of the poorest 50 percent of the people, whose income averaged less than $300 a year in the late seventies. Annual per capital rural incomes varied from $90 to $225 by region. The Somozas alone controlled a quarter of the country's agricultural land, as well as the national airline, a bank, the two television stations, a pharmaceutical firm, and more than forty of the country's largest companies.

The economy of the Pacific region was closely linked to the United States, which bought most of its exports and supplied almost all of its imports. Despite its agricultural economy, Nicaragua is one of the most highly urbanized countries in Latin America[11] (Table 1–1). About a million people are believed to live in Managua, whose population has more than doubled since the earthquake of 1972.[8] About a million more live in other cities and towns, and another million live in villages and rural areas.

Table 1–1   Demographic data for Nicaragua, 1990

Population	4.1 million
Infant mortality rate	62 per 1,000 live births
Under five years old mortality rate	95 per 1,000 population
Crude birth rate	42 per 1,000 population
Crude death rate	9 per 1,000 population
Population growth rate	3.4 percent per year
Life expectancy at birth	63 years
Percent of rural population	43
Total average births per woman	5.8

MEDICAL BEGINNINGS

A hundred years after conquistadors first established settlements in the Pacific region, the San Vicente Hospital was established in 1624 in the early capital city, León. Medical training began in 1798 and moved to the newly established university in León a few years later. The practices of European healers were probably inferior to those of the indigenous people, who used herbal medicines, simple surgery, cautery, and midwifery. Hospitals functioned more as objects of philanthropy, charity, and comfort than cure for Hispanic Catholics of the period. Medical leaders in the late nineteenth and twentieth centuries often trained in Europe, and religious orders from Europe supplied nuns to staff the hospitals. Mexican and Panamanian orders also provided staff and assisted in training.

The Rockefeller Foundation initiated a hookworm control program in Nicaragua in 1915. A malaria control program began in 1922 (later converted into a national eradication program in 1958), and initial public health administration began when the General Health Administration was created in 1925. An earthquake and subsequent U.S. military occupation in 1931 brought U.S. military doctors and civilian nurses, who directed many institutions and helped develop what was to become the Ministry of Health in 1946. Baptist and Moravian church missions built hospitals, and the Social Security Health system was established following the growth of an urban working class after World War II.

Health Revolutionaries

Despite the presence of some charity and religious hospitals, many doctors were part of the political and social elite of the country. Some, especially leaders of the *Colegio de Medicos* and Ministry of Health, were vociferous supporters of the regime. Many others took a stand against the system. One of the first was Oscar Danilo Rosales, a highly respected young pathologist. In July 1967, he resigned his post as director of the Department of Pathology at the Medical School in León to join the Sandinista guerrillas. In his letter of resignation to the rector of the university, he explained:[12,13] "In view of the current political situation in Nicaragua . . . I believe that it is the responsibility of all intellectuals . . . to join the ranks of the army of Nicaragua, according to the ideals of the immortal Sandino and under the flag of the FSLN."

A month later, he wrote what was to be his last letter from a mountain hideout: "Tomorrow everything will be different. New airs will be breathed in our country, an aura of justice will prevail and we'll end hunger and misery, malnutrition, ill health, illiteracy, and lack of liberty, from which our people suffer."

On 27 August 1967, in one of the first battles between the FSLN and the National Guard, Rosales and several other guerrillas were killed in an aerial napalm attack. Twelve years later, the new Sandinista-led government renamed the León Medical School in his memory.

Alejandro Davila Bolanos was another early medical revolutionary. Bolanos was a physician, naturalist, anthropologist, literary critic, linguist, and poet. He made a lifelong study of the history, languages, and medicines of the indigenous peoples of Central America. He collected 3,000 texts on these subjects while he worked with peasants and their organizations in the north of the country. A surgeon and father of eight, he was a respected social figure in Estelí. His home was a hub of local literary and political activity.[14]

Pamphlets that Bolanos published in the sixties for peasant farmers reflect the conditions of deprivation with which they coped:

> Good food, housing, money and employment contribute to maintaining health . . . If your boss doesn't give you meat, demand it or ask for eggs in its place . . . Give your children all the milk they want. . . . A garden, however small it may be, is better than a doctor . . . If you have a well, cover the top. . . . Struggle to improve your salary . . . When the children are sick give them boiled water . . . Bathe daily with soap, including the private parts. . . . Improve your house by separating the sleeping and cooking areas and putting in big windows. Separate the place for animals from the food storage area. Send your children to the nearest school and keep yourself informed of their progress. Get together with other *campesino* men like yourself and discuss how to improve the school. Alcohol will make you poorer, more unhappy, and a disgrace. If you are an honorable man, marry the woman with whom you live. . . . When your woman or children are ill, care for them. Don't spend your money on witchcraft or false cures. A pregnant woman needs more milk, vegetables, and meat than normal. If your woman has more than two days of pain in labor and still has not given birth, take her to a hospital. If there are a lot of mosquitoes where you live, sleep under mosquito nets. Demand better roads and communications from the government. Don't sell the land where you live, as you must depend on it for your livelihood.

Bolanos worked closely with the Sandinistas. When a general strike broke out in August 1978 in Estelí, he and seven other leaders were arrested and brutally tortured by the National Guard. His precious library was destroyed as "subversive." He wrote about the experience:[14] "My head moves constantly while the blows continue. They kick me in the chest, face, head, and back . . . I breathe quickly, superficially. The movement of broken ribs torments me more."

Released after three months, Bolanos was back at work in the Estelí hospital when the final insurrection began in April 1979. He was one of several doctors who stayed in the hospital night and day to treat those injured as Somoza's planes bombed the city. The National Guard stormed the hospital, seized Bolanos, and burned his body in front of the hospital. Three months later, the National Guard was defeated and the revolution for which he gave his life became a reality.

Health Status

When the Sandinistas came to power in July 1979, health status in Nicaragua ranked alongside that in Honduras and Bolivia as the worst in continental Latin America. Average life expectancy at birth was estimated at fifty-three years.[15] This low life expectancy was mainly a result of deaths in the first year of life. One in ten babies died before reaching one year of age. The main causes were diarrheal disease, pneumonia, tetanus, measles, and whooping cough. Malnutrition affected more than half of all children. Polio epidemics occurred every few years, leaving hundreds of children permanently disabled.[16]

Some of these problems were beyond the reach of the doctors, nurses, and midwives. Their roots were social and economic—poverty, landlessness, inadequate food supplies, illiteracy, poor housing and sanitation, and lack of clean drinking water.[17]

The health services themselves, though, bore much of the blame. The country's health system was uniquely inefficient and inequitable. Paradoxically, and in contrast to what some critics have suggested,[18,19] a lack of funds was not the main problem. The system was relatively well endowed with funds (including foreign aid), as well as doctors and hospital beds. But the system was severely imbalanced. There were close to 5,000 beds in about forty hospitals, but there were less than 200 health centers in the entire country.[20] Some of these health centers were well designed and lavishly equipped, but most operated at under 50 percent of capacity. The system was riddled with corruption and geared almost exclusively to the needs of the affluent.

It was estimated during the seventies that 90 percent of Nicaragua's health resources were directed to a mere 10 percent of the population.[21] Most of the affluent or medically insured lived in Managua and the second-largest city, León. They controlled most of the country's land, commerce, and industry and consumed most of the health resources. Among these groups, child deaths were about as low, and life expectancy almost as high, as in the United States.

Administrative Chaos

Before the 1979 revolution, Nicaragua's health system was deeply frag-mented. Four separate national institutions and nineteen semiautonomous local agencies were responsible for health services. Because each institution and agency functioned independently, chaos was the norm, with salaries, record keeping, and working practices differing from one town to the next.

The most powerful health institutions was not the Ministry of Health but the National Institute for Social Security (INSS), which provided curative health care to salaried employees. With its own hospitals and clinics in Managua and León, the INSS controlled half of all health expenditures but provided service to only 8.4 percent of the population.[22] Health expenditure per person was more than ten times greater for the insured than the unin-sured. In 1977, insured patients had more than eight times as many outpa-tient visits and prescriptions filled as the rest of the population.[23]

The Ministry of Health, although responsible for preventive care throughout the country and curative services in rural areas, controlled only 16 percent of health expenditure—and 75 percent of this was spent in Man-agua.[24] The National Guard also ran its own hospitals and clinics, providing high quality care to soldiers and their relatives. Private insurance groups, charitable organizations, and local health agencies accounted for most of the remaining health expenditure.

Only 28 percent of the Nicaraguan population had effective access to modern health services. An estimated 60 percent of all health resources were concentrated in Managua, where 25 percent of the population lived.[25] Others, especially those in rural areas, remained dependent on traditional healers *(curanderos)* and birth attendants *(parteras)* for health advice and treatment. They might see a doctor only if they were to sell their blood to the "Plasmaferesis" laboratory in Managua.

Whatever public health care did exist under Somoza was curative, except for malaria control. Alta Hooker, a nurse for the Atlantic coast, recalls conditions before the revolution:

> People were afraid to come to the hospital because they would have to pay. When symptoms started, they took home remedies. By the time they realized they needed help, it was often too late, because they would have to travel for days to reach the hospital. Patients used to appear at the hospital on a home-made stretcher, with a blood pressure of 40. This meant shock, deep shock. I remember one patient who had a ruptured appendix for ten days—that's how long it took them to reach us.

For landless laborers working on private owned farms and plantations, health care was virtually nonexistent. Luis Mendoza, who now works on a state farm, remembers:

> Before the revolution there was no place to go if somebody got sick. We just tried whatever we heard would work. A doctor would have been better, but how? The boss paid a doctor to care his animals but not for us. Why should he? He could always find more workers if we died.

Polio vaccination "campaigns" were carried out only after epidemics. Such campaigns received the patronage of First Lady Hope Somoza, but their function was essentially symbolic. They were "too little, too late" to have an impact on transmission of the disease.

Curative care was dispensed largely on an ability-to-pay basis. In Estelí Hospital, for example, a three-tiered system existed. Those who paid a small fee were admitted to large, open wards and received irregular attention. Those who could pay more went to semiprivate rooms and were visited daily. Those who could pay well had private rooms and round-the-clock medical attention. Dr. Fernando Silva, the first Director of the "La Mascota" Children's Hospital in Managua, remembers:

> There was care available to the poor, but there was never much and it was of very poor quality. It had all the limitations of charity care—bad doctors, worse medicine, and lack of consideration. Treatment at health centers was even worse. There was always a heap of people waiting around. When the doctor arrived he would begin writing and handing out prescriptions, one after the other. All that mattered was that people got a prescription.

Foreign Aid

Many foreign organizations set up hospitals and clinics after President John F. Kennedy set up the Alliance for Progress in the early sixties.[26,2] Many donors were religious and other nongovernmental organizations. The biggest donor was the United States Agency for International Development (USAID). Loans and grants from USAID were used to build rural health centers, set up a mobile rural health program, train doctors, build hospitals, stimulate community participation, and improve sanitation. Despite financial incentives and technical assistance, the anarchic, paternalistic, and profit-oriented nature of the Nicaraguan health system defeated USAID's reform efforts. A USAID evaluation in the mid-seventies found:[24] ". . . a combination of poor physical plant, lack of equipment, uncleanliness, and poor quality medical attention. No provisions were made to provide these [health] centers, once built, with adequate personnel, supplies, and management support. . . . The average health center operated at about 40 percent capacity in terms of patient visits per medical hour . . ."

The major stumbling block to reform was the political and economic system of the country. The evaluation summed up, in a cautious understatement, the effects of the Somoza dictatorship on the health system[24]:

> The long history of one party rule in the country . . . resulted in a centralized decision-making process with limited delegation of responsibility and authority, which often required the President to personally intervene in issues affecting even small amounts of sector resources. Thus the health sector and many health sector personnel lacked the motivation and innovative-experimental approach necessary to make a major impact on the enormous health problems facing the health agencies. . . .

Private aid was sometimes more effective. The Evangelical Committee for Aid and Development (CEPAD) was set up by the Protestant church after the 1972 earthquake in order to bypass the government in channeling development assistance to rural areas. CEPAD established and still runs more than twenty clinics in isolated rural communities. Their focus on home gardens, latrines, water systems, breast-feeding, and health education has been exemplary.

USAID and other international donors nonetheless continued to encourage reform within the government. The major result of this effort was a 1977 meeting of health leaders in Chinandega, which developed a blueprint for reform. Plans were made for unifying the various public health agencies into one ministry, coordinating the care provided by hospitals, building more clinics and improving their utilization, and starting a variety of rural health programs.

Such reforms, however, threatened powerful leaders and might undermine the Somoza system of control. None of the major urban programs called for in Chinandega were initiated. Rural programs begun because of the Chinandega initiative were wholly supported by foreign moneys and were subverted to help defend the dictatorship against growing support for the Sandinistas among peasants. In short, as long as the Somoza dynasty remained in power, efforts toward reform of the health system were condemned to failure.

Somoza Bombs Hospitals

Health workers were considered likely subversives by the Somoza regime because they dealt with a popular concern that the government ignored. The government carefully limited the number of doctors and nurses trained. FETSALUD, the health workers' union formed in 1974, organized several strikes in hospitals to oppose Somoza. By 1977, FETSALUD was one of the largest and most important trade unions in the country. The National Guard was reluctant to attack hospital workers with the same fury with which it destroyed other trade unions. The very doctors and nurses they might shoot today could well be needed to care for their own families tomorrow.

In August 1978, FETSALUD, encouraged by the proletarian branch of the FSLN, which believed that the urban working class would lead the revolution, led a hunger strike against the dictatorship.[13] As Somoza's position weakened, so did his restraint. Union leaders were jailed, murdered, or simply "disappeared." Many health workers, especially nurses, left the country because of political harassment or lockouts. Finally, the Guard turned its fury on the hospitals themselves. During the last months of the war, four of the country's public hospitals were destroyed and five others were damaged in air or artillery attacks by the Somoza government.[28,29]

The Sandinistas Organize

Meanwhile, growing numbers of doctors, nurses, and medical students abandoned hospitals, private practices, and universities to join the Sandinista guerrillas. For years, doctors had secretly treated wounded FSLN combatants. Clandestine networks were established to move injured or ill guerrilleros out of the country for treatment. Doctors and nurses (including twenty-one doctors from Germany, Costa Rica, Honduras, and Mexico) also trained medical orderlies who were attached to Sandinista combat units. In neighborhoods of León, Estelí, and Managua, where the National Guard had already lost effective control, the FSLN established clandestine hospitals where doctors operated on the war-wounded. Many health workers lived a dual life—an official one working in a government hospital or clinic and a secret one treating FSLN guerrillas and their families. It was a perilous existence. Dr. Fernando Silva worked with the FSLN in Managua:

> We would collect needles, syringes, penicillin, gauze, and other medical supplies to send to the countryside and the fighters. I remember the day when the medical director came to the Social Security clinic where I was working. He said he was convinced I was working for those sons of bitches the Sandinistas. This shook me because my white jacket was bulging with a pistol. I was in the habit of traveling armed because I was treating guerrillas. "After you finish with these patients, come to my office so that we can talk," he said. I didn't know what to do. I needed to get rid of the gun. I was trembling in fear that I would be shot because of the gun. There was a man nearby, holding a baby in his arms covered by a blanket. He touched me. "Don't worry," he said. He took the gun and put it under the blanket. I was saved from certain death. That night they attacked my house, but I had already fled.

Growing numbers of health professionals became deeply involved in the revolution. Medical students were recruited to treat wounded guerrilla

fighters in the mountains. Physicians went underground in the cities to coordinate protests. Former Minister of Health Dora María Tellez lived both
lives: "To go underground in the city was always very hard. At times there
were *compañeros* who spent months shut inside a single room. Life in the
mountains was physically very hard, but there was the advantage of being
together with others."

In the mountains, the second branch of the Sandinistas, the Guerra Pro-
longada Popular (prolonged people's war) group, encountered health problems for which they were wholly unprepared. Omar Cabezas was a guerrilla
fighter when he found white dots that grew into ulcers on his legs:[30]

> . . . Around the white dot it was red, red, red . . . I figured they would give
> me a shot to knock it out, because they had a fair supply of medicine [at
> camp] . . . It took three people for my treatment. A *compañero* would cut a
> couple of branches. They put one in each of my hands and another in my
> mouth so I wouldn't yell . . . The gauze came out all covered with pus and
> blood and chunks of flesh . . . Poor Flavio was always in his hammock, de-
> pressed because he couldn't figure out what it was. One afternoon he came
> running up: "It's leishmaniasis, leishmaniasis!" like somebody crying out,
> "Land, land!"
>
> "What's leishmaniasis?"
>
> "Brother, it's what you've got. It's mountain leprosy, that's leishmaniasis"
> [a disease of the skin and mucous membranes caused by a parasitic proto-
> zoan].

By early 1979, activity at the government health facilities, which had been
woefully inadequate under normal conditions, ground to a halt. Elizabeth
Perez Ode worked as a physician that year in Muy Muy, Matagalpa: "We
had to close the clinic because of the war. All the people were afraid to
come out. All we could do was register the dead after the National Guard
had finished 'interrogating' suspects."

Hospitals ran out of supplies and had to turn away patients. Many doctors
and nurses, fearing attacks by the National Guard, simply stopped reporting
for work at hospitals and health centers. In government-held areas, only
the Red Cross was able to provide emergency relief—and then only sporadically.[31] The National Guard often prevented the Red Cross from assisting the civilian population, and murdered several Red Cross workers who
defied their orders.

In neighborhoods supporting the Sandinistas, food, water, and other basic supplies ran out as the government attempted to starve the people into
submission. The third branch of the FSLN, the *terceristas* (third way), who
believed that popular organizations would rise up in a general strike to overthrow the dictatorship, responded by organizing Civil Defense Committees,
which acted as provisional local governments, storing and distributing

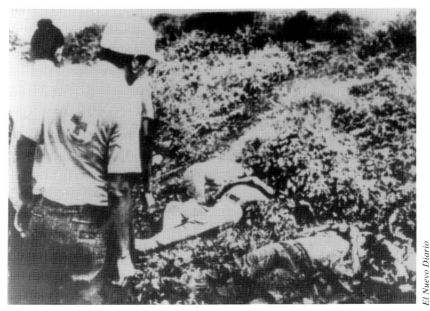

A site in Managua where the National Guard dumped the bodies of torture victims in 1979.

food, water, and essential commodities such as kerosene and cooking oil. The Committees also threw up street barricades, deployed lookouts and messengers to support the guerrilla fighters, coordinated health volunteers, trained orderlies to treat the sick and wounded, and organized the burial of the dead and the disposal of household refuse.

In effect, the National Guard obliged the Sandinistas to create a cadre of dedicated volunteers working in "liberated" communities.[32] By July 1979, when more than four decades of Somoza rule finally came to an end, the Sandinistas had established a makeshift system of widespread community involvement in health care.

MONTHS OF CRISIS

Even before a health ministry was formed, the Sandinistas had to deal with a national crisis in health. After months of intense fighting and the virtual collapse of health services, hundreds of thousands of people urgently needed medical care.[33] Many had scarcely eaten for weeks.

Reopening hospitals and health centers was another urgent priority. As medical supplies began to arrive at the Managua airport, some health workers also began returning to their posts. Community groups helped the effort by dismantling barricades blocking the roads and reconnecting water sup-

Timeline: 1979

JULY 17: Somoza flees Nicaragua for Miami.

JULY 18: A provisional "government of national reconstruction" is established in the city of León. In their proclamation, they announce plans to form a "unified national health service."*

JULY 19: The Government of National Reconstruction takes control of Managua.

JULY 26: The first Cuban medical brigade arrives.†

AUGUST 1: The newly appointed Minister of Health asks, via *La Prensa* newspaper, that hospital directors send information on employees and their salaries. Health workers have not been paid for three to six months.

The health ministry announces that vaccination campaigns will be started in a few days with the help of equipment donated by the West German government.

AUGUST 2: The Interamerican Development Bank and the Organization of American States pledge, respectively, $20 million and $500,000 in emergency food relief.

AUGUST 5: Headline in the new *Barricada* newspaper: "The Job in Health Will Be Gigantic!"‡

AUGUST 6: The health ministry announces that medical brigades have arrived from Mexico, Cuba, Germany, Panama, Costa Rica, Argentina, and Honduras.§

AUGUST 10: The new Ministry of Health (MINSA) is inaugurated.

AUGUST 17: MINSA announcement in *La Prensa:* "The permits given to exhume cadavers of those fallen in the insurrection are suspended immediately as a hygiene measure."

AUGUST 20: The Government of Reconstruction proclaims that all INSS (Social Security) hospitals and clinics will be opened to the public. Private rooms in public hospitals are similarly abolished.

AUGUST 27: The vice-minister of health announces: "Damage to the health system has been great, but we still don't know how great."
USAID announces a further increase in aid as 2,000 tons of food arrive.

AUGUST 31: Health is proclaimed to be a right of the entire population. It is announced that there will no longer be a fee to fill prescriptions.

*MINSA. Que es el sistem nacional unico de salud? Circular No. 1. Managua, MINSA, 1980.

†Anonymous. Brigada medica Cubana a Puerta Cabezas. MINSA Boletin Informatica No. (24 October 1979)

‡Anonymous. Sera gigantesca labor de salud. *Barricada* (5 August 1979), p. 1.

§Anonymous. Medicina rural y las brigadas internacionales. MINSA Boletin Informativa No. (17 September 1979), p. 1.

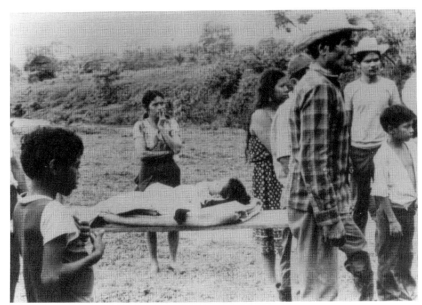

La Prensa

A typical scene after the revolution: peasants bring an ill child in for care while a worried mother looks on. They may have carried their make-shift stretcher for days to reach the clinic. Before the revolution, they probably would not have sought care.

plies. They also removed rubble, cleaned out bombed hospitals and health centers, and organized outpatient care.[20]

The first foreign health team to fly into Managua was a brigade of sixty Cuban doctors and nurses who arrived six days after the Sandinistas came to power. Within twenty-four hours, they set up an open-air clinic next to a bombed hospital in Matagalpa. The contrast between their operation and that of the health team that played volleyball and treated Somoza supporters behind the walls of the U.S. embassy after the 1972 earthquake could hardly have been more striking. Hundreds of patients queued up for treatment day and night. Within one month, the Cuban team had used up medicines they expected to last for three.

By late 1980, some 200 Cuban doctors and nurses were working in Nicaragua.[34] Many found the experience shocking. Patients suffered from diseases that had disappeared from Cuba, such as polio and neonatal tetanus. Malnutrition made the symptoms of measles so severe that the Cubans had difficulty recognizing this as the same disease that, in their country, had been controlled through mass immunization and improved nutrition. Pedro Azcuy, a member of the first Cuban health team, remembers: "I recall a very small town where there were ten or twelve children, of whom six died of measles . . . It was amazing to see how within ten days they began a vaccination campaign."[35]

Within months, the food crisis in the cities abated. Health workers began to take services to rural areas.[36] Most nurses and doctors in Managua had never before seen or dealt with people living in rural areas. They were shocked to find people who had lived for years from hand to mouth without a roof over their heads. Concepcion Huete, later MINSA director of nursing, recalls: "We went to a plantation and said: 'We are nurses from the Ministry of Health and we are here to vaccinate your children.' The people said to us: 'What is a nurse? What is vaccination?' I didn't know how to explain it to them. If somebody has never heard of a nurse, what can you tell them?"

2

A Health Service for All: 1979–1983

> The Sandinista People's Revolution . . . will provide free medical assistance to the entire population. It will set up clinics and hospitals throughout the national territory.
>
> *The Historic Program of the FSLN,* 1969[1]

Once in power, the Sandinistas moved fast. Within three weeks, they inaugurated the Unified National Health System.[2] This gave the new Ministry of Health (MINSA) control over most hospitals, clinics, and the National Social Security System. It was a historic step for the new government, one that raised their popularity even higher. As we discuss in future chapters, in time this act may have created more problems than it solved. But in these initial days of the new regime, more immediate questions demanded attention.

The Sandinistas had yet to decide how to make the new health system function. What would be the roles of doctors, nurses, and other health professionals? Would there be a role for private medicine? How would the public service be financed? How might the political commitment to community participation take shape?

These vital questions were not much discussed by political leaders during the hectic summer of 1979 when the new government was formed. Health was awarded a high priority, but it was considered mainly a "technical" issue, to be determined by leading revolutionary doctors. Besides, the main issue during 1979–1983 already seemed obvious: The health system had to expand radically to respond to the newly enfranchised majority.

Dr. Antonio Jarquin, one of the architects of health policy, admitted: "The Sandinistas were specialists in destroying dictatorships, but none of us knew how to construct a government."[3] The challenge was to select strategies and technologies that would be appropriate to Nicaragua's stage of social, economic, and political development. One possible model was Costa Rica, where close coordination between the Social Security system and the Ministry of Health, with substantial funding over a thirty-year period, had brought dramatic improvements in health.[4-12] Also at hand was the example of Cuba, where a nationalized health service with a high concentration of doctors had raised overall health standards to the level of most industrialized countries.[13–19] The presence of hard-working Cuban health workers in Nicaragua also lent prestige to their model.

A massive national literacy campaign had already begun. According to Jarquin,"When you teach people to read and write you are also giving them knowledge that doctors exist, hospitals exist . . . it was like a bomb exploding." Nicaragua had neither the time nor the funds to emulate the models of Costa Rica or Cuba.[20] Examples of simpler, less-expensive health systems were put forward by the World Health Organization, the Pan American Health Organization, and the United Nations Children's Fund.[21–24] One such example was China, with its focus on health campaigns and paramedical workers called "barefoot doctors." International organizations were also beginning to promote the "primary health care" strategy.

Elaborated in 1978 at a World Health Organization meeting at Alma Ata, primary health care was designed to make basic preventive and curative care universally available. Such care would be provided at the first level of contact with the health system. Underpinning the primary health care approach was a commitment to equality. In developing countries, this meant providing basic services for the whole population rather than focusing on high quality, specialty care. The specific elements of primary health care were to include the following:*

education to prevent or control common health problems
promotion of food supply and adequate nutrition
safe water and basic sanitation
maternal and child health care, including contraception
immunization against major diseases
prevention or treatment of common diseases and injuries
provision of essential drugs

A commitment to establish universal access to these basic services was embodied in the slogan "Health for All by the Year 2000."

*WHO. Declaration of Alma Ata: Report on the international conference on primary health care. Geneva, WHO, 1979.

The primary health care strategy seemed to fit well with the Sandinistas' political values and health objectives. Yet the practical implications of planning and implementing it throughout the country presented enormous obstacles.

Within MINSA, Sandinista leaders with strong trade union links argued that the health system should be oriented to the organized work force; private medicine should be prohibited and all health professionals should be employed by the state.

Revolutionaries who had fought in the mountains, on the other hand, believed that the peasantry was at the heart of the revolution. They argued that the government should give top priority to those in rural areas. Some wanted to follow China's example and downplay the role of urban hospitals and fully trained doctors. Organized medicine, for its part, favored a "pluralistic" approach to preserve private practice and respond to the interests of the urban middle class. New public health programs staffed by auxiliary nurses and volunteers could be developed for the poor and rural populations.

All three groups were represented in the political coalition that brought the Sandinistas to political power, and all three took part in the compromises needed to establish a national health policy at the end of 1979. MINSA's main focus was to be urban and rural laborers and small-scale farmers, particularly women and children.[25] These were the groups that had been the most disenfranchised under the Somoza regime.

While initially preserving the private medical sector, MINSA would attempt to orient the entire system, including the doctors and hospitals, toward rural areas and urban slums.[26,27] Revolutionary rhetoric emphasized preventive health care, health education, and community participation.[28,29] Vice-ministries in these and other areas were quickly established within MINSA.

This policy contained the seeds of conflict. On the one hand, the government proclaimed the need for low-cost, community-based, preventive health services. On the other hand, it also promised to provide wide access to curative care in modern hospitals. This well-intentioned commitment to sophisticated medical care was inconsistent with the primary health care approach. It was medically unnecessary and financially overwhelming. Yet pressure from the population, promises from leading revolutionary doctors, and a belief among political leaders that the "best" care should be available to all probably made this choice inevitable.

These contradictory views led to lively and sometimes acrimonious debates in MINSA. A leading figure in the debate was Dr. Adolfo Chamorro, an opponent of the high-tech, hospital-based approach. A military commander during the revolutionary war, Dr. Chamorro helped initiate a paramedical program involving 15,000 volunteers in the country's National Literacy Crusade of 1980.[30-32] He also advocated workers' health schemes as part of self-management.[33-35] Frustrated with both the government bureaucracy and the conservatism of the medical establishment, Dr. Chamorro went back to the army when the Contra war intensified in 1982. As one of Chamorro's supporters later reflected: "Adolfo was just ahead of his time."

REACHING THE PEOPLE

After 1979, doctors and nurses were suddenly posted in rural and poor urban communities. This expression of the government's commitment also brought complications. Dr. Leonel Arguello did his social service in the remote Atlantic coast town of Rama in 1980:

> Peasants would walk for days to reach the town because they had heard that there was a doctor. But they had no idea what to do when they got there. They would stand silently, with stoic pride, on the other side of the path in front of the clinic. If I didn't go out to ask them about their problems and invite them into the clinic, they would simply return home after a few days. They still weren't convinced that they had a right to health care.

Another young doctor, Roberto Valle Gonzalez, summed up the situation with a touch of wry humor: "We feel a need to rescue them from their backwardness, but they don't necessarily see this the same way we do."

Soon, however, even in remote areas, confidence in the new health services grew and they were used *en masse*. In the towns and cities, the demand for free health care created early morning lines at clinics that snaked down the street in the hot sun as far as the eye could see. Hospitals were also deluged with patients. Alta Hooker worked as a nurse in the regional hospital of the Atlantic coast town of Puerto Cabezas:

> Before the revolution, we never filled the twenty-seven beds in the hospital. About two months after the war of liberation, I attended a two-month anes-

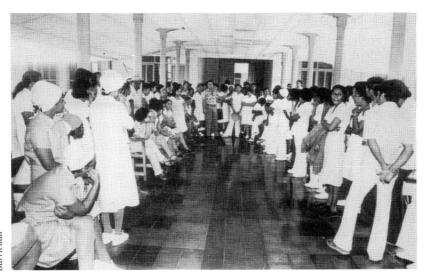

Barricada

An assembly of health workers in a regional hospital in 1980. The advent of the Sandinista government brought with it workplace democracy and union participation in management.

thesia course in Managua. When I got back I found lots of sickness in and around the hospital, because the people were really starting to come in. It became impossible to work—you'd nearly walk on the patients lying on stretchers or on the ground between beds. The Ministry of Health told us that we'd have to be patient, that it was the same everywhere, and we'd just have to wait our turn. We increased the number of beds from twenty-seven to sixty-nine in that first year, and in 1985 we got a new wing with twenty-two more beds.

This new access to care brought out a shocking legacy of long neglect. Antonio Dajer examined a woman who had what appeared to be a growth the size of a volleyball on her abdomen.[36] She said that it had been the size of a marble fifteen years before, and now caused her to vomit constantly. "What could it be? If it was lower intestine, she shouldn't be vomiting. If it was strangulated upper intestine, she would have died years ago. The books didn't help at all." It turned out that her entire stomach was in a hernia outside her abdominal muscles. Her recovery was uneventful after a simple operation.

FRENETIC BUILDING

The years of 1979 to 1981 were marked by frenetic construction of new health facilities. In 1979, there were fewer than 200 centers and health posts in the country. This was far too few for the Sandinistas to fulfill their promise of providing services in even isolated areas. A massive building program was needed, but some advised caution. Dr. Giorgio Solimano, a Chilean who had worked in the health ministry of the Allende government in Chile, was one of these: "The people's expectations were enormous and grew day by day, fueled by pronouncements by officials of the new government. How they were going to meet those expectations was anybody's guess."

By 1982, more than 300 new health posts had been built.[37] This provided the physical infrastructure needed for primary health care throughout the country[38] (see Figure 2–1). Only about half of these new facilities were constructed by the government. The remainder were built by the communities themselves. Leonel Arguello helped to build the health post in the Atlantic coast township of Punta Gorda:

Before the revolution, the Moravian church was used for all types of social functions, and once a year a pastor came to perform weddings and baptisms. We started by giving medical attention in the church as well, and then talked to the people about how it would be to have a clinic. One person brought his boat to transport materials. Another offered his services as a carpenter. Doctors, nurses, and the community people did the labor. Whenever we ran short

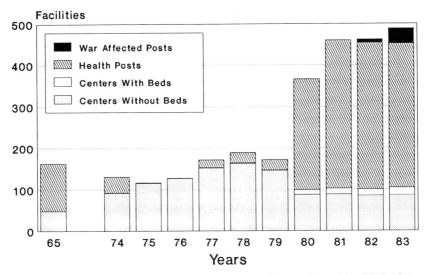

Figure 2–1 Primary care facilities, 1965–1983. The number of health facilities rose rapidly following the 1979 revolution as new health posts were established. This increase had a far greater impact than the construction of facilities with USAID funding in the 1970s.

of materials, people put out a call for donations or raised money to buy what was needed.

In many places, existing buildings were converted into health centers or posts. In the town of El Cua, a notorious prison was converted into a health center with beds. The elegant homes of Somoza supporters who had fled the country in 1979 were turned into spacious health centers in many small towns. In Waslala, the first revolutionary health service was staffed by a physician captured from Somoza's retreating army. He was convinced to work for the Sandinistas on the promise that following a year of public service he would be exempted from prosecution. One of Managua's better-designed health centers was once a brothel owned by one of Somoza's colonels.[39] When the revolutionary government proposed turning it into a prison, community groups persuaded the government that the building, with its rows of small cubicles, would be put to better use for medical consultations.[40]

Where health centers or posts could not be set up, mobile units, moving by truck or boat, visited weekly.[41] MINSA was not alone in this effort. Newly established state farms were assigned health workers who served as focal points for care to peasants living in the area.[42] Social Security clinics and hospitals, formerly restricted to insured workers, were also opened to the public. With the huge surge in building, the government's biggest task became staffing these facilities.

Training for Rural Health

In many remote parts of the country, the first health workers to arrive were young volunteers *(brigadistas)* with only two weeks' training in health care. Beginning just eight months after the Sandinistas came to power, the National Literacy Crusade recruited close to 100,000 volunteers—mostly high school and university students—to teach basic literacy skills to 400,000 adults between March and September of 1980.[43] MINSA trained 15,000 of these literacy *brigadistas* in first aid, sanitation, and malaria and diarrhea control at the newly formed Polytechnic Institute in Managua.[44] Apart from teaching literacy skills, these young men and women also worked as rural health aides, collected information on local herbal medicines and folk healing practices, and helped to construct health posts.

When the literacy campaign ended, the Polytechnic Institute began to train thousands of auxiliary nurses, as well as laboratory and dental technicians. The Institute was unprepared for this task. Students received instruction in open pavilions while the walls were being built.[45]

Meanwhile, medical students near the end of their courses were rushed into service, doubling the number of new graduates in 1980 and 1981. Overcoming long-held traditions and prejudices, a second medical school was opened in Managua to help reach the target of 500 new doctors a year by 1985. The Managua medical school was created almost from scratch and functioned virtually without teaching resources during its first three years. The León school was not much better off; its class size had tripled while the number of classrooms, teachers, and books remained the same.

Professional nurses were trained in similarly shortened courses, thus increasing their numbers by 1981. But the greatest increase in health personnel occurred among auxiliary nurses, who were trained *en masse* between 1979 and 1982 in nine- or twelve-month courses. The number of auxiliary students increased fivefold.[46]

A RATIONAL HEALTH SYSTEM

Building a rational health system on the imbalanced base of existing facilities was a daunting task. It was made doubly difficult when health officials of the old regime were encouraged to stay on. In a reconciliatory gesture and to avoid the loss of personnel with rare administrative skills, only the highest or most corrupt Somocista health authorities were dismissed.

It took MINSA several months just to determine how many clinics and hospital beds existed. Health officials worked with three different estimates of the number of doctors in the country. As the organizational dust settled, a three-tiered national health structure emerged.

The Structure of Health Care

The health service in 1980 was reorganized according to the three levels of technical sophistication of its institutions: hospitals, health centers, and health posts.[47]

The most technologically advanced care is provided at seven national-level hospitals in Managua and Leon and three foreign-run hospitals in Managua and Chinandega. These include surgical, pediatric, and gynecological specialty hospitals. Other nationally run hospitals include those providing long-term residential care for patients with leprosy or other skin diseases, tuberculosis, rehabilitation needs, or psychiatric problems.

Structure of the public health system

	Population	Facilities	Personnel and administration services
Nation	3,600,000	National referral hospitals (14)	Rehabilitation specialty and subspecialty care
Region (6)	10,000–100,000	Regional hospitals (16)	Surgery and basic specialties
Area (97)	5,000–20,000	Health center or post (104)	Graduate nurse and basic specialties: Gynecology, pediatrics, internal medicine, obstetrics
Sector (500)	1,000–3,000	Post or community center (417)	Visiting doctors, auxiliary nurse, malaria worker, brigadistas, health educator

The system is subdivided into six *regions* and the Zelaya Autonomous Zone on the Atlantic coast. The regions administer twenty "secondary care" hospitals staffed mainly by social service physicians and foreign volunteers. They usually have local doctors and several specialists as well. A doctor is present twenty-four hours a day. Eight of Nicaragua's nine private hospitals and the twenty-three private clinics with beds are also at this level of technical sophistication. Nine of the best regional hospitals are also teaching facilities with interns and medical students working in them.

Within the regions and the autonomous zone are health *areas*. Each region contains ten to twenty health areas. The country has a total of ninety-seven health areas, each covering 20;000–30,000 people. Primary care is provided at health centers and health posts in the areas.

Health centers are found in larger villages, towns, and cities of 5,000–15,000 residents. Patients can be referred to a health center from a health post, but most come on their own. There is at least one doctor present whenever the center is open. Health centers provide gynecologic, pediatric, internal medicine, and obstetric care. Larger centers may have four or more doctors, including older local physicians who work part-time and specialists who visit periodically. Some laboratory services are available, some clinics have a pharmacy, and a few even have X-ray machines. Many offer dental services and some have beds for overnight care.

Health posts are usually located in villages with less than 5,000 residents, though there are several posts where local communities have established them within the city of Managua. Rural posts are usually staffed by a nurse or auxiliary nurse and are visited once or twice a week by a doctor. They deal with common illnesses, prenatal check-ups, well-child visits, and minor first aid. A post usually doubles as an oral rehydration center. There is no clinical laboratory, although in some posts laboratory samples can be taken.

In more remote rural areas, health volunteers provide basic care in makeshift clinics or out of a knapsack. A health post or center functions as the nucleus for health activities in the area. Each area employs a health educator. The key to local health promotion is the subdivision of the area served by the health center or post into three to six *sectors*. Each sector has 1,000–2,000 residents, should be served by an auxiliary nurse and one or more local health aides, and is supervised by a physician at the health center. The auxiliary nurse monitors community health, helps coordinate and promote health campaigns, and provides preventive care to people in the sector.

PROBLEM HOSPITALS

When the Sandinistas came to power, work had begun on four of five new hospitals designed and financed by USAID. Work ground to a halt, however, when USAID funding declined following Ronald Reagan's election in 1980 and was completely cut off in 1981. Signs with the familiar handshake logo and the inscription "Funded by the people of the United States" were belatedly removed from construction sites. This represented an important turning point to many Nicaraguans. After a century of political and economic dependence on the United States, how would the country manage?

These new hospitals were seen as symbols of the government's commitment to provide care to all. Indeed, since health posts were staffed by new graduate physicians, hospitals became increasingly important. Self-referral and physician referral to out- and inpatient care in hospitals became common, even for simple problems. Ironically, as the primary care system developed, hospitals took on increasing importance as the backbone of the health system. The completion of the new hospitals, then, became a matter of great political importance. The Nicaraguan government took responsibility for all further construction. Unfortunately, serious prior errors in planning and construction resulted in long delays. The new hospital in Bluefields, on the Atlantic coast, was built by a foreign construction firm that failed to include the contracted structural supports under the building. By the time the hospital was due to open in 1985, it was already sinking into the sandy soil. Its opening was delayed for a year and construction costs doubled while the necessary improvements were made.

The Matagalpa hospital, designed as a large modern complex with a commanding view of the city, was situated so far from residential areas that new bus routes had to be established to make it accessible. When it was found that the municipal water system lacked enough pressure to raise water to the hilltop site, the opening was postponed for 12 months to allow for the construction of a new water system.

Funds for the construction of the hospitals fell under the budget of the Ministry of Construction rather than MINSA. Partly because of this, it was not immediately apparent that spending to build such modern hospitals would weaken the ability to provide needed maintenance to older hospitals or improvements to health centers and posts throughout the country.

REDUCING INEQUALITIES

In 1980, Managua had a doctor for every 1,000 people. In some remote regions there was a doctor for every 10,000 residents. The gap in geographic coverage of nurses was also huge. The best-endowed region had one graduate nurse for each 3,000 residents; the worst region had one nurse for each 20,000 people. As large numbers of health workers were trained and assigned to facilities in rural areas, geographic inequalities decreased dramatically.[48] By 1983, the best and worst health regions had only a two-fold difference in coverage of nurses and doctors.

The growth in access was most dramatic for basic curative medical care. In 1971, 12 percent of the country's doctors, 11 percent of the nurses, and 9 percent of the auxiliary nurses worked in primary care. By 1981, as a result of the large influx of health workers into rural areas after July 1979,

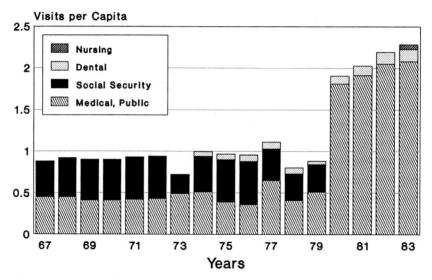

Figure 2–2 Medical, nursing, and dental visits, 1967–1983. Per capita medical and dental visits fell during the years of the insurrection and rose explosively following the revolution. These data are for public institutions; no data are available for private medical and dental consultations.

36 percent of the doctors, 30 percent of the nurses, and 30 percent of the auxiliaries—including almost all new graduates—worked in primary care.

Public health programs for rural areas, maternal and child health, and occupational medicine expanded enormously after 1979. Outpatient care and prescriptions—the curative services most lacking for the general population prior to 1979—showed the most dramatic increases. From 1977 to 1983, hospitalizations and surgical procedures rose more than 50 percent, outpatient medical visits tripled (see Figure 2–2), and the number of vaccinations increased more than fourfold.

By 1982, at least 70 percent of the population received some medical care from trained staff. This was a dramatic increase over the 28 percent getting modern health care prior to 1979.[46] The number of visits per capita to a doctor more than doubled. The northern Zelaya zone on the Atlantic coast had the highest rate of doctor visits, with more than three consultations per capita each year. Nonetheless, towns and cities were still better served than most rural areas. Residents of Managua in 1982 averaged 55 percent more medical consultations than people in the rest of the country.

Losers under the New System

This meteoric expansion in services partially hid the fact that for some groups, access to health grew poorer. The most obvious of these groups was the rich. They no longer enjoyed private beds at the major government hospitals. This was not greatly missed. When not seriously ill, the rich still had private clinics and hospitals to cater to their needs. When seriously ill, they generally went to Miami or Houston for care; the advent of the revolution simply made this option relatively more attractive.

The middle class also lost privileged access to care following 1979. The poor might be content to wait for hours in the sun to see a doctor at a government health center. The middle class was not, and began visiting private doctors. Yet even private medicine was subject to shortages of equipment and supplies. Amid complaints about empty pharmacy shelves, relatives and friends living abroad were increasingly relied on for medicines unobtainable in Nicaragua.

The largest and most powerful group to lose preferential access was the unionized work force. Representing about 26,000 people before 1979, union ranks swelled to more than 100,000 in 1980. The single largest organized group of workers was composed of government employees, who represented about a third of the unionized work force. Many unions opposed opening Social Security clinics and hospitals to the general public. This meant a rapid decline in the amount and quality of care they could obtain for their members. Unions repeatedly petitioned the government to reestablish preferential access to care.

Although unions were given minor concessions for several months, their privileged system of care was not reestablished and workers threatened to strike. In the end, however, opposition faded because so many unionists depended directly or indirectly on the government for employment.

For several years, the Ministry of Agriculture continued to operate an independent health service on state-owned farms. It was only in 1983 that the last Social Security hospital, at the Ingenio Julio Butriago sugar mill, was finally brought under direct MINSA control.

HEALTH LEADERS

The first minister of health was a respected pediatric neurosurgeon, Dr. Cesar Amador Kuhl. The selection of Dr. Kuhl, a political independent popular with most doctors, seemed a cautious step for a revolutionary government. His political neutrality, however, made him more acceptable to people from a wide political spectrum, both within and outside the country. He brought unity to the new ministry and played a leading role in obtaining international assistance. But his lack of political and administrative expertise put him in a weak position to lead such a complex organization. In early 1981, Dr. Kuhl returned to private practice, university teaching, and leadership of the *Colegio de Medicos*.[49]

His replacement was Lea Guido, a thirty-two-year-old Sandinista activist and lecturer in sociology who had studied at the University of Lausanne in Switzerland. Ms. Guido had led the national women's organization, and was the first minister of social welfare in 1979. She had no medical qualifications but was known as an effective administrator.

Although her youth was no bar to such a high office, she would have to operate in an environment in which *machismo* still flourished and conservative medical attitudes were deeply ingrained. Inevitably, her appointment caused consternation among doctors, who feared political interference in medicine. The stage was set for a trial of strength between a Sandinista health minister and the medical establishment. Although it was not seen at the time, the change in leadership created a window of opportunity for changing the focus of the health system. Until now, the government had tried to please everyone by simultaneously developing primary and secondary medical care and concentrating on urban, rural, maternal, child, and occupational health concerns. Tough choices would soon have to be made, and not everyone would come up a winner. Much of this battle would be fought over issues of community involvement in health.

3

Community Participation

I don't know much about science, but a doctor doesn't know this neighborhood like I do. When we work together, the doctor and I can make democracy a reality in health. But democracy isn't always easy.   ROSA GARCÍA, health volunteer

The mass organizations do not know, nor have any way to know, the true importance of various illnesses. They had big theories . . . but actually used the community as informers.
"The León Document,"
by a group of opposition party physicians.

A basis for community participation was laid during the revolutionary insurrections of 1978 and 1979. But when the Sandinistas came to power in July 1979, they had yet to formulate a plan. How could participation be organized so that it was genuinely local and spontaneous, rather than imposed from above? How could such participation be spread throughout the whole health system? And in what ways would the people want to participate? There were no ready-made answers available to respond to these questions.[1-8] This chapter describes the still-evolving structures and issues for community participation.

Perhaps the only clear plan in 1979 was to avoid a return to the token participation of the seventies. A national program to involve traditional birth attendants (TBAs) in family planning and health care, for example, had failed because of a lack of community interest and involvement. Corruption and poor leadership had resulted in high costs and poor efficiency in a USAID-sponsored sanitation project, where administrative costs amounted to 60 percent of the total budget.[9,10] Some of these programs were little more than window dressing for an unpopular regime. Several projects were reportedly located in areas of high guerrilla activity in order to collect strategic military information. All suffered from a lack of credibility and community involvement because of the narrow interests they represented and unpopular political regime they served.[11,12]

The first organized activities following July 1979 involved food distribution and the most successful vaccination campaign in the nation's history, achieving 70 percent coverage against polio in some areas. Measles and diphtheria-pertussis-tetanus vaccination programs soon followed.

The immunization campaign also brought to light the limited understanding people had of diseases and their prevention. Many parents were suspicious and refused to bring their children to vaccination posts. Some, never having seen a doctor or nurse, and fearing that injections would make their children ill, simply hid from vaccination teams.

It became clear that massive public education was needed.[13] Families needed to learn about immunization, sanitation, nutrition, and common diseases. But how could large numbers of barely literate people be motivated to learn about health? In 1980, MINSA experimented with teams of health educators who promoted "health literacy" by using socio-drama, role play, puppetry, and participatory theater. The task turned out to be far beyond the capacity of these small teams. A method was urgently needed for training large numbers of community members in a short period of time. Once trained, these people could then spread health knowledge and organize their communities to carry out activities to prevent diseases.

The National Literacy Crusade of 1980 provided direction. The Crusade had trained a core group of literacy teachers, who in turn trained tens of thousands more through a "multiplier" strategy in which each trained volunteer became a trainer of others. Adapting this strategy to its own needs, MINSA trained 100 health educators, then 1,000 multipliers, and finally 30,000 health volunteers called *brigadistas*.[14] The *brigadistas* made house-to-house visits and gave talks to small groups to educate and motivate their neighbors in health matters. In a little over a year, thousands of health volunteers were active in neighborhoods and villages throughout the country[15] (see Figure 3–1).

To support this massive effort, MINSA developed illustrated, comic-style booklets. According to a training manual, the objective was to develop "content and methods which corresponded to popular needs, [making education] a liberating process."[16] Newsprint booklets were distributed throughout the country. They covered a wide range of topics, including immunization, hygiene and sanitation, rabies, tuberculosis, breast-feeding, first aid, nutrition, diarrhea, dental care, food handling, water supply, and insect control.

Designed to promote an understanding of the causes, prevention, and treatment of major illnesses, the booklets also related health problems to their social and political context.[17] The booklet on breast-feeding, for example, discussed the role of international corporations in promoting powdered milk, as well as the cultural biases that downgrade breast-feeding as "uneducated." The booklets were widely used by neighborhood and church

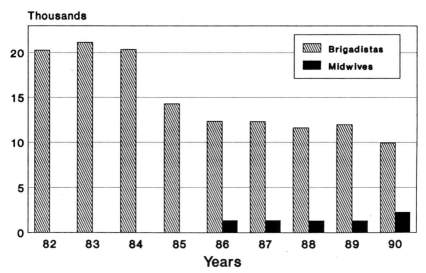

Figure 3–1 Health volunteers trained, 1982–1990. The number of volunteers trained to take part in health campaigns declined by 1985, as many experienced volunteers avoided repeat training. By contrast, the training of midwives slowly increased. No data are available for the total number of active volunteers.

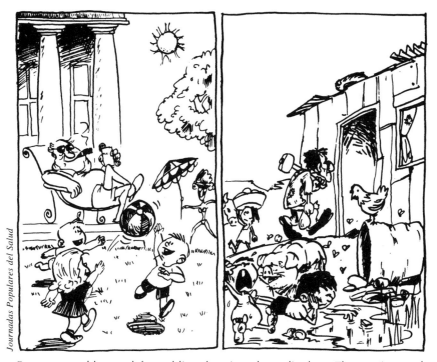

Journadas Populares del Salud

From a pamphlet used for public education about diarrhea. The caption read, "Analyze and discuss these drawings. Which children are more likely to suffer from diarrhea? Why?"

groups, trade unions, cooperatives, women's groups, literacy classes, and schools.

Health educators and *brigadistas* studied the booklets in groups in order to stimulate discussion and analyze health problems. By 1988, over two dozen booklets had been produced and more than 3 million copies had been distributed.

As more experience was gained with health campaigns, and as local groups gained the self-confidence to criticize national programs, it became clear that the original booklets had serious limitations.[18] The drawings, for example, were too abstract for many *campesinos,* and the handwritten texts often proved illegible to people who had only recently learned to read. Simpler drawings and typewritten texts were used in subsequent booklets, but many of these still proved too hard for the target audience to read and understand.

The release of a booklet was often timed to coincide with the popularization of a health slogan and a practical action. Radio, television, newspapers, and other media were used to promote health messages.

The prevention and treatment of diarrhea—the single most common cause of death—was a focus of particular attention. Special programs and advertising spots on radio and television explained the causes and dangers of diarrhea, and what families could do to prevent and treat the disease.

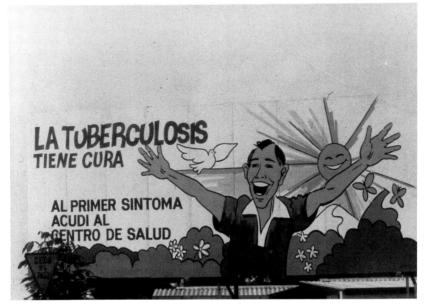

Roadside poster: "Tuberculosis can be cured. At the first symptom, go to the health center."

Roadside billboards, newspaper comic strips and advertisements, and posters in health centers were also widely used. The first slogan concerning diarrhea was: "A child with diarrhea can die. Take yours to the nearest oral rehydration [a solution containing needed electrolytes and sugar] center (URO)" (see also Chapter 8).

PEOPLE'S HEALTH COUNCILS

Educating for action required a system for involving communities in planning, implementation, and evaluation. In July 1980, the government established People's Health Councils in order to "mold the aspirations of the people into concrete programs" and to "channel the activities and concerns of the people in a coordinated manner.[19]

The first health councils consisted exclusively of community organizations.[20] The most important of these were neighborhood associations known as Sandinista Defense Committees (CDS). Also active were the national women's organization (AMNLAE), the farm laborers' union (ATC), the workers' union (CST), the teachers' union (UNE), the youth movement (JS19S), the children's association (ASN) and the health workers' union (FETSALUD).

Some of these organizations—especially the CDS—were already involved in organizing health campaigns and carrying out health education.[21] Previously, however, their involvement had been unofficial, spontaneous, and seemingly anarchic in character. Through community health councils, these organizations were recognized as having the right—and the responsibility—to participate in health matters.

Councils were established at local, regional, and national levels to parallel official MINSA structures. The councils took responsibility for organizing People's Health Days, campaigns to combat particular health problems.[22] In 1980, for example, an estimated 30,000 volunteers took part in a series of Health Days focusing on polio, measles, dengue, and environmental sanitation. On each occasion, volunteers attended weekend training sessions and made door-to-door visits to explain the purpose of the forthcoming Health Day. For the immunization campaigns, the volunteers also carried out a census of infants and children in their neighborhood who required vaccination. Each campaign was followed by regional "Analysis and Summary" meetings involving doctors, nurses, and health volunteers.

In 1981, the councils mounted four campaigns: vaccinations against polio and measles, an environmental sanitation campaign, an antidengue campaign, and—most ambitious of all—an antimalaria campaign involving about 200,000 voluntary workers[23] (see Chapter 4). Within MINSA, the department dealing with campaigns, the Office for Popular Health Education and Communication (DECOPS), became so large and active that other, more conservative offices were alarmed. It was even feared that DECOPS might take over the Division of Preventive Medicine.

Both conservatives and radicals were concerned about the meteoric growth in health campaign activities. Conservatives lacked trust in the *brigadista* program because it threatened to replace medicine as the heart of the health system. Radicals were concerned that the volunteers might weaken the push to reorient the physicians toward the poor majority. The "appropriate technology" of volunteers and preventive campaigns might therefore free doctors from the pressure of public service to continue "business as usual" with their urban, middle-class clientele.

Organized Communities

CDSs in most areas became the most active community groups. A CDS at the level of the urban "block" or rural neighborhood consists of 50–200 people. A group of about ten blocks makes up a *barrio,* and about five *barrios* make up a zone of the national CDS organization.[24] Most blocks and neighborhoods have a CDS: As many as 8,000 CDS committees have functioned at the zonal level, covering about 5 percent of all urban neighborhoods in the country.

Rural CDSs often have two subcommittees: one for welfare (including health) and another for production and defense. More elaborate urban CDSs have had as many as five subcommittees: organization, defense, education, health, and production. A local CDS may organize health activities as it sees fit. Locally initiated campaigns include environmental cleanups, first aid training, civil defense drills, and—in isolated areas—the training of volunteer paramedical health workers. A CDS may be involved in many health-related activities.

The Volunteers

Despite the wide popularity of the new government, many people wanted to avoid direct political involvement. Participation in health was a less overt, and therefore more acceptable, way to help rebuild the country. To political leaders, on the other hand, volunteer health activities were a way of attracting people into a commitment to the revolution's social and political goals.

Rosa García's story is typical.[25] In September 1978 she gave refuge in her home to a young guerrilla fleeing Somoza's National Guard. Soon she opened a stand near the entrance to Ciudad Sandino, where she sold fruit drinks. There she observed the movements of the National Guard, chatted

Health Activities of a Sandinista Defense Committee (CDS)

Some activities of the CDS in the working-class neighborhood Ciudad Sandino, on the edge of Managua, during the mid-eighties:

Social support:* Don Lencho, an elderly man suffering from leg ulcers and unable to care for himself, lived alone. A CDS meeting decided to ask a physician to examine him. The doctor explained that Don Lencho's poor health was due more to abandonment than medical causes. In response, CDS families took turns preparing an extra plate of food for the old man at mealtimes. A nurse from the clinic also came to his house to dress his ulcers—a job later taken over by a local health volunteer.

Disaster relief:† When a flash flood washed away 60 homes and damaged 160 others, the CDS evacuated families to local churches and school buildings, distributed food and clothing, and successfully petitioned the government for new plots of land and permission to build new houses.

Community health services:‡ When the Evangelical church set up an oral rehydration unit, the CDS recruited six health volunteers from each of the zones to help staff it.

Distribution of consumer goods:§ Among the many consumer goods in short supply were baby bottles and nipples, resulting in exorbitant prices for these items on the black market. The CDS persuaded the Ministry of Interior Commerce to make them available at guaranteed prices for women who brought their prenatal cards to the government distribution stores. This action resulted in 60 percent higher attendance of pregnant women at the prenatal clinic.

Sanitation: ‖ A single mother with several young children, living in a shack with no latrine, was reduced to using a chamber pot to empty family waste in a neighbor's latrine. Upon hearing that MINSA would give the base and seat for a latrine to anyone willing to dig the hole, the CDS decided to help the woman. One Sunday morning, a group of volunteers dug a hole, installed the latrine, and constructed a small shed to provide privacy for the woman and her family.

*Woznica, C. Community participation in health as an empowering process: A case study from Nicaragua. Ph.D. dissertation, University of Illinois, Chicago, 1987, p. 190.
†Ibid., p. 189.
‡Ibid., p. 241.
§Ibid., p. 196.
‖ Ibid., p. 191.

with the Guardsmen who purchased drinks from her, and later passed the information on to the FSLN. She had always been interested in health, but at the age of twenty-eight she was still illiterate. She learned to read in the National Literary Crusade in 1980 and became active as a health *brigadista*. The following year she led sanitation and antimalarial campaigns in her neighborhood. In 1982, her neighbors chose her to coordinate local health activities and to represent them on the board of the health center.

Like Rosa García, most *brigadistas* are part-time activists. Their work is greatest immediately before and during the People's Health Days, which may be held four times a year. They come from a wide spectrum of Nicaraguan society. A survey of the 30,000 volunteers trained for a sanitation campaign in 1982 found that most were young[26]: Seventy-five percent were under twenty-five years of age, and 20 percent under fifteen. Although most were literate, only a minority had finished primary school. At least two-thirds of *brigadistas* are women; most of them are urban housewives or students.[27] Most male *brigadistas* are rural farmers or urban students. About 20 percent of all *brigadistas* are either salaried workers or self-employed.

The drop-out rate among part-time health *brigadistas* is high, like health programs in much of the world.[28] Many volunteers are students who move, marry, or take full-time jobs. After participating in campaigns for several years, many volunteers lose their enthusiasm. Especially with the decline in living standards of recent years, the demands of day-to-day survival make volunteerism more difficult.

Recruitment and training methods for part-time health *brigadistas* have gradually changed.[29] Until 1983, they were recruited and trained separately for each campaign. This method proved inefficient. Many *brigadistas* were trained in previous campaigns and had the necessary skills and experience. There were also frequent conflicts between the need for volunteers for the health campaigns and other mobilization efforts such as coffee harvesting, tree planting, community cleanups, and participation in local militias.[30] In addition, the expanding health system reduced the need for some of the original activities of *brigadistas*.

In response, in 1986 MINSA began to provide more intensive, ongoing training in a few areas. These *brigadistas* were trained for one or two weeks in order to assume ongoing responsibilities, rather than be trained for only one day for short-term campaigns. Despite the stated popularity of this more responsible role, it had caught on only in a few places by 1989. People continued to believe that the government would provide more and better services than could local volunteers. Thus, while MINSA provided *brigadistas* with nonmonetary rewards such as scholarships, identification badges, and diplomas, their status in most communities remained marginal except for short-term MINSA-run campaigns.

Some critics argue that the government was responsible for this attitude.[29] Anna Quiroz, from the nongovernmental health education group CISAS, believes that more responsibility and training should have been given to the *brigadistas* when the war escalated in 1983: "That was the moment to strengthen community participation, not neglect it."[31] Remuneration for health volunteers, in cash or in kind, remained controversial. Some believed it unreasonable to ask volunteers to work for years without some type of payment. The dominant view within MINSA, however, was that paying *brigadistas* would be an untenable financial burden. It would also undermine the spirit of voluntarism, which has helped to stimulate widespread community participation.

In the south of the Atlantic coast and northern border regions, however, the sparse population, difficult terrain, and lack of communications means that there is a clear need for full-time paramedical workers at the community level. The regional MINSA office trained full-time health *brigadistas* to provide curative and preventive health services.[32] They use canoes as ambulances to ferry seriously ill patients to health centers. *Brigadistas* are relatively well supplied with basic medicines despite shortages at many health centers and hospitals. This was a marked contrast to the situation in many other developing countries, where the community health worker is at the end of the supply chain and loses credibility because of a lack of basic drugs and supplies.[28]

WHO DECIDES?

Community participation involves more than labor in Health Days. Above all, it means having a say in what sort of health care is made available.[33–35] This was one of the main reasons for establishing Peoples' Health Councils in 1980. Donahue argued that this participation was very successful.[17] In 1981 the membership of Health Councils was broadened to include health professionals—a decision that many later felt discouraged autonomous community initiative. Religious missioner Celine Woznica lived in Ciudad Sandino at that time:[36] "The overriding problem with the People's Health Councils is the dominance of the Ministry of Health. This stands in the way of broad and effective community participation."

Lacking the authority and funds for independent initiatives, many community health leaders feel weak in relation to doctors and health officials. Guillermo Sanchez, a former school teacher, became a full-time health organizer in Estelí:

> We want our communities to be healthy, so we carry out health campaigns. But the local doctor where I live doesn't like it—he feels we are taking his

> business away or showing disrespect for his position. I have to take this into
> consideration, because he is the only doctor in the area. What will I do if my
> children fall ill and he won't provide treatment? And what if the doctor goes
> to Managua or leaves the country? Even a reactionary doctor is better than no
> doctor at all.

Many community leaders, however, feel less inhibited by the authority of
local officials and doctors. But when communities take charge of their
health care, conflicts are inevitable. In Ciudad Sandino, for example, the
local CDS repeatedly asked the health center director to replace the ambulance, which broke down beyond repair in 1982.[37] The director refused to
pass on the request to MINSA, giving as his reason the lack of personnel
to run the ambulance or determine which patients genuinely needs its services. Two years later, to the director's great annoyance, the CDS took its
request directly to the regional MINSA office.

Dissociating himself from the request, the director decided instead to
seek funds and authority for the construction of a small hospital for mothers and children. This proposal, however, was rejected by MINSA as
too costly. Community leaders finally were able to put their request directly to the president and the minister of health during a televised, open-
air "face the people" session in 1984. This bold move finally resulted
in the health center receiving a new ambulance donated by a foreign
organization. Two years later, an obstetrics wing was added to the health
center.

Financial conflicts are common. In 1981, for example, the CDS of Ciudad Sandino decided to collect one cordoba as a "voluntary contribution"
from patients waiting to see a physician.[38] The purpose of these collections
was to buy medical equipment, construct benches and chairs, and support
community health activities. Because the policy of the government was to
provide health care without charge, the CDS obtained special permission
from MINSA for these collections. By 1983, such collections had become
common in many parts of the country.

In 1984, however, the regional MINSA office ordered the CDS to stop
collecting money from patients.[39] With national elections scheduled for November of that year, the official policy of free health care assumed greater
political importance, overriding the issue of local autonomy. The CDS in
Ciudad Sandino did not challenge the directive even though it meant the
loss of its only regular source of income. Left out of the decision-making
process, the CDS slipped into a more passive role. Attendance of *brigadistas* at CDS meetings fell off and more dropped out of community health
activities. Similar dynamics occurred when community groups lost control
over MINSA-owned weighing scales used for well-baby checkups and food
supplement distribution.

THE WAR ON PARTICIPATION

The country's economic troubles were probably not as great of a deterrent to participation as was the Contra war. In the war zones, hundreds of *brigadistas* and community leaders stopped volunteering for fear of reprisals by the Contras (see Chapter 5). In 1983, as the Contra rebels increased their attacks on the civilian population, community participation moved onto a war footing.

Many People's Health Councils, especially in areas directly affected by the Contra war, trained *brigadistas* in first aid. When petroleum storage tanks in the port of Corinto were set ablaze by a Contra attack, *brigadistas* were able to treat the injured and helped to organize a rapid evacuation. In areas where Contra activity made it dangerous for families to travel to health facilities, *brigadistas* carried out immunization on a door-to-door basis. They played a leading role in preventing or containing outbreaks of diseases such as diarrhea, malaria, and leishmaniasis among those forced to abandon their homes by the war. They remain the backbone of the People's Health Days, which took on added importance where regular health services were disrupted.

Recent Trends

New forms of community participation in the late eighties replaced or supplemented the old. On Saturday mornings, about 100 mothers in Ciudad Sandino started to take part in health classes. The classes are organized by the women's organization AMNLAE, the nongovernmental agency CISAS, and the local health center. On returning home, participants are asked to pass on their knowledge to neighbors and friends. The emphasis is less on mobilizing volunteers than on educating the community as a whole.[40]

The structures for participation are changing. The national People's Health Council was abolished in 1986 because, as one MINSA leader put it, "it had become an empty, bureaucratic organization with no particular function." In 1989, a new type of national council was established in order to promote the Campaign to Defend the Lives of Children (see Chapter 8).

As the health system decentralized, community participation was able to respond better to local conditions.[41] In Managua, for example, MINSA encouraged the formation of neighborhood health commissions when high rates of clinic or hospital attendance for preventable conditions were noted. Doctors were then sent to make door-to-door visits to identify cases. In this context, *brigadistas* take ongoing responsibility for up to twenty homes each in target areas.

By 1988, the CDSs, which had increasingly become predictable mouth-
pieces for the FSLN, generated progressively less community participation.
In that year they were freed to become autonomous groups, and new activity flourished. *Brigadistas* are now more often housewives, church activists, or chronic disease patients rather than students. Their bravery and motivation provide great inspiration. Jorge Rodriguez was a *brigadista* in the
rural north. In January 1988, he was kidnapped by the Contras and has not
been heard from since. His nineteen-year-old daughter Olivia completed
her training in April to take his place. Asked why she would take on such
a dangerous task, she replied, "For the health of Nicaragua's children and
in memory of my father." An elderly rural birth attendant, when asked why
she risked her life, replied, "Because I'm tired of seeing my children and
the children of this country die of diarrhea."

After the new Chamorro government took power in 1990, participation
began to wane. There were 1,200 *brigadistas* in Managua's Villa Venezuela
in the late eighties; in 1990, only 800 could be found and many of these
were less active. The center-right UNO coalition even organized some of
its own health committees and volunteers! At the same time, many poor
communities are organizing local health activities to defend themselves
against what they consider a hostile national government. Many more are
demanding ongoing *brigadista* training in anticipation of a withdrawal of
the government-sponsored system to station social service physicians in
local health posts. Ironically, the populists who wanted volunteers to take
more (and doctors, less) initiative in health are now seeing their dream
come to fruition. When the government was controlled by the Left, community groups put more emphasis on pressing the state to respond to their
demands. Now that the Left is out of power, they feel compelled to defend
themselves from the government through developing greater self-reliance.
The Movimiento Comunal, for example, was training 7,000 permanent *brigadistas* for regions 2, 3, and 4 by late 1990. USAID views such efforts
with suspicion, as they may be closely allied with the FSLN and its efforts
to reestablish a political power base. For its part, the new government supports the concept of participation, but is seeking to generate the participation of wider, less politically motivated sectors of the population.

Community participation has become a major feature of the Nicaraguan
health system. Walt's review of similar projects concludes, "Large scale
volunteer programs will only be possible under [certain] enabling conditions . . . even then, they will suffer from high attrition and low activity
rates.[42] Heiby in Nicaragua viewed these problems differently. Referring to
prerevolutionary community health programs, in 1981 he described them
as "independent of the actual health services provided and the type of community agent selected."[43] This seems little more than an apology for the
failed health programs of the seventies. Attrition and inaction have indeed

been continuing problems, but important enabling conditions came into existence with the revolution. These include strong support for *brigadistas* from local communities, regular consultation and frequent supply of medicines from health authorities, and a political environment that encouraged voluntarism.

Regardless of the regime, the enormous force of community participation in Nicaragua has run up against serious political, financial, and administrative constraints. It is still an open question whether education and popular campaigns have led to empowerment. Early efforts in health promotion seemed to work so well that leaders thought they had hit upon "the" right formula, which was thereafter followed rigidly. It was assumed that mobilization was equivalent to empowerment. At the same time, resources crucial to independent community efforts were disappearing. Under these conditions, even the best approach to health education would likely bring only limited results.

Emerging new forms of participation described above will likely place more power in the hands of *brigadistas* despite their weakened political position relative to the new post-Sandinista government. Nonetheless, it is clear that the roles of such volunteers have been carefully circumscribed to reduce conflicts with health professionals. The one-day health campaigns described in the next chapter were a shrewd way to build the system by motivating volunteers while limiting the threat to doctors.

4

Mass Mobilizations

We do not believe that health institutions will make people healthy. The protagonists of health are the people themselves.

DORA MARÍA TELLEZ, minister of health

Our community is sick. The cure is the people.

JUAN ROSADO, community health organizer
Acajualinca barrio, Managua

SCENE: The health center in Ciudad Sandino, a township about ten kilometers outside Managua.[1]

TIME: About 1:30 in the afternoon on a People's Health Day.

Nearly 150 children have been vaccinated since the health team arrived at 8 A.M. Now the pace has slackened. Most mothers are home feeding or bathing their children, or rocking them to sleep in hammocks.

Jimena puts a vial of polio vaccine back into a thermal flask and sits down on an empty bench. On the far side of the room, two other health volunteers have begun dancing to American pop music playing on the radio. Others are chatting with the nurses or tidying up after the hectic morning. Some of the *brigadistas* are medical students. A few are fifteen- or sixteen-year-old high school students. Others are housewives with part-time jobs. Jimena, who is responsible for organizing this vaccination post, normally runs a refreshment stand from her home.

Five stocky, middle-aged women wearing frilly white aprons now file through the doorway. One carries a huge bowl of rice on her head, another a bowl of coleslaw and fried pork rind wrapped in banana leaves. A third brings a plastic bucket filled with a sugary fruit drink. The women immediately set about serving the *brigadistas* and nurses, laughing and joking with them as they eat. When Jimena and the others have finished, the women move on to the next vaccination post at the local primary school.

At about 3 P.M., a dozen children take to the street, banging pots and pans and yelling: "Parents! Bring in your children to be vaccinated! We don't want any cases of polio in our *barrio!* Vaccinate them! Every child deserves to grow up healthy!"

A few stragglers arrive, but Jimena's records show that two babies from the neighborhood have still not been brought in. She sends off two *briga-distas* to vaccinate them at home.

Finally, around 5 P.M., Jimena checks her records for the last time: Every baby and young child in the neighborhood is now up to date with its measles and polio vaccinations. She picks up a megaphone and goes out into the muddy streets, shouting, "It has just been learned that Block 8 has been liberated from the scourges of polio and measles. The children are victorious!"

This happy story is an appropriate opening to the chapter about this innovative and important subject. But mass mobilizations involve more complex issues. Who should control them? What difference can they make for health? How are they manipulated by political groups? What are their limits? And finally, when might other approaches work better?

We address these questions following a description of mobilizations for immunization-preventable diseases and malaria. Related efforts to reduce diarrhea morbidity and infant mortality are discussed in Chapter 8.

CONQUERING POLIO

Three times a year, between January and March, some 20,000 *brigadistas* immunize children in health posts, community centers, schools, and homes. Before 1979, immunization coverage was pitifully low. Fewer than 5 percent of young children were immunized against diseases such as measles, polio, tetanus, whooping cough, diphtheria, and tuberculosis.[2] Sporadic campaigns led by First Lady Hope Somoza left the great majority of children unprotected against these diseases, which killed hundreds of children each year and left many more disabled.

In late 1979, a series of epidemics swept the country: First polio, then measles, and finally whooping cough. Doctors and nurses responded by organizing weekend trips to immunize children in rural areas, where they met with some resistance. People opposed to the Sandinistas and their health initiatives (including some doctors) spread scare stories about the harmful effects of immunization. A particularly imaginative tale was that the fluids for injection were not vaccines at all, but Fidel Castro's urine. Most doctors resented what they saw as an incursion onto their "turf." "I won't say anything now," said one, "but these people have no right to come into this neighborhood and interfere. They think medicine is all politics. But what will they do when they get sick once they have destroyed the medical profession and there are no more doctors?" In any case, weekend trips by volunteers would not succeed in immunizing more than a small minority of young children. Nor would the formal health system, with its limited personnel and facilities, be able to rapidly accelerate immunization coverage. A new way had to be found to make immunizations more accessible and to convince parents to take advantage of them.

Once again, it was the Literacy Crusade of 1980 that showed the way forward. In some areas, literacy volunteers started polio immunization campaigns. The oral polio vaccine was cheap, safe, and easy to use: Volunteers could easily be trained to administer two drops into a child's mouth. Mexico and Brazil had already followed Cuba's example of organizing polio vaccination campaigns involving tens of thousands of volunteers.[3,4] In late 1980, MINSA decided to organize a national polio vaccination campaign during the first few months of 1981.[5,6]

The campaign proceeded in six steps: Volunteers were first recruited by community organizations and trained in a one-day workshop. They next made a census of all families in their area to identify children who should be vaccinated and to explain to parents why vaccination was important. Third, national publicity blanketed the country with information just prior to and during the campaign day. Fourth, on a People's Health Day, volunteers set up temporary vaccination posts in community centers, schools, health posts, or private homes (one post for every 100–200 residents) and vaccinated as many children as possible. Fifth, within three days they car-

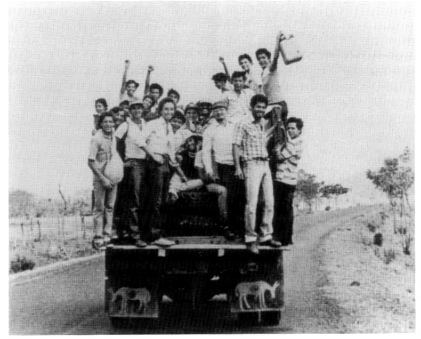

Volunteer vaccinators going to rural Jinotega in 1980.

Richard Garfield

ried out a "cleanup" campaign, going from house to house to vaccinate children not brought to the vaccination post. Finally, they filled in reporting forms that showed how many children in need of vaccination had been covered and how many were still unvaccinated.

The plan seemed to make sense, but would it work? In other countries, such campaigns had many problems. Would competing demands on people's energies limit the number of volunteers available? Would the low educational levels of volunteers leave them unable to vaccinate correctly? Would the government's poor organization lead to inadequate vaccine supplies? And would the trust and motivation of parents be enough to bring the children to the vaccination posts? In most countries, unpaid volunteers quickly lost interest in preventive health programs. Could Nicaragua find a way to keep people involved?

The 1981 campaign turned out to be highly successful. Estimated coverage with oral polio vaccine rose from about 24 percent to 70 percent among all under-one-year-olds[7] [increase as reflected in MINSA's estimates prior to each year's campaign]. The campaign also made apparent many weaknesses in the system. In the south, there were insufficient volunteers and large numbers of children went unvaccinated. In the north, there were enough volunteers, but many parents failed to bring their children to vaccination posts because they had not been properly informed about the benefits and safety of immunization. Many volunteers lacked the training or maturity to carry out their tasks effectively: Census information, for example, was often incomplete or inaccurate. There were also logistical problems: In many places the amount of vaccine available was insufficient; in other areas there was not enough "cold-chain" equipment to keep the vaccines potent until use.

In hundreds of meetings throughout the country, health workers and community leaders met to evaluate the 1981 campaign and plan the campaign for 1982. Health education activities were stepped up, volunteers were retrained, regular health workers were trained, and logistical systems were improved. The results in 1982 were even better and by 1983 the system worked better than anyone had dared imagine. Polio coverage reached 80 percent of children under five years old, with most doses being given on the three People's Health Days between January and March (see Figure 4–1).

Even more important, the campaigns were being planned and implemented by People's Health Councils with only technical assistance from MINSA. By 1983, most parents understood the importance of immunization against polio and wanted it for their children. "We don't see immunization campaigns as a medical question," said Lea Guido, then health minister, "but as a demand which comes from the people."

No cases of polio were documented in Nicaragua during 1982–1990 (see Figure 4–2). Cases were reported near the northern border in January

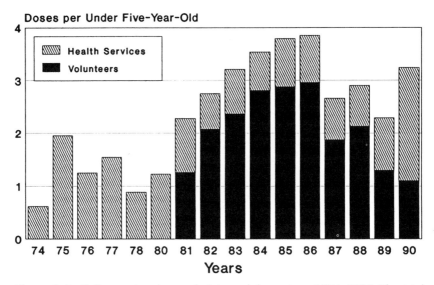

Doses per Under Five-Year-Old

Figure 4–1 Polio vaccine doses administered, by system, 1974–1990. The total number of polio vaccine doses administered exceeded the amount needed during the early 1980s. This "overkill" helped insure adequate population coverage. While the health care system continues to administer vaccines, all of the increase in doses was due to volunteers in health campaigns.

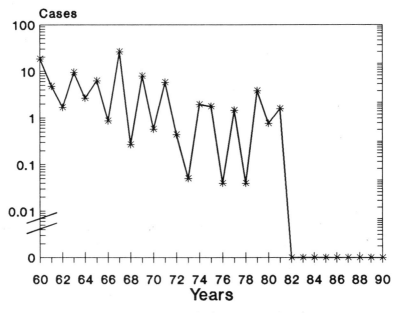

Logarithmic Scale Used

Figure 4–2 Polio cases reported per 100,000 population, 1960–1990. Incomplete reporting from past decades shows a slow decline followed by a rapid disappearance in the number of reported cases. Through 1990 no new polio cases were reported.

1989,[8,9] but these turned out to be other illnesses. Still, the often-made claim of "eradication" of polio seems overly optimistic. Cases are still being found in nearby countries, and low immunization coverage in some areas shows that a potential for outbreaks still exists.

BROADENING THE CAMPAIGN

Enthusiasm for this approach was so great that, in 1981, MINSA administered measles and diptheria-pertussis-tetanus (DPT) immunizations on People's Health Days. Since new skills were needed to administer these injectables, volunteers were given additional training.[10] Health education activities within the community, however, were sadly lacking. As a result, many parents objected to their children being vaccinated against two or three diseases in a single session. Waiting times at vaccination posts were also longer because of the increased workload on volunteers and staff. Even with these limitations, measles coverage doubled to 40 percent,[7] with volunteers providing 55 percent of all vaccine doses (see Figure 4–3). DPT coverage also increased, but only to a level of 22 percent. In 1982, DPT was dropped from the campaign, as it was thought that clinics and health posts could do the job better. Continuing low levels of DPT coverage led to its reintroduction in the 1986 immunization campaign (see Figure 4–4).

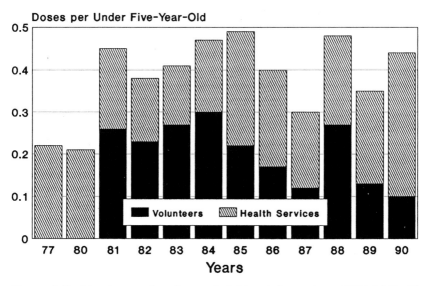

Figure 4–3 Measles vaccine doses administered, by system, 1977–1990. Although the number of doses of measles vaccine doubled after the revolution, coverage was still inadequate. The rise in doses administered is due both to the professional health system and volunteers.

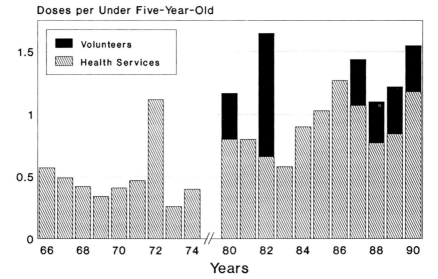

Figure 4–4   Diphtheria, tetanus, and pertussis vaccine doses administered, 1966–1990. A marked rise in DPT vaccine doses administered is due both to the professional health system and volunteers.

Measles coverage rose to 58 percent in 1985 but declined in subsequent years. The proportion of all immunizations provided by campaigns also fell. This decline was related to the war. Communities in areas under the threat of Contra attack were unable to organize effective health campaigns. Several years without access to vaccines created a large pool of vulnerable children. Under these conditions, one case of measles can lead to an epidemic.

Such an epidemic occurred in the war zones of regions 1 and 6 in 1985 and 1986, where nearly 500 cases were reported. Greatly improved reporting of vaccine-preventable diseases helped control the epidemic, but makes direct comparisons with prerevolutionary case-reporting data impossible (see Figure 4–5). Special teams made emergency forays into the war zones to provide measles vaccine. By late 1986, the epidemic was brought under control. Efforts made in subsequent years to raise immunization coverage throughout the country may be the reason why few cases and no deaths were registered in Nicaragua during a region-wide epidemic in 1989 that killed hundreds of children in Guatemala, El Salvador, and Honduras.

But by 1989, signs of another impending epidemic grew. A growing proportion of the cases reported in 1990 occurred among children over five years of age. This suggested that many of them had received ineffective doses as small children or failed to receive the vaccine, as they were too old to be targets of the campaign. Ironically, infants were now more vulnerable than before the vaccination campaigns began in the eighties. If their

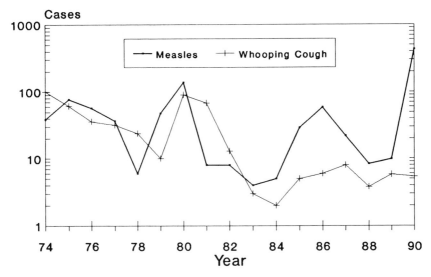

Cases

Logarithmic Scale Used

Figure 4–5   Reported cases of whooping cough and measles per 100,000 population, 1974–1990. Epidemics of whooping cough and measles were noted in the
year following the revolution. Levels then declined until 1985, when the cases in
war zones led to a rebound in the incidence of these diseases.

mothers had contracted measles in years past, they were protected by maternal antibodies during their first nine to twelve months. Now many mothers-to-be were immunized; their antibodies no longer offered protection to
infants. With only moderate vaccination levels in 1989 and a region epidemic underway, the dangers to Nicaragua were great.

The early months of 1990 passed uneventfully and the first MINSA mo-
bilization for measles vaccination reached routine levels of coverage. By
March, however, case reports started pouring in from around the country.
The first national epidemic in a decade had begun.

By the time of the second vaccination campaign on March 24, the UNO
government had taken over. Although most MINSA personnel retained
their posts, new leaders were unable to coordinate activities as efficiently
as the experienced Sandinistas. Publicity was scant and former volunteers
were not advised of dates for new campaigns. Vaccines in short supply were
administered on a first-come, first-served basis, without regard to their
prior immunization status or risk for contracting measles. New region 4
MINSA leaders reportedly gave the campaign low priority; an English solidarity group provided emergency funds to prevent the collapse of the campaign there. In region 1, syringes needed for the administration of vaccines
were diverted to provide care to contras returning from Honduras. Threats
from contras made brazen by the election lead to threats and the abandonment of the campaign in some areas. Diverting attention from weakness,

in MINSA's preventive activities, the new minister of health focused on traditional dietary practices, which tend to worsen measles cases among young children, and the importance of taking ill children to hospitals.

Worse still was the lack of cooperation from others in the government. In the middle of a campaign to discredit former Sandinista leaders, new officials claimed they were unable to lend vehicles as expected because the Sandinistas had stolen them. Municipal workers led reporters into parking lots at several ministries to show that, indeed, they were able but unwilling to cooperate. Only the army came to the aid of MINSA by supplying vehicles to mobilize vaccinators. But momentum had been lost, vaccines were missing or wasted, and the number of children reached fell. A volunteer from the poor Managua neighborhood Acajualinca complained: "When the vehicles and supplies didn't come, they told us to take people to the local health center. But there were only five doses of vaccine at the center, and we had hundreds of children to protect."

By the end of June, 6,000 cases and 190 measles deaths were reported. The third campaign went somewhat better and the epidemic had largely run its course by the end of the year, when 16,000 cases and 600 deaths had been totaled. By then, all that was left was to find a group to blame for this health disaster. Sandinistas pointed to the new government, which failed to mobilize community volunteers or utilize them effectively. Some, however, chose to blame the Sandinistas, who neglected preparations for the impending epidemic while spending lavishly on their reelection campaign.

Ironically, the positive example of Nicaragua has encouraged other Central American countries to organize community-based immunization campaigns in recent years. In El Salvador, a temporary truce arranged three times a year through the Catholic church and the Red Cross allows health workers and volunteers to vaccinate throughout the country. National or localized immunization campaigns are also organized in Honduras and Guatemala. It appears that vaccination campaigns combine the interests of volunteers and doctors better than any other preventive health technology. Volunteers can easily learn how to administer vaccines, governments can organize their efforts with relative ease, and doctors usually do not oppose them. Such campaigns in most countries, however, have achieved neither the high rates of coverage nor the same degree of community involvement as in Nicaragua.

Even the rightist "León Document" following the 1990 election gave a backhanded compliment to the Sandinista health program: "The only effective collaboration was the popular health campaigns for vaccinations."[11] Perhaps because of wide social agreement to encourage vaccination campaigns, MINSA wants to extend these campaigns. Such additional efforts are likely to bring diminishing returns to the country. Most of the deaths from immunization-preventable diseases had already been eliminated in the early eighties (see Chapter 8). What is most needed is continuous monitoring and rapid action when an epidemic is beginning.

MOBILIZING AGAINST MALARIA

Malaria control was the only public health program in Nicaragua that achieved broad rural coverage prior to 1979.[12,13] Funded primarily by international donors since the fifties, the program consisted mainly of periodic pesticide sprayings in houses to kill the malaria-transmitting *Anopheles* mosquitoes. Communities were not actively involved in these activities, which were carried out by technicians unrelated to the rest of the health system. The initial results of the malaria control program were quite dramatic. As in many other countries, however, the mosquito's astonishing ability to develop resistance to new pesticides meant that large-scale outbreaks of the disease continued to be common.

Antimalaria activities ground to a halt during the insurrection against Somoza. By July 1979, the malaria control system was in complete disarray and the number of cases reached epidemic levels not seen since antimalaria campaigns began in the fifties. As the demand for an effective response grew, the government searched for solutions. Campaigns were organized to clean up places where mosquitoes bred, but these achieved little.

Health planners began to reevaluate their strategy. Previous efforts had concentrated on attacking the mosquitoes to protect the people. But people were the only known reservoir for the disease. What would happen if they tried instead to eliminate the malaria parasites carried in the blood of infected people? If this were done on a wide-enough scale, a whole generation of mosquitoes might live and die without becoming infected, thus breaking the chain of transmission.

An extremely ambitious plan for a campaign, called the Final Offensive Against Malaria, was developed to administer antimalarial drugs to the entire population above one year of age during three days in 1981. It was a massive undertaking. Hundreds of thousands of volunteers were needed to inform every family and to distribute the right quantities of tablets to every person in the country. Once again, the "multiplier" strategy pioneered by the National Literacy Crusade provided the organizational basis.[14] A "core" of 120 malaria health educators were trained. They each trained ten volunteers as multipliers.[15] These, in turn, trained and supervised a total of 73,000 health *brigadistas,* who were responsible for educating their own communities according to their guiding principle, "Only the people can educate the people."

In September, six weeks before the campaign began, community groups, government workers, and school children began packing 35 million anti-

Some Sandinista activists saw the antimalaria campaign as a test of revolutionary faith, and the FSLN leadership had to quash an attempt to pass legislation that would have outlawed opposition to the campaign. In the end, the right of individuals to choose not to take part in the antimalarial campaign was upheld.

In the final week of the campaign, a total of 240,000 health volunteers and their helpers distributed antimalaria tablets from house to house throughout the country. Tallies showed that more than 8 million doses of chloroquine and primaquine had been distributed to 1.9 million people—70 percent of the total population.

During the next four months, the number of confirmed cases of malaria dropped dramatically: The campaign is estimated to have prevented at least 9,200 new malaria cases.[17-20] But by March 1982, transmission of the *Plasmodium vivax* malaria parasite returned to the level of previous years. The more serious *Plasmodium falciparum* specie of malaria was suppressed below expected levels for an additional three months.

The campaign did not succeed in eradicating the disease. It did, however, lay the basis for a new, more effective approach to combating malaria through community-based activities. It also succeeded in promoting widespread public awareness of malaria's symptoms and treatment. In addition, it created a new spirit of optimism and determination among community leaders and many thousands of new health volunteers.

It also succeeded in shaking up the government's routine malaria control program and in involving other government ministries and community groups in the program (see Table 4–1). The postcampaign antimalaria strategy involved many health volunteers in seeking out cases, taking blood samples, making a speedy microscopic diagnosis, assuring complete treatment of each proven case, and searching for further cases nearby. Under this strategy, the number of blood samples taken by health volunteers doubled from 1981 to 1984.[21]

The new approach brought dramatic results. Between 1983 and 1985, the number of malaria cases diagnosed in areas not directly affected by the Contra war—and inhabited by just over half the total population—dropped by 62 percent. An estimated 11,000 malaria cases were prevented between 1983 and 1986 in these areas. More importantly, the more serious *Plasmodium falciparum* parasite dropped by 88 percent, nearly disappearing in the peaceful areas. Thus, for the first time, and almost without using pesticides, malaria fell to low levels for more than five years in large parts of the country.[22,23]

In the war zones, where few malaria control activities could be maintained, thousands of people continue to suffer from this debilitating disease (see Figure 4–6). Movements of refugees and Contra troops along the borders also spread the disease in Honduras and Costa Rica. War-related de-

Table 4–1 Participants in the antimalarial campaign

Community Groups
    CDS: Block associations
    AMNLAE: Women's Organization
    JS: The Sandinista youth group
    MPS: The civilian defense militia
Labor Organizations
    ATC: Rural Workers Association
    CST: Federation of Sandinista Unions
    UNAG: Farmers and Ranchers Association
    ANDEN: Teachers Union
    FETSALUD: Health Workers Federation
    UNE: Office Workers Union
Govermental Bodies
    MINSA: Ministry of Health
    MED: Ministry of Education
    INRA: Ministry of Agriculture
    EPS: Army
    JRM: Municipal Governments
    MINCONS: Ministry of Construction
    INAA: Water Ministry
    IRENA: Natural Resources Ministry
    INTURISMO: Tourism Ministry
Other Groups
    Christian and other religious groups
    University and other student groups

Source: Garfield, and Vermund, SH. Health education and community participation in mass drug administration for malaria in Nicaragua. Soc Sci Med 22(8):869–77, 1986.

terioration eventually led to wide effects. In 1988 and 1989, vehicles, equipment, and aggressive case-finding for malaria control deteriorated throughout the country and the number of cases rose. The goal for 1990 was to "contain the deterioration" throughout the country.

Controlling other infectious diseases has resulted in similar dynamics. Dengue is a virus carried by another mosquito, the *Aedes egypti*. Dengue became an enduring problem throughout Central America with cases reported in each year of the eighties. Campaigns helped prepare for and limit the impact of epidemics, but were ineffective in replacing ongoing, routine attention to case-finding, public health education, and sanitary engineering.

Tuberculosis is a growing problem in much of the developed and developing world. It is estimated that 1 to 1½ percent of all Nicaraguans are infected yearly. The combination of campaigns and routine health services have helped make the tuberculosis control program in Nicaragua highly successful. Vaccinations delay the onset of infection and may reduce the

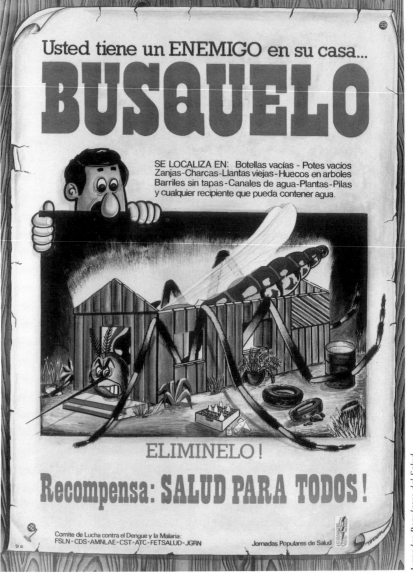

A poster used to motivate sanitation activities against the *Aedes egypti* mosquito imitates a 'wanted' poster from the old west: "You have an enemy in your house. WANTED. You will find it in empty bottles, ditches, puddles, old tires . . . and any other water-holding container. Reward: Health for ALL!"

severity of symptoms. Public education and the use of volunteers to search for cases and provide treatment has helped raise the proportion of all cases to receive treatment. An expanded search for cases, started with volunteers in 1988, has increased the number of cases diagnosed by about 10 percent (see Figure 4–7). A majority of diagnosed cases in recent years successfully

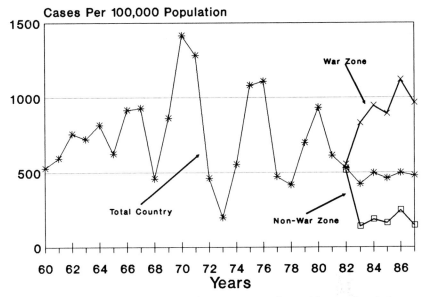

Figure 4–6 Malaria cases diagnosed, 1960–1987. The incidence of malaria varied greatly from year to year in the decades prior to the revolution, largely because of changes in insecticides used. A more stable national rate since 1981 masks a marked divergence in incidence rates in the war and non-war zones of the country.

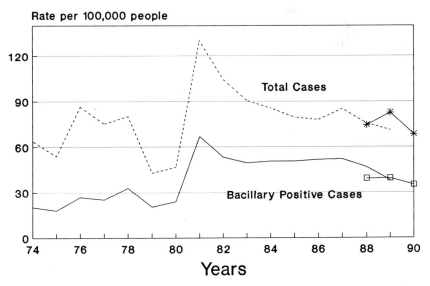

Figure 4–7 Reported tuberculosis cases, 1974–1990. Improved reporting of tuberculosis cases following the revolution masks a gradual decline in the incidence rate during the 1980s. A new reporting system, initiated in 1988, includes only physician-confirmed cases.

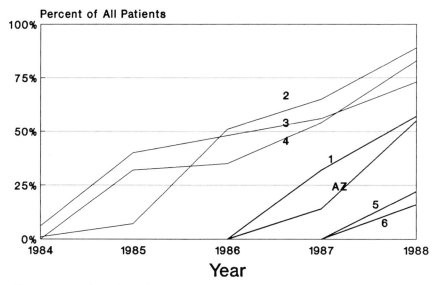

Figure 4–8 Tuberculosis short-course therapy, 1984–1988. Short-course therapy for tuberculosis requires more intensive administrative supervision of treatment. It was earliest and most extensively implemented in the non-war zone.

completed the twelve months of drug therapy required. A new short course of treatment yields even better results, but must be supervised. Begun in 1984, the eight-month short-course therapy by 1989 covered 64 percent of all those receiving treatment.[24] Even in the relatively unstable war zones, supervised therapy has become common (see Figure 4–8). With a guaranteed supply of medicines from the International Union Against Respiratory Diseases and careful coordination of volunteers with the professional health system, the tuberculosis control program has become one of the most successful in the developing world.

HOW USEFUL ARE MASS MOBILIZATIONS?

There is no doubt that the mass mobilizations against malaria and vaccine-preventable diseases gave a huge boost to efforts to control these serious health threats. They also succeeded in involving large numbers of people in health activities. Other mass campaigns—such as those against dengue and rabies—also appear to have had an important impact and involved tens of thousands of volunteers. Other campaigns, to improve sanitation among food handlers, to improve compliance among patients of chronic diseases such as hypertension, and to reduce smoking, have been considered.

But these mobilizations have drawbacks. The first is their short-term, periodic nature, which relegates ongoing health promotion to a secondary role. The malaria campaign, for example, led many to think that the disease was gone and could be forgotten about. Valuable time was lost before routine malaria control activities were reestablished following the "Final Offensive."

Short-term actions are easily manipulated when the outcomes will not be apparent for a longer period of time. MINSA, for example, was quick to take credit for averting an epidemic of dengue when no cases appeared following its massive 1983 antidengue campaign. When an epidemic did hit in 1985, resulting in 17,000 cases and 7 deaths, the political opposition attacked MINSA for failing to prepare for it with adequate beds and medicines for the sick.

Another drawback is the shift away from routine, ongoing health services that campaigns can cause.[25] According to Carolina Siu, formerly of the Division of Preventive Medicine:

> Mobilizations can raise our level of immunization coverage rapidly, but they should not be idealized as the best solution. Many children are missed in these mobilizations or receive vaccines before or after the optimal age. Immunization is only one component of the health needs of a child, and it should not be treated in isolation from the others. We must continue the campaigns to raise coverage right now, but in the long run our efforts to build up the basic health services will be more important, and will do away with the need for some campaigns.

A fourth drawback of mass mobilization is its tendency to alienate the medical profession. In the seventies doctors had become accustomed to lending their services on a charitable basis to short-term campaigns that did little to involve the general community. The status and power of the medical profession was thus reinforced rather than threatened. Many Sandinista activists had something very different in mind. They viewed community mobilizations as a way of demonstrating how much ordinary citizens could achieve *without* the help of doctors.

This often meant bypassing the medical profession. Oral rehydration posts were set up in community centers or private homes, volunteers were trained to give polio and measles vaccinations, and community leaders took responsibility for organizing People's Health Days. These were important steps in giving ordinary people the skills and confidence to take greater initiative in health matters. But they were perceived by many doctors as a threat to their professional status and power. Some tried to obstruct these initiatives. Others simply ignored them or refused to cooperate. Community-led initiatives probably contributed to the decision of some doctors to leave the country (see Chapter 9). Many viewed the situation like Dr. Mauricio Herdocia, who in a postelection article in *La Prensa* described the Sandinista health program as "based merely on preventive activities, irresponsibly marginalizing the curative sector."

The enormous influence of the medical profession on health policy cannot be long ignored. When organized medicine is openly hostile to the purposes or methods of mass health campaigns, passive or active sabotage is certain to follow. Yet doctors have the potential to make a major contribution to the success of such campaigns. They can assist volunteers with technical advice and skills, supply medicines and equipment, and organize training and evaluation sessions. They are also highly influential members of the community: The advice they give can be a critical factor in the success or failure of a campaign.

The model of the People's Health Days succeeded in involving thousands of people in health activities. But repetition of the same slogans and activities often became more of an act of political faith than a genuinely liberating process. According to Leonel Arguello, former director of the Division of Preventive Medicine: "To change someone's behavior by concentrating efforts on one day can help. But what about next month or next year? We need to pay less attention to slogans and put more emphasis on reaching a basic understanding. Only then will the people be in a position to take initiative, rather than just respond to MINSA requests."

According to Siu, "To bypass the doctors, we created vertical structures for health campaigns. What we need now is to foster an interdependence between doctors, community leaders, and volunteers." This interdependence seems to be a casualty of the 1990 election. The government is now less able to encourage health campaigns and collaboration between volunteers and doctors, as only the Ministries of Health and Defense lend their resources to such campaigns.

5

The War on Health

Stop your medical work or we will burn the clinic and you
with it.   Note left by Contra troops
for nurse in El Cedro, region 6.
[Three weeks later, on 18 March 1988,
the clinic was destroyed. The nurse fled to safety.]

Just before daybreak on the morning of 14 April 1984, Dr. Roberto Valle
Gonzalez woke to the clatter of small-arms fire and the crash of mortar
shells. Rushing out of the flimsy wooden house adjoining the health center,
he flung himself into a shallow trench. Moments later a child fell into his
arms, blood spurting from its mouth. It was, he later recalled, "the worst
moment I ever experienced as a doctor—watching that child die while I
was helpless to act."

They were under attack by Contras—the once-secret army of peasants
and former National Guardsmen organized by the CIA to weaken and overthrow the Sandinista government. Dr. Valle was marched away by Contras,
leaving behind a shattered health center and a burned-out ambulance. The
health center, built only a year earlier, had been the first ever in Sumubila,
a settlement in a remote area of the Atlantic coast inhabited by the Sumu
and Miskito peoples. Thirty days later, Dr. Valle managed to escape and
eventually found his way back to safety. Sumubila was left without a permanent health service until 1989.

The effects of the war on health in Sumubila were easily apparent to all;
the more subtle effects on the rest of the country were no less important.
This chapter reviews these effects and discusses their overall impact on the
health system and the country.

TARGETING THE HEALTH SYSTEM

Contra attacks on health and social services began soon after the Sandinistas
came to power. During the National Literacy Crusade in 1980, bands of ex-
National Guardsmen killed three young literacy volunteers near the Hon-

duran border in the north of the country. In 1982, a nurse and two Cuban schoolteachers were murdered by counterrevolutionaries. Following preparations in Florida, Contras equipped and supplied from bases in Honduras infiltrated northern Nicaragua in 1983 while others crossed the border from Costa Rica in the south. By the end of 1983, Contra forces were estimated to number between 12,000 and 15,000 troops.

Health facilities have been among the Contras' prime targets.[1-9] By the end of the war in 1990, 128 of the country's 600 health facilities had been closed, damaged, or destroyed (see Figure 5–1). The losses included one hospital, seven health centers, and 115 posts in six regions in the country. The construction of twenty-two others was abandoned because of the war.[10]

Whereas attacks took place over a wide area, they were particularly intense in regions 1 and 6, near the Honduran border in the north of the country. There were hopes that the Contra war would end after the five Central American presidents signed a regional peace accord in Esquipulas, Guatemala, in August 1987. But this long war was slow to intensify and slow to fade. Attacks decreased, but continue. In the twelve months that followed the signing of the peace accord, eight health workers were kidnapped, two wounded, and two killed in region 6.[11] A Red Cross ambulance was one of three attacked in the region during the same period. This was the first attack on the Red Cross since those by the National Guard in 1979. Two health centers and two child feeding centers were also attacked. Although such actions continued for several more years, their frequency di-

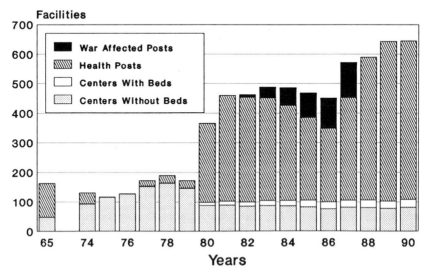

Figure 5–1 Primary care facilities, 1965–1990. The rapid rise in health facilities in the early 1980s was reduced in the late 1980s by the destruction or closing of health facilities in war affected areas.

minished as the Contra army slowly disintegrated and disbanded following the election of Violeta Chamorro.

Contras targeted health services as part of the social infrastructure established by the Sandinista government. They destroyed or damaged 67 schools and 125 social service centers serving 17,000 children and elderly people.[10,12,13] Another 503 schools and 800 adult education centers were closed due to threatened attacks, and 170 adult education teachers were killed. The government also halted the building of 2,000 rural homes and abandoned the construction of rural roads, water supplies, and sanitation facilities. By the end of 1985, close to 10 percent of the country's inhabitants and at least a quarter of those living in war zones—about 300,000 people—had lost access to health services because of the war.[1,14] Some facilities were destroyed and rebuilt several times. The health center in the township of Cerro Colorado, in region 6, was blown up for the fourth time by Contra troops on 21 October 1987. Before leaving, they gathered the social people together and told them: "As often as you rebuild this clinic, we will return to destroy it." It has not been rebuilt again.

In the small town of Mancotal, near the Honduran border, the health post was destroyed three times. On the first two occasions the people rebuilt it, despite contra threats of reprisal. After the third burning, health activities were transferred to the homes of three local *brigadistas*. Each took charge of a portion of the medicines to limit the risk to any one of them. In late 1988, they began to rebuild the health center again.[15]

Contras also raided government health services and *brigadistas* for medical supplies and equipment, especially in isolated rural areas. In the formerly neglected Atlantic coast region, where many new health facilities have been built since 1979, Contras robbed clinics at least thirty times since 1982. Dr. Domingo Vanegas was kidnapped from his social service post in south Zelaya and obliged to provide medical care to the Contras for almost a year:[16] "If I was short of supplies to attend to the Contra sick and wounded they would take me to the houses of *brigadistas* and say 'Take what you want, take everything if you need it.' The only reason they didn't kill the *brigadistas* was because they were a source of medical supplies."

DEATHS AND INJURIES

The Nicaraguan government reported a total of 6,760 people killed, more than 10,000 injured, and a total of 7,226 taken hostage or prisoner by Contra forces from 1982 to 1988[17] (see Figure 5–2). Almost 60 percent of the dead were civilians, including 455 children and 355 women (see Table 5–1). Apparently to dramatize the seriousness of the situation, many Ni-

Casualties (Thousands)

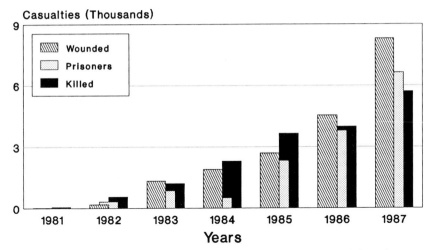

Years

Figure 5–2 Casualties, 1981–1987. The ratio of dead to wounded civilians is unusually high, reflecting the high intensity of this low intensity conflict.

caraguan and foreign observers have reported casualty figures as high as 12,000 dead.[8] They had no need to do so.*

The documented figure of 6,760 reflects a death rate of 0.2 percent. This rate is more than ten times greater than that for the U.S. population due to the Vietnam war.[18,19] It represents the proportional equivalent of 500,000 deaths in the United States. Less reliable estimates of Contra casualties suggest that close to 20,000 deaths have occurred among these forces.

Another common comparison is between those who die from war-related and non-war-related causes. Several investigators suggest that the war caused more deaths than occurred from polio, tetanus, and measles prior to the revolution.[20,21] In a more positive tone, MINSA promoted the slogan, "The revolution has saved more lives [through reduced infant mortality] than the Contras have taken." These comparisons are inaccurate or invalid. Some of the infectious diseases cited are highly visible, but are seldom causes of death. Yet these questionable comparisons were not needed to make the point; the war had far-ranging consequences for people's health.

Nearly one in every ten hospital admissions between 1983 and 1986 was for war-related injuries.[22] In the first two years of hostilities, 2,500 military personnel were wounded. Half of these injuries occurred among those under twenty-one years of age. Fifty-eight percent of those injuries were due to firearms, while 22 percent were due to bomb fragments.[23] Among survivors of Contra attacks, the most serious wounds are to the lower extremities as a result of fragmentation and explosion caused by mines or mortars.[24]'A third of all military wounds were to the legs. About half of those

*Part of the confusion concerning the number killed results from erroneous interpretation of the term "casualty." Casualties are defined as those injured or kidnapped in addition to those killed.

Table 5–1 Nicaraguans directly affected by the war,
1980–1988, in government-controlled territory

	Dead	Injured	Hostages, prisoners
Total	6,760	10,546	7,226
Age under 15 years	455	1,542	691
Seriously disabled		507	
Age 15–20 years	1,098	1,865	1,545
Male	6,405	8,943	6,363
Female	355	1,603	863
Military	2,961	8,507	1,060
Peasants	2,311	1,657	5,701
Professional, technical, workers, or students	1,488	382	465
Heath workers	48	26	32
Doctors	25	18	17
Nurses	9	7	6

Source: INSSBI.

injured are civilians. A typical incident occurred on the road from Pantasma
to Jinotega, in region 6, on 20 October 1986. A truck full of civilians hit a
Contra land mine. The force of the blast blew out the entire back of the
truck and killed four women, a seven-year-old girl, and a man. Among the
forty-three injured survivors, six had amputations on the spot and five more
had leg amputations within days.

Approximately 0.2 percent of the Nicaraguan population now has some
kind of physical disability. About half of these 6,000 people were disabled
in the Contra war. If the problem isn't a leg or foot amputated in the war,
it may be a missing hand or forearm from a homemade fragmentation bomb
during the 1978–79 insurrection, a deformity resulting from polio, or a
spinal cord injury from the 1972 earthquake. Treatment and rehabilitation
for these people are a heavy burden on the country's already overextended
medical and social welfare services.[25]

Many war deaths result from limitations in health services caused by the
war itself. American doctors Susan Cookson and Tim Takaro awoke on the
night of 2 July 1987 when a wounded government soldier was brought to
their poorly equipped health post near Matagalpa. Initially it seemed that
the young man had only a gunshot wound to the knee, but they soon real-
ized that he had abdominal injuries and was hemorrhaging. Hospital surgery was needed, but the army could not risk making the journey at night
because of the threat of Contra attack. "Our job," Dr. Cookson later re-
called, "became a race against the hemorrhage and time to keep him alive
until daybreak. The race was lost at 2:38 A.M."

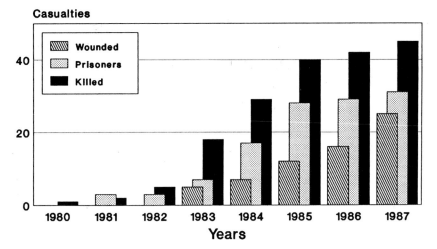

Figure 5–3 Casualties among health workers, 1980–1987. Health workers were in greatest danger in 1984 and 1985, before a revised MINSA strategy took many of them out of zones of conflict.

ATTACKS ON HEALTH WORKERS

By December 1987, a total of 48 health workers, including 25 doctors and 9 nurses, had been killed by Contras (see Figure 5–3). Another 32 had been kidnapped and 26 wounded.[18] Some of those kidnapped, including Dr. Gustavo Sequiera, vice-dean of the Managua Medical School, and Dr. Myrna Cunningham, governor of the northern Zelaya province, are high-ranking medical leaders. Most victims, however, are young nurses and doctors working in isolated rural communities.

In some cases, health workers were targeted and killed while carrying out professional duties. Such an attack claimed the lives of nurse Juana Cruz Padilla and ambulance driver Ambrosio Raudales Lopez, on 28 March 1983, as they were taking a patient by ambulance to Ocotal Hospital. Both were tortured before being killed.

Contrary to what has been reported elsewhere,[26] other health workers have been killed because they happened to be in an area under Contra attack. French physician Pierre Grosjean received a fatal shrapnel wound on 26 March 1983, during an attack on a village near Matagalpa where he was doing tropical medicine research. Nurse Marilu Reyes died in a Contra ambush in El Cua on 3 November 1984, when returning home after voting in the country's presidential election.

Brigadistas on the Firing Line

Nestor Castilblanco, a health *brigadista* in region 6, was abducted from his home in August 1986. He had already been kidnapped by Contras three

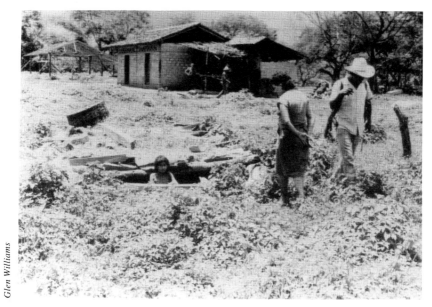

Santiago Arauz Cooperative, near the Honduran border, was attacked by Contras on December 31, 1984. Six people were killed. Several women and children took refuge in this shelter during the attack.

times before, and was warned each time not to take part in vaccination campaigns. This time they took him and three other male relatives. As his wife tried to follow, he yelled back: "I'm a dead man. " The next morning a search party found all four bodies, their eyes gouged out and testicles cut off.

The war took a heavy toll on the activities of health volunteers.[27] More than forty were killed and many more kidnapped. Hundreds have stopped volunteering because of death threats from Contras. Mary Elsberg, a health educator in south Zelaya, reported that the number of active *brigadistas* fell from 250 in 1983 to 60 in 1984. In 1986, when Contra activities lessened, the number of *brigadistas* increased to 120.

Health campaigns and educational activities in the war zones have suffered from the threats, killings, and destruction wreaked by counterrevolutionaries. Yet in many areas, despite a constant Contra presence, the government's health initiatives were carried out by volunteers. In order to avoid attracting the attention of the contras, health campaigns in war zones were often held prior to or following their announced national date. In some areas, vaccination campaigns were held on a door-to-door basis so that families did not have to leave the relative safety of their homes.

MINSA trained *brigadistas* for the armed forces, and armed guards sometimes accompany volunteers in dangerous areas. Initiatives to reach the people cut off by the war came not only from the government. In some areas, progressive priests gave *brigadistas* church identification cards. This was believed to confer some protection to the volunteer if he or she were kidnapped.

The Contras see health volunteers as representatives of the Sandinista government. Dr. Manuel Alzugarey, a Cuban exile, was in charge of Contra "The Miami Medical Team":[28] "The *brigadistas* are working with the enemy. They are a legitimate target. These people should not be in the war zones. The Sandinistas are using them for propaganda . . . It's hard to instruct our troops on Geneva Convention rules when they don't even know where Geneva is."

Dr. Tim Takaro worked with health volunteers near the Honduran border: "Their number one fear is being killed or kidnapped by Contras. They try to keep good relations with both sides. I would say they are Sandinistas in one way or another. They see that the children now get medicine. They own land they used to work for someone else. They see and want to participate in the progress."

WAR-RELATED DISEASES

Contra attacks, lack of basic supplies, and disruption of food production forced about 300,000 people to move from their homes (see Figure 5–4). Most fled to Managua and other urban areas, placing a severe strain on the already inadequate social and economic infrastructure. At least 100,000

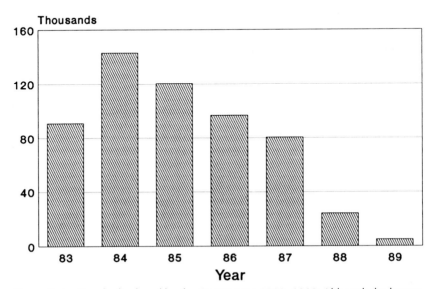

Figure 5–4 People displaced by the Contra war, 1983–1989. Although the largest group of people to flee their homes due to the Contra war did so in 1984, many more were displaced in the years which followed.

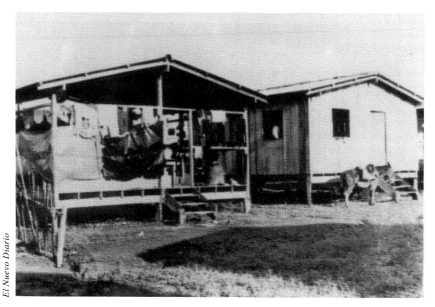

El Nuevo Diario

More than 100,000 people took refuge in resettlement camps after fleeing their homes during the Contra war. These houses, in La Esperanza resettlement camp, are being built by refugees.

settled in 145 new settlements established by the government in areas near their original homes.[29] A health clinic and a school are among the first buildings to be constructed in these new communities. Water supplies, sanitation, and food production invariably lag behind.

In the cities, marginal neighborhoods (called spontaneous or clandestine settlements) seemed to appear overnight. These neighborhoods have no lights, running water, or sewers. The epidemiology department of the regional MINSA office is responsible for identifying, visiting, assisting, and monitoring the health of people in these settlements. Forty-four of them were classified as unhealthy and nineteen as extremely dangerous in 1988.

These large-scale population movements—coupled with the inaccessibility of large areas due to Contra attacks—led to an upsurge in epidemics. The most serious and widespread of these was malaria. In the areas most seriously affected by the war, malaria control activities have been severely hampered. Malaria workers are hesitant to go into many areas, and visit war zones only briefly for cursory inspections. Regions 2 and 6 reported 70 percent of all malaria cases in 1986, compared with only 35 percent in 1983. Before the war, the risk of contracting malaria was almost equal in what were to become the war and nonwar zones. In the late eighties, the risk was ten times greater in war zones.[30] The worst malaria situation was found in new settlements, where poor housing, stagnant water, and overcrowding sometimes resulted in infection rates close to 100 percent.

Starting in 1983, some rural regions became inaccessible to immunization teams because of Contra activity. This breakdown in immunization coverage led to epidemics in those areas. In 1985 and 1986, the first measles epidemic since 1979 affected several thousand children. The great majority of cases appeared in regions 1 and 6, the two regions most affected by the Contra war (see Figure 5–5). In the department of Matagalpa, for example, the number of measles cases rose from 153 in 1985 to 956 in 1986.

There have also been smaller localized epidemics. In early 1987, for example, Drs. Cookson and Takaro diagnosed six cases of meningococcal meningitis in Jinotega. Four cases were from Abisinia, a Miskito area in a nearby war zone. Under normal conditions, health workers would have rushed to the area with antibiotics to treat the infected and halt the spread of the disease. Since health workers could not safely enter the area, however, the disease rapidly assumed epidemic proportions and lasted for several months. "The sick here," said Cookson, "are war victims whose number are not reflected in government casualty figures."

The war is also a major cause of malnutrition, due to the disruption of planting and harvesting and the difficulty of ensuring a regular supply of supplementary foods to new settlements.[31,32] Malnutrition killed two-year-old Gloria Rosales, the daughter of *brigadista* Pablo Rosales. Gloria suffered repeated bouts of diarrhea for several months. When Pablo was killed

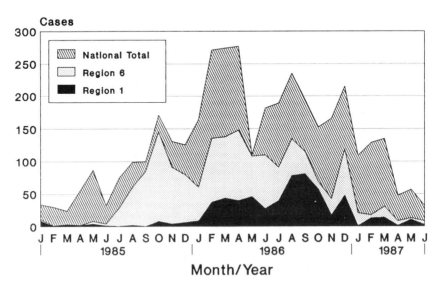

Source: Vigilancia Epidemiologica, MINSA

Figure 5–5 Reported measles cases, January 1985–June 1987. In the middle of 1985 a rapid rise in reported measles cases occurred in region 6. The epidemic soon spread to region 1. These two regions account for most reported measles cases during 1985 and 1986.

by Contras, along with U.S. volunteer Ben Linder, the family's income and plantings declined, reducing food availability. Within six months, Gloria died as an indirect victim of her father's work as a health volunteer.

Dr. Antonio Dajer saw a more alarming side of the picture of water-borne illness in five-year-old Kenia Calderon. "Her belly was tight as a drum and she hollered every time I put my hand on it." She suffered from intestinal perforation, a dreaded late symptom of typhoid fever. "We had heard of such cases but never seen one. With water systems breaking down from lack of parts and maintenance, it was no surprise that we finally had an epidemic on our hands." Kenia's story turned out to be a happy one. Following surgery, she overcame the odds and recovered.

Psychological Effects

The psychological impact of the Contra war is the most difficult aspect to quantify but may be the most far-reaching.[33-36] It affects three broad groups.

First are civilians living in war zones. Adults who see the results of Contra attacks on repeated occasions often wonder when death, torture, or injury may catch up with them or their loved ones. They tend to be preoccupied with the present and experience psychological problems stemming from a sense of insecurity and vulnerability.

The second group consists of civilians who live and work outside the war zones. They do not see the violence, but hear about it from friends, relatives, at meetings, or via the media. They often feel guilty about the im-

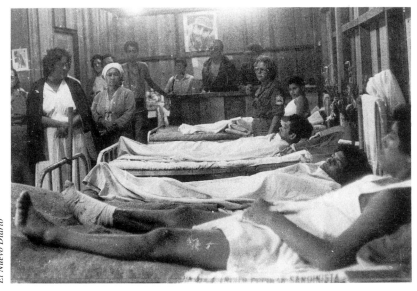

El Nuevo Diario

Mothers visit at the frontline military hospital in Apanas, region 6.

mense sacrifices made by those in the war zones and feel helpless and depressed about their inability to do anything to change the situation.

The third group consists of military personnel, including conscripts and militia, both in and outside the war zones. They experience the same problems as other soldiers who do not know when or where they next will have to place their lives at risk. Nor—despite the concerted international efforts in 1987–1988 to achieve peace—were they able to foresee an end to the hostilities. Battle psychosis, paranoid behavior, and depression are common.

Children living in war zones are particularly vulnerable to psychological trauma as a result of the war. In May 1988, an assessment team from CARE estimated that 40,000–50,000 Nicaraguan children suffered some degree of trauma.[37,38]

A museum in the town of Estelí exhibited children's art. Such art can reveal children's feelings, preoccupations, and inner thoughts. Asked to draw whatever she liked, twelve-year-old Marbelli Palacios Blandon had drawn a house with many people, small and large, going in and out. In the doorway was a coffin, and in other parts of the picture there were drawings of a garden, some flowers, and a heart. The child explained: "They took my Daddy, dragged him away, and killed him. Also, I painted the garden where we played with my Dad." Around the heart was written: "My heart is not quiet because they tortured my Daddy." And on one side: "This is my community, my Daddy they took away, dragged him, but I cried, screamed, and I want peace to come. Goodbye Daddy, I said while crying."

The meaning of a particular drawing depends on an understanding of the symbolic meaning and experience of each child. Common themes in this exhibit included fear, loss, and insecurity. These seem reasonable responses to the environment in which these children lived.

Terror invoked by sporadic death and destruction can devastate one's sense of autonomy. Dr. Antonio Dajer reflected, "It is so easy to forget the attrition factor when war is looked at from a distance. Every time the electricity went out, every time an extra shift of guard duty had to be done, every additional queue that wasted time, sapping people's energy and morale, made them less able to rebuild the country. For the civilians, it was the sense of impotence, of waiting to see where the Contras would strike next, that was so demoralizing."

Grief can also become overwhelming. Dr. Dajer observed that many of the patients at Somoto Hospital, just outside the war zone, were relatives of fallen soldiers. "Their grief kept them from eating, so they were brought in for IV fluids. One grandmother especially broke my heart. She was eighty-five, all wrinkles, and repeated with her raspy voice, 'Why couldn't I have died instead?' I tried everything: vitamins, saline, pep talks, and placebos, but nothing worked. By her fifth visit I wanted to escape out the back window rather than face the depth of her sadness again. My books say there is a natural limit to grief, but what do American psychiatrists know about the effects of interminable war?"

Effects of Embargo and Financial Boycott

Claiming Nicaragua to be a "serious and immediate threat to the security of the United States," the Reagan administration imposed an economic embargo in 1985. The embargo is commonly blamed for shortages of essential drugs, medical supplies, and surgical equipment.[38] This has only occasionally been the case. In 1984, for example, a shipment of raw materials to produce drugs was delayed for three months due to the mining of Nicaragua's ports and patrols by U.S. gunboats.[39] Some U.S. companies have refused to sell to Nicaragua for fear of breaking the law. Medical and relief supplies, however, were exempted from the embargo.[40] The lack of foreign exchange is a far more substantial reason for the shortages. This can be seen in the shortages of medical supplies, which grew worse in 1990, following the Chamorro election and the ending of the embargo.

More insidiously, basic materials needed for training and development of health programs are in short supply. For each dollar of value destroyed by the Contras, three dollars in funds for development were lost to a withdrawal of credits, loans, and shifts to defense spending.[41] Paper shortages meant that medical students could not copy their class notes to make up for the medical books that are unavailable. Lack of reagents led to cutbacks in the number of laboratory tests and X rays provided by the health services. In Puerta Cabezas, Dr. Kevin Cahill reported a "bizarre conversation with a German-born surgeon who firmly refused 'to operate any more without anesthesia; they move too much, I just can't do it.' "[42] Shortages of pens, felt-tip markers, slide projectors, and posterboard restricted health education activities. Journals, medical texts, and spare parts for equipment were in critically short supply.

Lack of finance meant fewer scholarships in the medical and allied health training schools. The economic downturn and the war led many health professionals to leave the country or seek private practice rather than government service. From 1984 to 1987, about a quarter of all MINSA employees left their posts each year, making continuity of programs impossible. In these and similar ways, the war was felt every day throughout the country (see also Chapters 11 and 12).

LOW INTENSITY WARFARE

In military terms, the Contra war was of "low intensity."[43] This is reflected in a comparison between 6,760 deaths among Nicaraguans in this war and 35,000 deaths during the insurrection of 1978–79.[44] But damage to the country's social and economic infrastructure has been devastating. Living standards and the quality of services have declined sharply since the war intensified in 1983. It is estimated that more than $3 billion worth of loss has occurred.[45] This is the result of a U.S. policy aimed at undermining the government rather than confronting it in conventional, land-based territorial warfare. The same policy was applied throughout the eighties in "low-intensity" wars against progressive regimes in Angola and Mozambique[46] (see Table 5–2).

Low-intensity warfare, according to Colonel John Waghelstein of U.S. Army Special Forces, is "total war at the grassroots level," involving "political, economic, and psychological warfare, with the military being a distant fourth."[47] The United States' objective is not to defeat the Sandinistas militarily, but to bring about their political downfall. Zeno Bisoffi, an Italian doctor working in the north of the country, described the Contras' motivation in this way: "Some of them lost power or money with the advent of the revolution. They want to come back to their areas and punish their neighbors for the improvements these people now enjoy. Others want to deny social benefits to the population because services increase the population's support for the Sandinistas. Somehow, they seem to feel that they can terrorize the peasants into passive submission, like in the old days of Somoza's rule."

The protagonists of low intensity warfare use disease as a political metaphor. The Reagan administration repeatedly referred to Nicaragua as a "virus" or "cancer" that had to be surgically removed.[5] Former White House spokesperson Patrick Buchanan called Nicaragua a "malignant tumor" threatening the health of the whole Western Hemisphere: "There can be no negotiating with a cancer. Surgically precise military strikes are the necessary remedy." This political "diagnosis," however, has given rise only to remedies that make the "patient" suffer more.

Table 5–2 Low-intensity wars in the eighties: A comparison of Nicaragua and Mozambique

	Nicaragua	Mozambique
Heath workers killed	48	21
Health workers taken prisoner	32	45
Ambulances destroyed	10	20
Health posts attacked or closed	131 (22 percent of all)	484 (25 percent of all)
Destruction of health facilities (millions)	$6	$20
Health as percentage of all destruction	3	4

Source: Cliff, J and Noormahomed, AR. Health as a target: South Africa's destabilization of Mozambique. Soc Sci Med 27(7):717–22, 1988.

The Contras do not fit the classical model of a guerrilla army.[49] Rebel forces fighting wars of national liberation in countries such as Angola, Mozambique, and Zimbabwe enjoyed the support of the majority of the population. They attacked government forces by surprise but usually left civilians in peace. They had a broad, coherent political program. The Contras, by contrast, attack civilian targets and avoid engagements with the Sandinista armed forces.[5] Their political agenda involves little more than trying to return to the prerevolutionary status quo.

The Government's Response

Three programs involving health volunteers were mounted to mitigate some of the most harmful effects of the war. The first, a first aid training program, prepared 25,000 volunteers in wound management, resuscitation, evacuation of the injured, and patient assessment. The second, building refuges to protect civilians from attack, came from the experience of the FSLN during the insurrection of 1978–79. A refuge in this case consists of a hole about five feet deep covered with logs and earth to provide protection against bomb and mortar attacks. Finally, fire control education and practice sessions are held periodically throughout the country to reduce damage caused by sabotage or enemy attack. This helped to reduce damage and speed evacuation of civilians following the Contra attack on petroleum storage tanks in Corinto in October 1983.

Paradoxically, the war also led to some positive changes in the health system. Among these were more efficient use of resources, better organization, the setting of clear priorities, and increased administrative decentralization.[26] According to former Health Minister Dora María Tellez: "The tighter things are, the better we have to organize things so as to obtain maximum usage of our resources." While concentrating formerly scattered rural communities into new settlements quickly led to localized epidemics, it also made it much easier for health workers to reach families with preventive and curative services.

But the war also distorted the way in which health and social services developed. When the Contras started losing the war in 1986, land mines were used more intensively. This resulted, late in the war, in a rise in the number of amputations performed in Managua hospitals and a rapid rise in the number of permanently disabled citizens (see Figure 5–6). The government was forced to invest heavily in rehabilitation instead of other health programs. Similarly, social welfare is focused on the 10,000 orphans caused by the war, neglecting other children in need of care.

The deaths of a French and a German physician early in 1983 brought a sobering reassessment of the roles of foreign health workers in primary health care. Responding to the concerns of Western European governments,

MINSA moved foreign health workers in areas with frequent Contra activity to safer places. In 1986, foreigners were further restricted to living and working in the capital cities of regions with frequent military activity. This caused many rural health and development projects to come to a halt. Ironically, of the foreign doctors, this left only the Cubans and Americans to work in war zones. The Cubans were there because of the close political alliance between their government and Nicaragua's; the U.S. citizens could remain there since their government was already so hostile, it had little influence.

In many rural areas, the government halted construction of health facilities due to the war. Nevertheless, new hospitals, health centers, and health posts were built in the war zones. These facilities, usually located in areas close to main roads and therefore more defensible, now form the backbone of the health system in these areas. The town of Jalapa, for example, is only five miles from the Honduran border and was twice put under siege by the Contras. New operating theaters were added to the government hospital there in 1986, making it a more independent regional center.

Hospitals in border regions functioned on a war footing.[49] The hospital in La Trinidad, near Estelí, for example, has become exclusively surgical, serving as the main curative center for war-related injuries in the north. A new surgical army hospital was built at Apanas, in the north. In other hospitals in the north, up to 25 percent of all patients suffer from war-related injuries. These hospitals maintained empty beds in order to receive the war-injured on short notice. Even the major hospitals in Managua had contin-

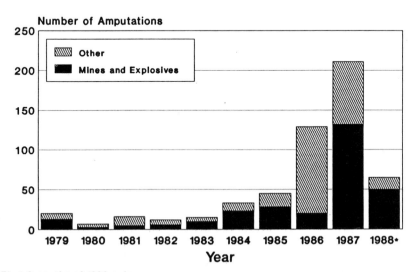

•First 6 months of 1988 only

Figure 5–6 Amputations performed, 1979–1988. A shift in military tactics to hit-and-run attacks and the widespread use of mines toward the end of the Contra war was associated with a dramatic increase in the number of amputations carried out in Managua hospitals.

gency plans to handle up to three times their usual number of patients if necessary.

In war zones, army doctors treated large numbers of civilian patients in order to fill the gap left by the destruction or closure of health centers and posts. This was made possible through the recruitment of more physicians into the army, the mobilization of civilian doctors (see Figure 5–6), the creation of teams of medical students in health brigades of three to eight months' duration, and close coordination between the civilian and military medical authorities in the war zones.

Health as a Bridge to Peace

In May 1988, 500 health workers took advantage of a sixty-day cease-fire to reestablish contact with people in areas controlled by the Contras near the Honduran border. They started to enter the war zone in March, before the cease-fire, under the protection of the Red Cross and the Catholic church. In May they fanned out across a vast area in pairs. In most communities the presence of health workers was welcome. The teams' goal was to learn what were the greatest health needs after five years of isolation. Dr. Alvaro Ramirez, who organized the teams, saw this as a chance to rebuild. He said, "When peace comes, MINSA will be a purely social institution, so we are trying to get a new image now. We want to talk less about the revolution and do more for it."[50] Dr. Amado Gavidia, a team leader, added, "We must think about building health for the future, because we are not always going to live at war."

Predictably, they found a population that was sicker and poorer than in other rural areas. Only 6 percent of the people had latrines, 70 percent of children were malnourished, and 80 percent of pregnant women were at high risk for poor birth outcomes. Tuberculosis, diarrhea, and respiratory diseases were common. Surprisingly, immunization coverage was good. As immunizations were the only long-lasting protection mothers could secure for their children during occasional trips into Sandinista-controlled territory, they had carefully sought them out.

The teams trained *brigadistas* to staff four abandoned health posts and established twenty new ones. These volunteers will form the core of a rural health service. Private organizations also must be involved in the efforts. Private organizations also must be involved in the efforts. The most important of these is probably CEPAD—the major Protestant social service organization in the country. CEPAD's health branch PROVADENIC runs dozens of exemplary clinics, as well as programs to feed the displaced, rebuild houses, and construct latrines and piped water systems.[51]

Volunteers treat the local population, as well as patients who have brought medical records (complete with Contra insignias and flags) back with them from Honduras.[52] They hope to continue building this rural health network as the war winds down. According to Dr. Gavidia, "We have to create the peace now." This work isn't easy. Contra supporters bring back with them heavy burdens of tuberculosis, typhoid, sexually transmitted diseases, malaria, and malnutrition. They present an enormous new burden to the health system, as well as a threat to the health of other Nicaraguans.

ENDING THE WAR

Following the 1990 election, the Contras were asked by President-elect Chamorro to lay down their arms, return to Nicaragua, and reintegrate into civilian society. This included at least 70,000 people. Some 30,000 of them were indigenous people who slowly trickled back to northern Zelaya starting in 1988. The 40,000 others were Hispanics: 20,000 were Contras, and 20,000 were refugees who accompanied them. The UN set up the International Verification and Support Commission (CIAV) which, through PAHO, established health services at eight reception centers to facilitate their return, assure the destruction of their arms, and initiate their reintegration during the spring of 1990. But they didn't come. "We set up clinics at the reception points. Day after day we sat and waited," according to Dr. Julio Caldera, former director of several military hospitals and current head of the CIAV medical service. President-elect Chamorro met repeatedly with Contra leaders, but still there was no action.

Part of the problem was organizational. Disintegration of the Contra military command structure during the last years of the war left no one with whom to negotiate effectively. Some Contras had already trickled back. The main problem appeared to be psychological. After so many years of fighting, the peasants who made up the Contra forces knew no other way of life and were hesitant to give up familiar weapons for an uncertain future. That's why medical services were considered key. A familiar, friendly, neutral-looking station might elicit their voluntary return; an authoritarian police or army structure would not.

The reception centers were set up in consultation with Contra physicians. Their main sources of care in Honduras had been a Contra family clinic in Danli and a military base hospital in the jungle near Yamales. These centers sometimes provided good care, but suffered from unstable administration and routine robbery of supplies. In one case, a stock of soy milk was rushed to Danli to respond to the desperate malnutrition among young children that followed the reduction of adult food rations. The milk was found for sale the next day in nearby Honduran food outlets. Thus, little was known about the health conditions of those who were to return. How sick would they be? Would referrals to be accepted at appropriate civilian hospitals? And would they lay down their arms, or were doctors at the reception posts putting themselves in danger? Four tense weeks went by with hardly anyone crossing over. When Sandinista leader Umberto Ortega was reappointed minister of defense by Chamorro, there was renewed talk of fighting and reception centers considered closing.

Following further negotiations, things finally started to happen. Radios linking the reception centers started squalking: "Four real soldiers appeared this morning." Other small groups appeared sporadically. "Look, there really are doctors, it's not a trap," they whispered among themselves. They received medical exams, AIDS and laboratory screening, immunizations, and health education. Then larger groups appeared. From April to June 1990, more than 2,000 Contras were processed at the demobilization centers.[53] By the end of the year, about 20,000 people passed through the centers. While only a small number of venereal disease and HIV-positive cases were found, conditions prevalent in jungle environs were common. A third of those processed were children. They had a rate of malnourishment (18 percent) similar to that of the general population. Only 6 percent of them had a complete set of immunizations. Of the 2,000 individuals screened, 125 children had severe caloric malnutrition and 129 women of fertile ages had dysmenorrhea. Skin diseases were rampant, and tuberculosis, leishmaniasis, and malaria were common. More than half of the adults had never attended school.

The women especially had suffered. Many had lived under plastic sheets in almost complete isolation except for when the male combatants to whom they were attached came to visit. Many had little relationship with these men, and kept the appearance of a relationship to maintain access to U.S.-supplied food rations. There was often little attention to the children, who were semiabandoned.

Even after passing the reception centers, the ex-Contras and their dependents remained isolated. Rather than staying at reception sites in the northern Nicaragua cities, they set up camps of their own several miles outside of the towns. Their main contact with the world was via field radios, which they were allowed to keep.

If medical care had facilitated their return, it didn't assist the planned settlement of "development poles." Plans for new health centers and rural hospitals were shelved when people trickled away to their communities of origin throughout north and central Nicaragua. Instead, new or augmented clinical services were scheduled for areas where they became a major burden on existing services. These take advantage of the 1,200 Contra military medics in the system of *brigadistas* for rural areas. By late 1990, some of the medics had started training in maternal-child care along with local volunteers in short workshops in El Cua. In addition, plans were developed for rebuilding a hospital on the Atlantic coast at Bilwascarma for the indigenous peoples.

Whereas malnourishment and malaria were expected, measles was not. Many young children had received almost no medical attention in their Honduran base camps. Many of those who were vaccinated had received the immunizations just before returning. As a result, the vaccines didn't have time to take effect. These unprotected children contributed to and were victims of the epidemic then engulfing northern Nicaragua.

PRIMARY CARE VERSUS HOSPITAL CARE

Commenting on a health system in Afghanistan, structured like Nicaragua's to maximize scarce medical resources, doctors observed that "unfortunately, such a [sophisticated] system is vulnerable to political instability and war."[54] The war in Nicaragua greatly increased the need for highly skilled surgical care and rehabilitation, which can be provided only through expanded and improved hospital facilities. Until 1983, Nicaragua's health budget increased the share for primary health care and reduced the proportion for hospital care. Since 1983, however, the proportion allocated to hospital care increased in order to cope with the influx of war-related injuries requiring hospital surgery, and to reduce the deterioration of hospital services.

It appears that the war led to a retreat from community-based, primary health services with an emphasis on prevention. Greater reliance on the skills of hospital-based surgeons and other medical specialists became the norm. Yet where doctors cannot provide modern curative care, as in the war zones and other remote areas, a renewed reliance on volunteers and preventive activities occurred. A two-tiered system of care emerged with the war. The rural system was run by *brigadistas* at the primary level; the urban system was led by surgeons and other specialists needed for war-related pathologies.

While the curative hospital system was being strengthened in cities, the resources of the entire health system were being stretched to the breaking point. The military and economic war against Nicaragua had, by the mid-eighties, plunged the health system into a deep economic and organizational crisis.

6

From Expansion to Crisis Management: 1984–1990

> The truth is that we have made errors. One of these was the big expansion plans we had for the health sector. It was right to bring health services to the whole population, but not to try to do it all immediately, overnight.
>
> PRESIDENT DANIEL ORTEGA, 1985[1]

When there was a national shortage of light bulbs in 1985, hospital nurses on their nightly rounds carried a bulb with them from ward to ward. It seemed that everything—supplies, equipment, spare parts for vehicles, fuel, and food for patients—was either in short supply or not working. Articles in local newspapers denounced the theft of medicines by MINSA officials. Articles started to appear in the international press about the collapse of the health system.[2] It hardly seemed possible that this was the same country that, in 1982, was provided priority funding and attention by UNICEF and the World Health Organization (WHO) for the development of its primary health system.*

WHO's investment was fitting acknowledgment of the momentous changes that occurred during the first years of the Sandinista revolution. Between 1980 and 1983, government health expenditure in Nicaragua averaged forty dollars per person annually—triple the level of spending prior to 1979.[3,4]

Hospitals were opened to the entire population, hundreds of health posts were constructed, thousands of health workers were trained, and nationwide prevention programs were begun. Community organizations set health priorities and carried out programs.[5] Tens of thousands of volunteers organized health activities. Yet these initiatives were often anarchic in character, leading to waste and inefficiency.[6-8] They added to the already considerable pressure exerted by the people on the health system, and created new de-

---

*This was widely misreported as an award that Nicaragua won from WHO for its achievements in primary care. In fact, no such award exists.

mands without satisfying old ones. A way was urgently needed to bring them together in a coherent national primary care program. The years from 1984 to 1990 can be readily viewed as the period in which such a system slowly emerged.

PIASS

In April 1983, PIASS, "The Integrated Program for Activities in the Health Area," was launched. PIASS was an attempt to take clinic-based services into the community.[9] MINSA hoped that this would foster community participation in, and demand for, health services. PIASS was also expected to relate to literacy promotion, combat childhood diseases, improve housing and nutrition, and generally raise the quality of people's lives.[10]

PIASS had four distinctive features. First, it aimed to assure that doctors would be available at health posts so that professional health services could extend from the clinic to neighborhoods and villages. Second, PIASS programs would be carried out by interdisciplinary teams of health workers. The primary health program was to involve a total of eighteen disease- or risk group-specific activities. Third, health volunteers (including trained birth attendants) were to be members of the team at the health center or post. Finally, the program was to emphasize the importance of living conditions (housing, water, sanitation, hygiene) as determinants of health. PIASS (along with DECOPS; see Chapter 3) was expected to help communities examine the cause of ill health in the social and political context of their communities in order to motivate local efforts for change.

The program began in Estelí, where the revolution had strong support and community organizations were very active. It was further tested in five of the seventeen health areas of Managua in early 1983. Later that year, despite warnings from some health leaders to avoid hasty implementation, it was proclaimed the nationwide program for primary care.

Health leaders hoped that the enthusiasm with which PIASS had been taken up in pilot areas would be replicated nationally. The economy was growing, the health sector was still relatively well endowed with funds, and the Contra war was only starting to drain the country's limited resources. Health and community leaders were also euphoric about the recent participation of tens of thousands of volunteers in mass campaigns against malaria, dengue, polio, and measles (see Chapter 4). It seemed that anything could be done.

The scheme captured the imagination of many health professionals, community leaders, and volunteers. It soon became evident, however, that PIASS made impossible demands on the country's limited resources. They

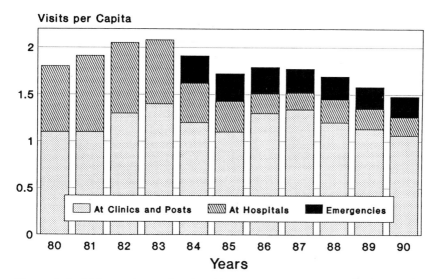

Figure 6–1 Visits to doctors by site, 1980–1990. Per capita medical visits declined from 1982 to 1985. They rose again in 1986 when new efforts in primary care were made. The war and survival economy continued taking its toll on the health system, resulting in declining visits per capita through 1990. Throughout the decade, the proportion of all visits to take place at hospitals declined.

believed that the improved health PIASS would engender would reduce demands on the curative care system. Instead, it led to new demands and expectations for doctors and medicines that the health system could not meet. In 1983, the year when PIASS was launched nationally, the average number of visits to a doctor per person was just over two per year (see Figure 6–1). This was three times higher than the average number of per capita visits prior to the revolution, but a continuing rise in visits could not be sustained without more doctors and funds (see Figure 6–2).

In 1985, the average number of visits to a physician fell to 1.7. The decline in medical visits was partly a result of the closing or destruction of facilities by contras. But the haste with which PIASS was introduced, with insufficient resources or planning, also limited the chance of success. With inadequate training and little information about the new system, many health workers did not even fully understand how it was supposed to work. By 1984, with the Contra war draining government resources and the economy beginning to decline, PIASS faltered. The program was thus one of the first major casualties of the Contra war.

Yet the program may have contained the seeds of its own demise. As the Health Plan for 1987 admitted,[11] "[PIASS] was planned on the basis of international norms without consideration of the national reality. It was planned to implement an endless number of programs, each of high priority,

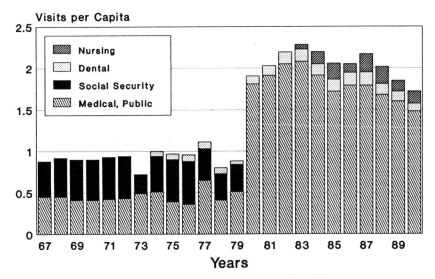

Figure 6–2 Medical, nursing, and dental visits, 1967–1990. Despite a rise in visits to doctors following 1985, population growth prevented a return to per capita rates of two visits per year.

in the health areas, without careful consideration of the fact that, at the present time, only nursing personnel are available at this level [the health post]."

The critical weakness of PIASS was the assumption that there would be enough revolutionary doctors and funds to operate a high-quality system of primary medical care. As shown later, neither the doctors (see Chapter 9) nor the funds (see Chapter 11) materialized. Primary health care continued, but services were less accessible, less community-oriented, and less preventive than was envisioned in the program. the PIASS name fell into disuse after 1985.

QUALITY OF CARE

During the early eighties, Nicaragua's political leaders encouraged the public to expect free health care as one of the fruits of the revolution. It was therefore hardly surprising that people demanded more and better health services, especially at hospitals. By 1983, the country's health leaders recognized that the *quality* of the health services was often poor and getting worse. Former Health Minister Amador Kuhl observed, "In preventive medicine, I think we have come a long way. . . . But curative medicine is a disaster. The hospitals are in terrible shape and doctors do not have the tools for even the most basic diagnosis or treatment."[12]

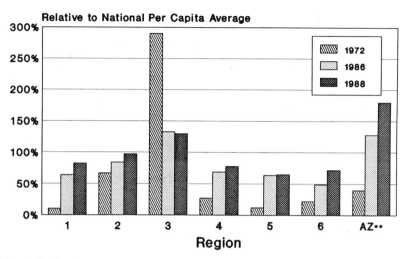

Relative to National Per Capita Average

*National Per Capita Average = 100%
**The Autonomous Zone, Atlantic Coast

Figure 6–3   In 1972 health funding was highly concentrated in the capital city of Managua. By 1986, per capita spending was far more equitable.

From 1979 to 1983, MINSA allocated increasing resources to primary care. This resulted in a much fairer distribution of health resources between Managua and outlying regions (see Figure 6–3), except for medical care to infants, which remained far more accessible in Managua (see Figure 6–4). The inevitable result was that hospitals, which had already suffered from neglect during the Somoza regime, declined more rapidly, especially in Managua. Staff salaries were frozen and little incentive for educational advancement existed. Chronic supply shortages became more severe, and long neglect of maintenance led to the deterioration of physical plants.

Many hospitals had running water only part of the day, electricity failed during surgery, and backup lights broke down. On three separate occasions in a single year, a surgeon in Estelí was left in the dark with a patient's abdomen wide open during a gastrointestinal operation. Whenever the electricity failed or respirators in an intensive care unit broke down, a nurse had to maintain the oxygenation of the patient by hand for up to twenty-four hours.[13]

Dr. Antonio Dajer helped perform an operation for retained gallstones and an infected gallbladder under these conditions. "Without cautery, intraoperative X rays, or even the right-sized drain, we plunged in. I could barely tell the gallbladder from the liver or small intestines, the scar tissue was so thick. The operation lasted five hours. Halfway through, the power went out. An emergency generator kept a light on, but there was no air conditioning. Beneath heavy surgical gowns, sweat soaked my underwear.

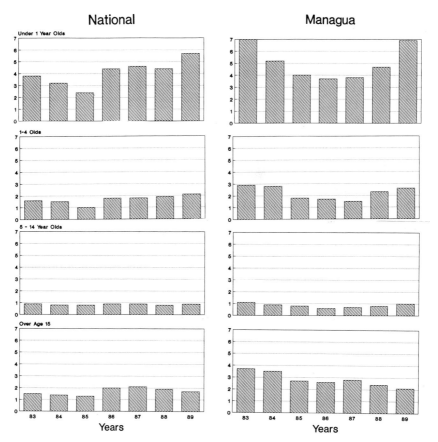

Figure 6–4 Per capita medical visits, by age, 1983–1989. Infants had by far the highest rates of health service utilization. Among most age groups, Managua residents enjoyed higher rates of health service utilization than the national average.

My glasses threatened to slide off my nose. The scrub nurse fainted, but the patient's vital signs remained steady.''

Some of the older hospitals had a medieval atmosphere about them. The wards were long, dark chambers, in which two patients often had to share a single bed. Psychiatric patients wandered freely across dirt court-yards, dogs and children scavenged in garbage heaps, while laundry-women scrubbed blood-stained hospital laundry over open-air concrete sinks.

Three of the worst hospitals were closed when five new ones came into service between 1981 and 1984. Financial constraints made it necessary to shelve plans for other new hospitals and clinics. Instead, emergency repairs were carried out to keep old facilities in use. Hospital salaries were also increased in 1983 to attract larger numbers of qualified doctors and nurses.

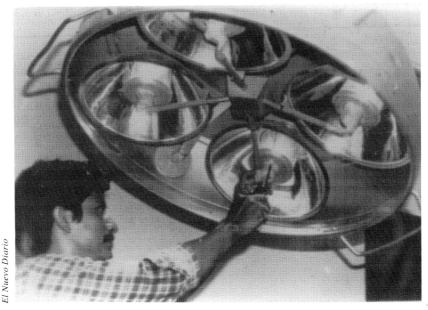

El Nuevo Diario

Because of a shortage of high intensity surgical light bulbs, ordinary bulbs are being adapted for use.

Personnel and resources were shifted from primary care to hospitals in the hope that the quality of hospital care would improve within two or three years. The war intervened, however, depriving the health system of human and material resources, and giving a further twist to the downward spiral in the quality of hospital care.

With rapid population growth and no new hospitals being built, the bed-to-population ratio fell below the rate of population growth (see Figure 6–5). The PAHO goal of 4.5 beds per 1,000 population slipped farther and farther out of reach. Yet, remarkably, utilization of the hospitals and the clinical service they provide continued to expand (see Figure 6–6). Lack of funds to buy or repair equipment meant that even investments in the new hospitals sometimes did not translate into more or improved care. At best, the shift in funding from primary care to hospitals slowed the deterioration.

To make matters worse, many people continued to use hospitals as primary health centers. Doctors contributed to this: The limited skill of new doctors led many to treat their health posts mainly as referral pathways to the health centers and hospitals. Consumers quickly became aware when hospitals once again received a greater share of health funds. As a result, the increased funds were used to keep up with increased demand for services.

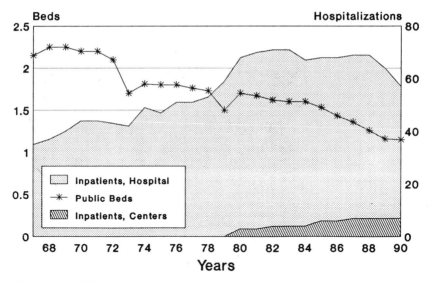

Figure 6–5 Although the rise in hospital beds has not kept pace with the rise in population, beds are being used more intensively, and the rate of hospitalizations has increased over most of two decades.

Doctors commonly saw eight patients per hour in hospital clinics. This gave them a chance to do little more than write prescriptions and make a short note in the chart. It started to look disturbingly like the charity system of care described by Dr. Silva before the revolution. The moneys and time needed to fix the buildings and improve the quality of care at hospitals never materialized. Yet while patients with routine illnesses started queuing up outside hospitals at 3 A.M., urban health centers and posts sometimes were without clients. Despite the rhetoric of primary care, referral hospitals remained the backbone of the health system.

Matters came to a head in June 1985, when President Daniel Ortega, along with the ministers of health, finance, and transport faced 500 doctors in a lively question-and-answer session in Managua. The doctors voiced grievances concerning salaries, taxes, housing, vehicles, supplies of medical equipment and drugs, and the deplorable state of public hospitals. President Ortega was frank in admitting the failures of the new health system: "We spread out to build hospitals in every direction . . . without taking realistic account of our human and financial limitations . . . The hospitals we build are open, but without the staff to make them work, they are functioning only at 20 percent or 30 percent capacity."

Finally, public confidence in MINSA was shaken by the discovery in 1985 that several officials in Managua had stolen valuable pharmaceuticals to sell on the black market.[14] Morale was low and solutions to pressing problems in the health system seemed elusive.

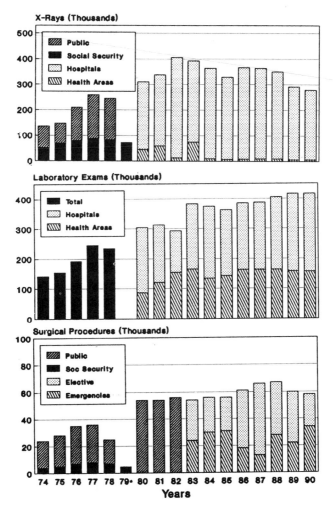

Figure 6–6 A rise in the number of clinical services paralleled the rise in the number of medical and hospital visits in the 1980s. The most expensive service, X-rays, fell the most during the economic decline of the late 1980s.

A CHANGE IN LEADERSHIP

It was against this background that, in July 1985, Health Minister Lea Guido was replaced by thirty-one-year-old military commander Dora María Tellez. Before joining the FSLN in 1974, Tellez had been a second-year medical student. An inspirational leader and efficient organizer, she rose quickly to become a high-ranking political and military figure. She seemed well suited to the challenges of restoring staff morale and overhauling the system of health administration. Many doctors, however, feared that she would impose military-style solutions on MINSA. The opposition news-paper, *La Prensa,* had more trivial concerns, twice pointing out in its first article on the new minister that she did not wear makeup during the inter-view.[15]

Tellez surprised and impressed her critics with a professional approach and clear sense of priorities. She tightened national administration through her personal involvement in many technical matters. Accountability im-proved dramatically. At the same time, many decision-making powers and personnel were transferred to the regions.[16] Most regional health directors established daily contact with the minister's office.

Tellez's tenure at MINSA began with a review of the previous six years' work. When the Sandinistas came to power in 1979, they promised free, universal access to doctors and hospitals. In the rosy afterglow of the rev-olutionary insurrection, this promise did not seem unrealistic. But it was a promise based on three crucial assumptions: First, that the economy would recover rapidly; second, that large-scale international aid would be avail-able; and third, that most doctors would remain in the country.

In practice, none of these assumptions proved true. The economy, after an initial recovery, declined rapidly after 1983. Large-scale international aid for health and development was limited after 1980[17] (see Chapter 11). Some 300 doctors, including many of the country's most highly qualified specialists, left Nicaragua by 1982, leaving gaps in specialty care. A fun-damental reappraisal of the sort of health system that Nicaragua could af-ford was needed.

In the first few years of the revolution, MINSA's policy was to provide the most advanced care available to the poor majority. Some argued for a cheaper and more limited approach to primary care based on low-cost tech-nologies, community participation, and an intersectorial approach to health. This "poor man's medicine" is often called "appropriate technology" in development circles.

Indeed, the revolution's most successful health programs—malaria con-trol, polio and measles immunization, and promotion of oral rehydration therapy—had used such low-cost health technologies and involved tens of thousands of nonprofessional health workers.

But many leaders, including those in MINSA, were suspicious of this approach. Jaime Wheelock, minister of agriculture, voiced these views suc-cinctly:[18] "We are not a country of appropriate technology, that would have as its philosophy the institutionalization of underdevelopment." Such sus-picions were reflected in the attitude toward the community health manual *Where There Is No Doctor,* the most widely used clinical reference text for auxiliary health workers in the developing world:[19] "We were told," re-called one young doctor, "to go ahead and use it if we wanted to, but officially speaking it was neither needed nor wanted. Our health leaders thought that such a simple, basic book was shameful in a top-notch public health system like ours."

By the mid-eighties, however, such attitudes had changed. Even without the drain on human and material resources caused by the contra war and the economic crisis, Nicaragua simply could not afford a health system based on highly trained doctors and sophisticated hospitals.

This realization led to a revised health strategy, more appropriate for a developing country with a rapidly growing population but dwindling resources. The Health Plan for 1987 stressed the importance of "the wider search for, and application of, low-cost simple, alternative technologies."[11]

In a speech to the National Student Organization in 1987, President Daniel Ortega went further: "We aren't thinking about medical care for a developed country, but about minimal care for our population. But we don't have even the resources to pay for the medicines, maintain the hospitals, and keep all the operating theaters and recovery rooms working. We have to create a survival economy in health."

By 1988, MINSA openly embraced the concept of low-cost health technology. The plan for the Campaign to Defend the Lives of Children, for example, stresses the need "to promote cost-appropriate water projects, especially in rural areas." Minister Tellez, addressing the need for latrines, said: "Any kind of latrine is better than defecating in the open air. If we don't have the resources to make latrines with good seats, even just a simple hole in the ground will suffice. We have to be ready to meet our needs with whatever minimal resources are available, and not wait for better conditions."

A "survival economy" approach to health did not mean a return to the choice between third-rate medicine or no medicine at all.[20] Instead, it attempted to adapt effective, inexpensive modern medical technologies to the country's most common and urgent problems. One example is the strategy for attacking cervical cancer, the most common cause of cancer deaths among adult women.

Nicaraguan cancer specialists have long wanted to build a specialty hospital to diagnose and treat a wide variety of cancers. Such a hospital would be enormously costly, but would bring only limited benefits since a long-term cure is still unavailable for most cancers. Cervical cancer, however, can often be cured if discovered early. It accounts for about 40 percent of the cancers diagnosed among Nicaraguan women and occurs most frequently among women in their reproductive years.

Rather than build a cancer hospital, MINSA built a pavilion attached to one of the hospitals in Managua to treat cervical cancer patients.[21] The specialized staff needed to read pathology smears were trained in Europe. Pap smears are being performed at many health centers and there are several regional units able to read the test. This is a far more modest project than

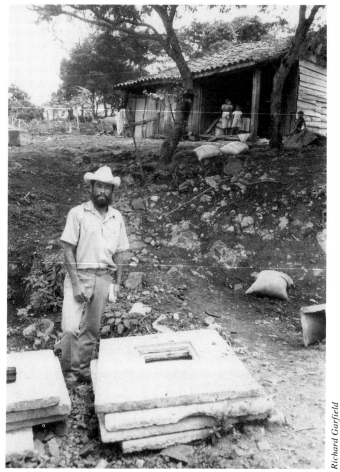

A health *brigadista* with latrines to be installed in his village. He has organized this area to provide the labor to build latrines, one after another, for each family. The *brigadista* was himself displaced two years earlier due to fighting in the Pantasma Valley, fifty miles to the north.

the originally planned cancer hospital. It is, nonetheless, likely to bring many of the same benefits, much sooner, and at greatly reduced cost.

Hospital Shopping

In 1986, medical students carried out a review of seven national referral hospitals in Managua. Their findings reveal the great difficulties under which care was provided.

Most patients treated at hospital emergency and outpatient departments could be treated better at health centers or posts. A study in Manolo Morales Peralta Hospital, for example, found that 70 percent of patients treated

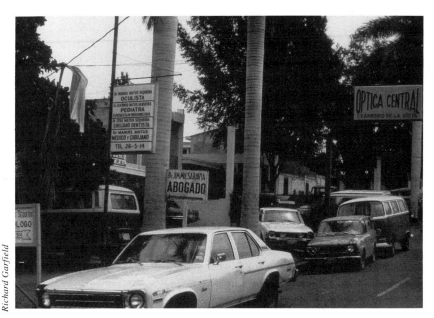

Richard Garfield

Private medical practice flourished throughout the 1980s in middle class Las Flores neighborhood in Managua.

private physician as a perk for employees. Dozens of church-run clinics and a Baptist hospital are also major sources of care.

The 1988 Health Plan reflected on this situation:[23] "At this moment, there is no health system in the strict sense. What exists is a combination of uncoordinated subsystems with diverse objectives, priorities, and technologies."

MINSA provided the administrative coordination to maintain these subsystems. Facilities in most health areas, whether public or private, depended on the government for transportation, coordination, supply, referral, and personnel. More importantly, only MINSA provided political and technologic leadership to shape and modify the subsystems, set priorities, and influence action on health-related issues in other sectors of society.

This started to change after the 1990 election. Where national MINSA had always provided leadership and supervision, a more laissez-faire approach became the norm. Some of the experiments in self-financing and establishing private wards in public hospitals came back to haunt the health system. Many cash-starved units began to charge for medicines and services that were supposed to be distributed free.

There was great talk about the 1990 election of a radical privatization of the health system, and many such projects were begun. In response, the new minister of health was interviewed in the *Barricada* newspaper: "Eighty percent of the population is extremely poor, 56 percent are under fifteen years of age and 24 percent are women of reproductive age. The

productive sector is very small and the country is suffering the consequences of fourteen years of continuous civil war. Anyone who's going to
establish a private health system here, under these conditions, not only will
go broke, but also has absolutely no notion of what is going on in this little
world called Nicaragua."[24]

Nonetheless, more new doctors seem to be oriented toward private practice and the system for distributing pharmaceuticals is de facto privatizing
(see Chapter 10). The new leaders need to reestablish their authority to
effectively coordinate the disparate and complex health system.

Health Information

> When you fill out this form you make it possible for Nicaragua
> to know her children so that she can care for them.
>   MINSA Vital Statistics Training Manual

Much information on births, deaths, and outbreaks of epidemics goes un-
registered, providing policy makers and planners with inadequate information.[25] Until 1983, for example, more tetanus deaths than total tetanus
cases were reported (see Figure 6–8)! Although MINSA trains and employs
registrants in all regions, the war has limited their effectiveness. Despite
the inauguration of a vital statistics system of national scope in 1983, the
percentage of the estimated total births that are actually recorded fell from
80 percent in 1980 to 68 percent in 1985 (see Figure 6–9). Similarly, the

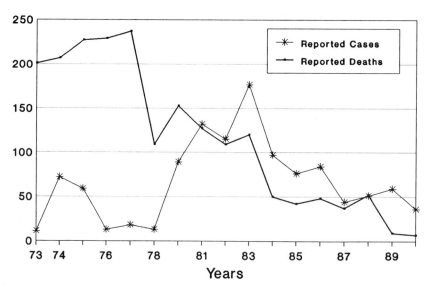

Figure 6–8 Underreporting of diseases in the 1970s was so bad that, unbeliev-
ably, more deaths from tetanus were reported than cases! Only after a new vital
statistics system was developed following the revolution were more cases than
deaths reported.

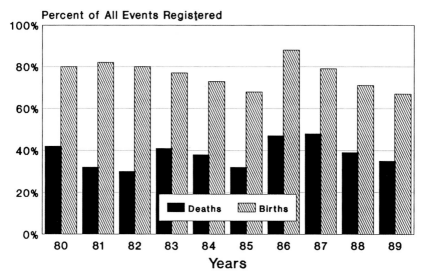

Figure 6–9   Births and deaths recorded are compared to the estimated number of births and deaths in the country. Reporting on births is much more complete than reporting on deaths. The quality of reporting for both vital events declined from 1983 to 1985. A large-scale effort to improve reporting is seen in 1986, but this effort was short-lived in the context of severe economic decline.

percentage of all deaths recorded by the vital statistics system fell from 42 percent in 1980 to 32 percent in 1985. This situation has improved since 1986, and information on the specific causes of death among the registered deaths has improved steadily. But there is often not enough paper or pencils available for staff to record vital events. Due to a paper shortage, annual summaries of health service data have not been published since 1983.

Most deaths occur among children under the age of five or adults over the age of fifty. It is among these groups that mortality reports are poorest. About half of all registered deaths occur in hospitals (see Figure 6–10).

Diarrhea and respiratory infections remain the first and second most common causes of death among children under five years of age.[26–28] Violence is the most common cause of death among the otherwise low-mortality groups aged five through forty-nine years. Circulatory diseases are the most common cause of death reported for those aged fifty and older (see Figure 6–11). While the projected death rate for each of these disease groups is higher in Nicaragua than in the United States, the difference in rates is particularly striking for diarrhea, respiratory diseases, perinatal conditions, nutritional conditions, and unknown causes; they are, in short, the diseases of underdevelopment (see Figure 6–12).

In 1983, the epidemiology office began to collect individual reports of a group of diseases with epidemic potential.[29,30] Each region reports suspected cases of diseases such as measles, malaria, tetanus, and typhoid at least once a week to the national office. An "active case-finding system"

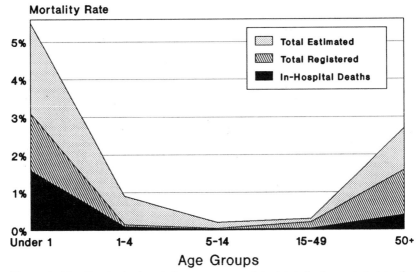

Figure 6–10 Deaths in hospitals are compared to total deaths reported in the country and the total number of deaths estimated to have occurred in 1986. Most deaths occur among those under one year of age or over the age of fifty. In each of these groups, a high proportion of all deaths occur outside hospitals and are not reported.

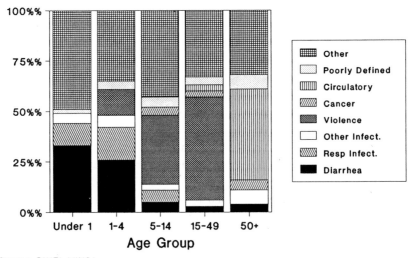

Source: DINEI, MINSA

Figure 6–11 Reported causes of death, by age group, 1986. A cause of death is recorded for most reported deaths. While diarrhea is a major cause of death among young children and circulatory diseases are a major cause of death among those over the age of fifty, serious underreporting of deaths in these age groups limits the utility of these data.

106

Deaths per 100,000 Population

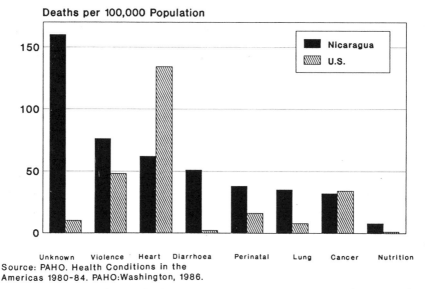

Source: PAHO. Health Conditions in the
Americas 1980-84. PAHO:Washington, 1986.

Figure 6–12   Age-adjusted death rates by major causes, Nicaragua and the United States, 1983. Death rates for diarrhea, perinatal causes, malnutrition, and violence are much higher in Nicaragua than the United States. The "diseases of development"—heart disease and cancer—are higher in the United States.

has been established among *brigadistas* to supplement the registration system for reports of deaths and births. The Campaign to Defend the Lives of Children (see Chapter 8) and infectious disease reporting systems have piggybacked on the *brigadista* reporting system to greatly improve health statistics for maternal and infant deaths (see Chapter 7), malnutrition, and tuberculosis. These "reporting by rumor" systems have greatly improved the availability of relevant information. Maternal mortality registration has nearly doubled, as did the number of deaths recorded for diarrhea in region 6. By contrast, improved tuberculosis reporting shows that almost all cases were registered before. Still, data received from some regions are not good enough. Health areas started to report to their regional offices in 1986, but 30 percent of them still do not provide regular reports for lack of telephones.[31]

The first microcomputers reached MINSA in 1985. They have since accumulated about a dozen 8086 and 286 chip systems. Sophisticated programs have been developed for recording and processing the data, some of which is now available in a more timely fashion. But few have illusions that computers will solve the problems of health information. As health planner Enrique Morales stated, "With the help of computers in the United States, you can provide instant statistics on the number of times a baseball player has struck out two batters in the seventh inning wearing blue socks. Here, we are still trying to figure out how many children are dying, and why."

Decentralization

MINSA began to reduce administrative centralization in 1982.[16] Each regional director was freed to determine how to optimize the use of available supplies, personnel, and funds. The setting of norms and targets, evaluation, and data collection remained a national responsibility. Decisions about how to meet the norms or respond to the evaluation were to be made at the regional level. In practice, the change from national to regional decision making was gradual. Decentralization received a big push in 1986, when many decision-making powers and personnel were transferred to the regions.

Although it was not apparent at the time, regionalization and the use of short (one- to two-year) rather than long (five-year) plans was key in reducing the destructive effects of the war and in motivating continued high levels of participation in health activities among volunteer health workers. Without such a radical decentralization, the flexibility to respond rapidly to local disease outbreaks or military attacks would have been lacking.

Improvements in the medical logistics system have greatly increased the availability of drugs and medical supplies at outlying health centers and posts. Since 1986, all health centers are staffed by a doctor twenty-four hours a day in order to improve the local accessibility of care.

An innovative experiment in decentralization was begun in 1988. Interministerial groups at the regional level began to set health priorities. Regional health authorities were made responsible for coordinating the actions of various government ministries and generating some of the resources for health programs. In this way, the resources of nongovernmental groups, including the church, private industry, and international aid organizations, were mobilized more effectively.

In 1988, budgetary authority was transferred from regional offices to local health areas. This pattern of decentralization seemed the best solution to the lack of national resources. MINSA continued to set norms and evaluate services at the national level, while local areas have more freedom to organize. This includes deciding which types of health personnel to train and utilize, what programs to stress, and which groups to mobilize. These "territorial health systems" have increased flexibility to determine how to relate to private medicine and promote community participation. The system has become most active in outlying regions, where regional governors and health leaders have a close working relationship. The main product of the territorial system in Managua was the "*barrio* doctor" program.[32]

Twenty new graduate physicians were sent to poor neighborhoods of Managua in 1987. Doctors were sent only into neighborhoods where a local resident offered consulting space. They provided ambulatory care in a local home during mornings and made door-to-door visits with *brigadistas* in the afternoons. Their presence attracted great interest among local residents. Not since PIASS was launched in 1983 had health professionals gone beyond the clinic door in reaching out to the community. Residents began to vie for the opportunity to host a doctor, local health councils organized the construction of health posts, and *brigadistas* took ongoing responsibility for families targeted due to special health needs. By 1989, 120 physicians were practicing in the "*barrio* doctor" program. Special care groups, including patients with diabetes, asthma, and hypertension, were set up in some neighborhoods. Some doctors who were completing their social service considered opening private practices in these high-need areas. This trend declined under the new Chamorro government. By the beginning of 1991 there were only 90 *barrio* doctors and 160 base houses; as of this writing their numbers were in decline.

Decentralization was greatly strengthened when budget cuts made MINSA reduce its spending by 10 percent in 1988 and 30 percent in 1989. In both *compactaciónes,* the major casualty was administrative staff at the central level. At its peak, national MINSA employed 1,000 people. By March of 1989, there were only 300. While many of those "compacted" left the health system, others were shifted to more useful technical duties. By the end of 1990, the actual number of MINSA employees had risen again to new highs.

The territorial health systems have seemed effective operationally but provided a poor fit administratively. Budgetary decentralization authorized by "Resolution 5" in 1989 created the opportunity for a final step to what are called "local health systems" at the municipal level. These systems, directed by a local health director as part of the mayor's office, have authority to set local priorities and generate resources in addition to those supplied by MINSA. This created more pressure for accountability of local elected officials and promoted coordination among the various ministries of the government that influence the health situation in the local government.

As part of this process of decentralization, local health centers were being equipped with beds to meet an increasing portion of patient demands without referral (see Figure 6–5). This reduced the demand for more sophisticated medical care at referral hospitals. In 1989, the rate of one hospitalization for every twenty-six ambulatory visits was still considered to be high. Better than the rate in the seventies, this figure had been stagnant throughout the eighties.

Such radical decentralization brought several dangers. First, the health system could disintegrate rather than decentralize. One does not have to look far for examples of this. The decentralization of latrine building and distribution in 1982 led to the rapid decline of that program. Anarchic and separate health administration in each department prior to the revolution could also euphemistically be called decentralization. Second, the increasing dependence on local initiatives meant that greater inequalities emerged. More affluent communities, those that give health a higher priority, or those that achieve better intersectoral coordination did better than those that are poorer, more disorganized, or where local government is unresponsive or fails to coordinate with the various ministry offices. Especially in the context since 1990 of pressures to privatize and limited supervision by the new national authorities, decentralization could lead to disintegration. Some believe such an outcome would have already occurred were it not for the dedicated, open, respectful, and clear-headed leadership of the new minister, Dr. Ernesto Salmeron.

WHERE TO GO FROM HERE

In contrast to the "glory days" of 1979–83, the health system suffered many real world problems during 1984–91. Former Vice-minister Ivan Tercero views these are "two very different stages. In the first, none of us knew just what to do. All of our efforts were tentative and revisable. By 1984 we had enough training and expertise to establish more stable administration and more comprehensive health programs. But the resources needed for this work have disappeared. This has forced us to make ever more careful choices."

Falling quality, rising dissatisfaction, and promising programs gone bureaucratic are among the signs that enthusiasm and good ideas are not enough. The health system did not create the economic crisis of the country, but it contributed to it, suffers under it, and must protect the population from it. Decentralization and appropriate technologies for dealing with the country's most common health problems are essential for coping with this crisis.

Another conceivable solution would be the nationalization of the entire health system and the elimination of private medicine. Such a solution was effective in Cuba,[33] but would probably fail in Nicaragua. First, it would be very expensive. No country has offered the massive funds that such a solution would require. Second, such a top-down approach would probably stifle many of the dynamic processes now at play in the health system. Nicaragua is better off mobilizing the wide variety of public and private resources already in place and making tough choices about health priorities in the new "local" municipal health systems. This process has breathed new life into some of the structures for representation that were particularly important in the first years of the revolution: local rural development committees and municipal government.

Officially, decentralization started in 1982. Some observers describe important restructuring of the national health system through PIASS by

1985.[5,34] This view may confuse rhetoric with reality, as substantive structures for budgeting and administration only began to change with the "survival economy" starting in 1986.[35] By 1990, limitations of MINSA's ability to finance health services effectively led to one of the most radical decentralizations of a public health service in the developing world. Can the country manage such a system, or has it gone too far? The answer may depend on the abilities of the 200 physicians trained in public health specialties since 1983. This is discussed in Chapter 9. The next two chapters explore how these dynamics translate into programs for the pressing concerns of women and children.

7

Women's Health

You can't say now, and maybe you will never be able to say,
that the problems of women have been solved. There are enormous problems which have been solved, but there are other
great problems which we have not yet begun to address.

DORA MARÍA TELLEZ, former minister of health

Imagine that you are thirty years old, extremely poor, have four children,
and your partner is off in the mountains somewhere. Being "off in the
mountains" could mean several things. He might be fighting with the army,
he might be with the Contras, he might be planting beans, or he might have
just dropped out of the picture. None of these situations would be unusual:
About 60 percent of Nicaraguan children are brought up in single-parent
families. You come into a hospital to have your fifth child. You look around
at all the people dressed in funny-looking surgical green pajamas. Which
is the doctor, which the nurse, which the cleaning woman? Finally you
approach the most sympathetic face and ask the question you've been re-
hearsing for hours: "Is it true I can have an operation to stop having kids?"
The sympathetic face belongs to a young intern, who looks at your chart.

"Thirty years old and five children. Yes, you meet the criteria. All you
have to do is write a letter to the director and get your husband to sign it."

A particularly painful contraction starts and you wait until it passes before replying: "He's not here."

"What happened to him?" the intern asks.

"He's in the mountains," you reply.

"Well, you can't get sterilized without his consent. I'm sorry." The intern smiles and moves on.

Until recently, such scenes were common in Nicaraguan hospitals. Many
women arrive with a barely legible note, supposedly written by a husband,
describing a litany of personal tragedies: twelve pregnancies, several stillbirths, deaths in infancy, children who were mentally ill or physically de-
formed. The note stresses that the family cannot possibly afford to feed any
more children, and that the woman will die if forced to bear another child.

"Please doctors," the note ends, "you must do something so that my wife won't have any more children."

The policy on female sterilization started to change in 1986. A male partner's signature is no longer always required. The interpretation of the new policy, however, varies widely from one hospital to another. Sterilization is only one of many subjects on women's health to explode into medical and social debates during the eighties. Here we review issues related to childbirth, contraception, abortion, sex education, and AIDS.

A NEW BEGINNING

Women's health is related to the oppression they have long suffered throughout Latin America. It is manifest in spoken and unspoken rules concerning sexuality and childbearing. When Spain colonized Central America, traditional informal marriage was condemned as immoral, while formal church marriages were available only to the moneyed classes. This left most women without property rights, a stable male partner, or full dignity.

The growth of export agriculture and increasing dominance by Hispanic culture further weakened women's economic and social position. A respectable woman did not work outside the home, though her partner might be absent for long periods of time to work on the plantations. Until 1979, any woman seen in public after dark might be considered a prostitute. The position of women was worst in rural areas, where most were illiterate and economically and politically powerless.[1] Domestic violence, rape, and abandonment were commonplace in both urban and rural areas. Prostitution was widespread and accepted, even expected, among the poor.

Male chauvinism—*machismo*—found its clearest expression in the area of sexuality. Women often are not even permitted control of their bodies, as *machismo* demands that men have as many male children as possible. Concern for the health of mothers comes last. Dr. Susan Cookson, who worked in a health center in Jinotega, often saw the results: "Last week I saw a twenty-year-old mother of four. She has been taking birth control pills for a year to avoid pregnancy, but she is terrified that her husband will find out. She asked for an intrauterine device [IUD], but insisted that I must cut the string too short. If she can tell that the IUD is intact, so can her husband. What should I do? She can't handle another pregnancy, but she would be beaten or abandoned if he knew she used contraception."

The revolution promised women a new beginning. The Maternal and Child Health program was the first long-range initiative announced by MINSA in 1979. It included activities related to care during pregnancy and delivery, the detection and treatment of cancer (mainly breast and cervical), fertility control, and sex education. Rapid increases occurred in medical

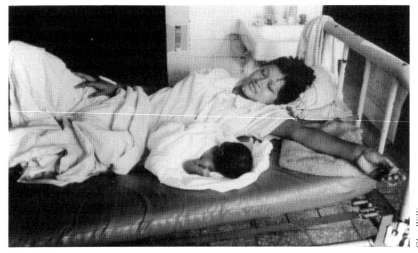

Maternity ward in Rosales Hospital, Leon. Many more births now occur in health institutions, but the percentage of all births that occur in such institutions has risen little.

services to women, including prenatal care, hospital deliveries and gynecological consultations. At the same time, social and legislative changes were implemented to defend and protect women. These included:

Direct payment of wages (rather than paying the woman's father or husband)

The institution of eight weeks' maternity leave and the right to breastfeed at the workplace

A law prohibiting discrimination against children born out of wedlock

A law specifying the financial responsibilities of fathers

The establishment of a legal office for women to inform them of their new rights and help them to pursue cases

New laws such as these are essential to improve the health status of women and children. But laws alone can do little. Major social changes are also needed to prevent oppressive and exploitive treatment of women. Since the mid-eighties, many feel that the pace of reform in this area has slowed.

WORKING OVERTIME AT THE BABY FACTORY

"After I had my baby, all I wanted to do was sleep," said Esperanza Soriano, who at the age of twenty gave birth at the Berta Calderon Hospital in Managua. "The nurses put me in a bed with my baby by my side and I was out like a light. In minutes I was awakened when another new mother and her baby were put in the bed. After a little while, a third mother and baby were brought in. 'What's going on,' I said, 'there's not even enough room for the babies, let alone us mothers!' We ended up leaving only the babies in the bed—there was just no room."

Double and triple bedding is common in maternity wards, and mothers are discharged after eight to twelve hours if there are no apparent complications. Berta Calderon Hospital, originally designed to handle twenty births a day, has handled forty to seventy a day since 1979.

Prior to 1979, the average woman gave birth to six children. In rural areas a total of seven children was average; in the cities, five was the norm. Following the revolutionary war, a baby boom further raised the birthrate.

In 1980, MINSA made a commitment to have doctors attend all births in hospitals within a decade. Before the revolution, 37 percent of births took place in hospitals. By 1983 the health system handled about 50 percent more births, but rapid population growth meant that the proportion of births in health facilities rose only modestly, to 43 percent. By 1985, further population growth and reduced access to health services brought the percentage of births in hospitals down to 38 percent of the total—almost the same proportion found prior to the revolution (see Figure 7–1).

Even in Managua, about half of all births still occur at home. In rural areas, about 65 percent of births take place at home. In part this stems from the inherited concentration of maternity services in cities, particularly Managua. There, the two hospitals that attend deliveries are located in the southwest corner of the city, a long distance from most inhabitants. Many women

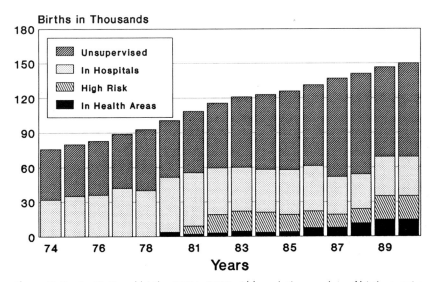

Figure 7–1 Institutional births, 1974–1990. Although the number of births to take place at health institutions rose throughout the 1980s, the total estimated number of births rose much faster.

prefer to give birth at home rather than travel long distances under difficult conditions when labor begins.

As the number of births in hospitals increased in the early eighties, the quality of care dropped. Berta Calderon Hospital came to be known as the "Managua Baby Factory." Hair-raising stories circulated of babies being born in the showers, in wheelchairs, and at the admissions desk. The hospital staff, especially interns and residents, worked under extremely difficult conditions. Stress levels resembled those in a disaster relief operation. Staff managed to keep their spirits up with the knowledge that conditions in the hospital were still better than those in most homes.

It was not until 1985 that serious reforms in delivery practices began. Health centers were equipped with more beds in order to attend births in both urban and rural areas. In 1986, health centers began to offer physician staffing twenty-four hours a day. Despite these energetic efforts, coverage of deliveries rose only moderately, to 41 percent of all births in 1986, while most women delivering at home did so without trained assistance.

Medical leaders finally admitted that the professional health system was unable to meet the demand for maternity care and accepted that there would be a long-term need for trained traditional birth attendants (*parteras empiricas*) to assist women who give birth at home.

The number of antenatal visits has similarly expanded rapidly since 1979, yet in the early eighties only about half of all pregnant women receive

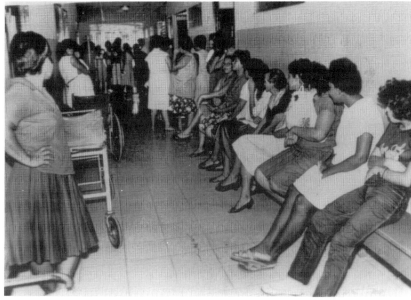

C. Dona/El Nuevo Diario

Waiting for specialty care at an out patient department in one of the major hospitals in Managua.

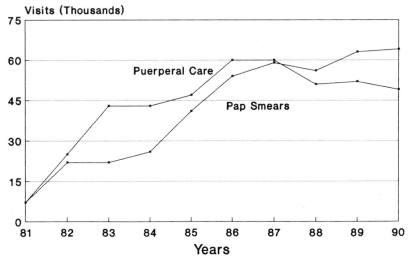

Figure 7–2 Women's health programs, 1981–1990. In the latter 1970s the health system continued to slowly develop the capacity to deal with women's medical needs.

any professional antenatal care.[2] Only a third of all first antenatal visits in 1987 occurred in the first trimester of pregnancy.[3] Among those who received antenatal care, an average of two visits was made. In 1985, a majority of those giving birth in hospitals and half of those giving birth outside hospitals received antenatal care. Many more needed it. Fifteen percent of those giving birth in Managua were under twenty years of age and 12 percent were over thirty-five. The percentage of high-risk births was higher in outlying areas. The number of antenatal visits nearly doubled from 1987 to 1988, and the percent of women initiating prenatal care in the first trimester rose to about 40 percent. A sentinel-site study found that three-fourths of all pregnant women received some kind of prenatal care. In 1990, under the new Chamorro government, decreased access to primary care led to a 30 percent decline in the number of first trimester visits, while the total number of visits remained stable.

Only a third of those giving birth in hospitals returned for follow-up care after discharge.[4] Improved access to postnatal care at health centers was to improve this situation, and it did (see Figure 7–2). It is not yet known if there will be a similar decline in postnatal care since the change in government.

Contraceptives—Now You See Them, Now You Don't

Some military and political leaders still regard contraception as part of a conspiracy by the rich countries to reduce the population and power of poor countries. Unfortunately, prerevolutionary fertility control efforts lend some credence to this jaundiced view. During the sixties and seventies about half of the international funds for health in Nicaragua were earmarked for fertility control. The pressure to show quick "results," combined with a lack of concern for people's needs and desires, led to abusive practices, including sterilizing women without their consent. A backlash was therefore inevitable. Upon entering Managua in July 1979, a Sandinista commander found a warehouse full of oral contraceptives and ordered them burned. Only an emergency petition from the women of the neighborhood prevented their destruction.

Despite greatly expanded access to primary care, most Nicaraguan women still do not have ready access to any effective method of fertility control. Although the number of contraceptive users grew rapidly during the eighties, only about one in four women of fertile age uses birth control. About 80 percent of them use oral contraceptives (see Figure 7–3). MINSA estimates that more than half of all women of childbearing age want contraceptives.[3]

Part of the problem is cultural. In this largely Catholic country, 38 percent of women interviewed in a national survey in 1985 said that family planning was against the will of God.[5]

Men have long been resistant to using condoms; it is believed that less than 5 percent of men in Latin America use them. *Machismo* prejudices men against condoms because contraceptives reduce the potential number

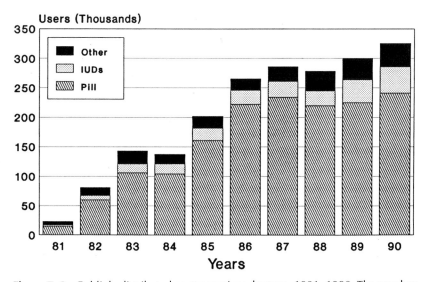

Figure 7–3 Publicly distributed contraceptives, by type, 1981–1990. The number of contraceptive users served by the government has grown rapidly. Most use contraceptive pills.

nesses characteristic of plans designed in one country and carried out in another. Only 768 *parteras* were identified and trained in two years.[18] Contrary to their tradition, the *parteras* were encouraged to sell medicines. By turning what had functioned as a community service into a business, the program reduced the attention given to health practices and emphasized the prescription of medicines and contraceptives. Only one day of the seven-day training program was devoted to well-baby care and referral of high-risk pregnancies. Most of the course focused on the promotion of contraceptives.

A variety of new attitudes toward *parteras* emerged among physicians following the revolution. One group, including some revolutionaries, wanted to pass laws making such work illegal. Others jumped on the populist bandwagon to speak well of *parteras,* while quietly working to restrict their activities and eventually eliminate them. A third group believed in the *partera* system so much that they thought doctors would have little to teach them, but much to learn.

MINSA was initially hostile to the idea of training traditional birth attendants. It was not until 1981, when the Matagalpa regional health authorities first began to identify, recruit, and retrain them, that the tide began to turn. Although it was proscribed by national policy, the program caught on and was implemented in Estelí as well. In 1982, national directives were changed to permit the training of *parteras,* thus according them tacit recognition. With the more recent shift to "appropriate technology" for the "survival economy" in health, the system is being actively promoted.

To many women, *parteras* are not just the most accessible type of maternity aide, but also the best. Says obstetrician Dr. Marta Norory,[6] "Someone who is in daily contact with a woman will know her problems, and will be the best person to bring health education to her home and to encourage her to go to her local health center for more specialized care."

Training of *parteras* now has three main objectives. First, it encourages safe, hygienic delivery practices and discourages potentially harmful ones. For example, while most *parteras* don't distribute medicines, an estimated 70 percent of women giving birth at home take some of questionable efficacy. Second, it opens a channel of communication with the professional system of care, facilitating referrals and improved coordination. Third, it involves *parteras* in promoting prenatal care, immunization, oral rehydration, and well-child home visits. Contraception is included in the training but is not its main focus.

As part of this new program, *parteras* are encouraged to maintain regular contact with the local health service and to participate in health campaigns. Starting in 1985, training included visits to the obstetric units of hospitals in order to observe institutionalized delivery practices. In some areas, *par-*

teras are even allowed to attend their clients in the delivery room of a health center. In Ciudad Sandino, on the outskirts of Managua, *parteras* are part of the local obstetric service.

Many *parteras* initially lacked trust in the government training initiative. They thought they would be punished or ridiculed if they took part. An early organizer of the program recounted her many difficulties:[19]

> When I arrived in Jalapa, MINSA had identified only eight midwives in the entire area of 9,000 urban and 23,000 rural inhabitants. I said that if that's all you can find, then there is a poor relationship between the ministry and the community. I went to the mass organizations and explained the program . . . I got the best help from the teachers and church workers . . . and it was beautiful how the mass organizations selected their *parteras* to attend the course . . . Within ten days the list went from eight to sixty midwives . . . and the communities organized child care so that they could come to attend the course.

By 1986, close to 6,000 of the estimated 10,000 *parteras* in Nicaragua had been trained. Their training manual states: "In bringing the traditional birth attendant into the heart of the health system . . . we are making her part of the health team of the area; we are giving her the right, which was formerly usurped, to manifest herself as a person; we are giving her the opportunity to be a participant in the solution of the health problems of her family and of her people."

Most traditional birth attendants are over fifty years old. In 1988 MINSA called for the development of a new generation of *parteras*. In the early days of the program, nurses were responsible for their recruitment and training.[20] Now *parteras* themselves take some of these responsibilities. In addition, other health volunteers and even members of the police force are given a six-day course and provided with a delivery kit. In this way a partnership between midwives and health professionals is emerging.

SEX EDUCATION

Visits to Nicaragua by feminists from Europe and the United States during the early eighties typically involved interviews with leaders of the national women's organization, AMNLAE. On many occasions, sex education books such as *Our Bodies, Our Selves*[21] were brought. AMNLAE staff looked at the explicit pictures and studied the frank texts with a mixture of curiosity and self-consciousness. "Thank you for the materials," the foreigners were told, "but they are not appropriate for us."

Until recently, it has been almost impossible for women to talk about sex in public. Their understanding of their own bodies has been severely limited. Ignorance of sexual and reproductive matters is still reflected in everyday conversation. Many women talk about men "having" sex and "giving" it to them. It is common for Nicaraguan women to say that the man "gave me a baby." Most health workers know women who have tried to use birth control pills by inserting them into the vagina. Others believe they should take oral contraceptives only after sexual intercourse.

A study on sexuality was carried out through a survey among 500 successive patients admitted to Berta Calderon women's hospital in 1986. Most of the women reported never or almost never experiencing orgasm. Many had no idea what the word meant. Most had their first baby before reaching the age of eighteen. A staggering ninety-five percent reported never having received any form of sexual education, and eighty-four percent denied using any form of contraception.

Yet attitudes are changing. Former Minister of the Interior Tomas Borge opened the debate in 1982 during a nationally broadcast speech by unabashedly proclaiming that, among other rights, women had a "right to sexual pleasure."[22] Mass media and nongovernmental organizations followed Borge's lead. In 1985, Sistemas Sandinistas, a government-sponsored television station, helped the national Sandinista youth organization produce a series of eighteen video programs covering topics from puberty to prostitution. It became the second most popular show on TV. The program on juvenile masturbation was highly praised by Nicaraguan youth camps. The day after the broadcast, however, angry parents flooded a call-in radio show with complaints. As a result, subsequent programs were broadcast later in the evening, and a nonjudgmental video on homosexuality was replaced by one scripted by military doctors, which presented homosexuality as a psychological illness.

Nongovernmental social service agencies also play an important role in sex education. One such organization, the Center for Information and Advisory Services (CISAS), provides a wide range of information on women's health to small groups at rural health posts, factories, churches, and schools. With the help of puppets, games, slides, and simple drawings, CISAS teaches women to examine their breasts for tumors, demonstrates the insertion of a diaphragm, and shows how a Pap smear is done.

By 1985, the word "sexuality" had crept into polite conversation. Not everyone, of course, is ready to discuss such issues openly. The Catholic church still believes that sex education should take place only in the home. By no means all of the Church's followers, however, feel confident about teaching their children about sex. "How can I teach my kids about sex?" exclaimed a father of three and a fervent Catholic. "They used to slap our hands when we were kids if they thought we were even thinking about it."

Conflicting attitudes over women's roles in society also leave unclear the best approach to sex education. Said obstetrician Marta Norory:[23] "In my opinion we can't have a sexual education campaign like the literacy campaign; you can teach people to read in a few months, but you can't change a whole culture. We need to reach many different layers of society at the same time. How are we to educate schoolchildren if their teachers are ignorant?"

Improvement will require changed attitudes and better information among the teachers. The government now plans to make sex education part of the secondary school curriculum. This will be useful, however, only if the health system also responds adequately to widespread demands for methods of controlling fertility.

AIDS

The AIDS epidemic is forcing health professionals to become more involved in issues on sexuality. Through the end of 1990, a total of twenty-eight Nicaraguans tested positive for the HIV antibody; twenty-one other positives in Nicaragua were members of a group of European ex–IV drug users. Two seropositives have been discovered among Contras returning from Honduras. About 60,000 blood donors and 27,000 other people have been tested for the HIV virus using the enzyme-linked immunosorbent assay (ELISA) method. Eight people with clinical AIDS cases have been diagnosed and have died. Data on Nicaraguans with HIV infection or the AIDS clinical syndrome who are diagnosed and treated outside of the country are unavailable.

Two of those with positive blood tests were hemophiliacs who got the virus from infected blood products; other Nicaraguans who tested positive had all engaged in high-risk sexual practices. Although there have only been a small number of cases to date, there is plenty of reason to worry. Intravenous HIV transmission is now unlikely, but opportunities for sexual transmission among homosexuals and bisexuals, prostitutes, and those with multiple sex partners are many. Other sexually transmitted diseases have become increasingly common among these groups, particularly in Managua and Bluefields. In Managua, reported rates of syphilis and gonorrhea were 14 and 121 per 100,000 people; actual rates were probably much higher, as only about a third of these cases are diagnosed and reported. If the HIV virus circulates among these groups, the number of AIDS cases will probably rise rapidly.

It is doubtful that cases are being underreported. An aggressive search for cases among prostitutes, those with tuberculosis, and blood donors have turned up nothing. By contrast, the other Central American countries have reported many more cases. The worst situation is found in Honduras, where more than 600 cases have been diagnosed. The disease also is growing much more rapidly there. The high number of cases in Honduras is probably associated with extensive contact with foreign military and other personnel. By contrast, Nicaragua's enforced isolation due to the Contra war and U.S. embargo probably spared them from the early stages of this epidemic. Ending the embargo and Contra war will likely lead to a faster rise in cases in Nicaragua in the coming years.[24]

A few leaders favor the Cuban approach of widespread screening and quarantine of all those who test positive. A conservative leader of a private medical society argued at an AIDS seminar in 1988: "It works for rabies, so why not do it for AIDS? We are medical professionals here, and we can tell who is and who isn't homosexual. If we round them all up, that will be the end to this problem."

There is far more widespread support for an approach that focuses on educating and organizing those at greatest risk. MINSA in 1988 began a campaign to convince men and couples to use condoms. Starting in March 1989, all motels routinely provided condoms to clients.

The approach to AIDS was surprisingly open. A "Collective of Popular Educators for the Prevention of AIDS" formed in 1987. With the assistance of funds and expertise from groups dealing AIDS in the United States, they have trained a network of twenty-five homosexual and prostitute volunteers on promoting safe sex. Members of this collective have been recruited to the group that sets MINSA policy on AIDS. Workshops on blood testing and safe sex have been held at schools, among prostitutes, and at parks and bars frequented by homosexuals. Television programs, health education pamphlets, and full-page ads in the newspapers openly discuss the means and prevention of transmission.

With the continued growth of HIV infection and AIDS, a new urgency has been given to condom use. Posters encouraging safe sex went up all over the country in 1988 and 1989, condoms were distributed widely, and women were encouraged to carry and use condoms in order to protect themselves from sexually transmitted diseases. Under the new Chamorro government, Catholic church doctrine gained great influence starting in 1990. Condom use was tolerated, but not encouraged. The schools no longer talked about sexually transmitted diseases, and Minister of Health Salmeron had the condom posters taken down. His slogan, "Every sheep with its partner," was to replace propaganda about safe sex. Archbishop Obando y Bravo continued to push the Church line aggressively, even equating all contraception with abortion and specifically condemning condom use. Minister Salmeron finally responded publicly that "God, in his infinite wisdom, has given man the intelligence to develop means to prevent infections like AIDS." MINSA's sex education and sexual disease prevention activities continued, achieving about 34,000 woman-years of protection from pregnancy. The private International Planned Parenthood Federation affiliate in Nicaragua, PROFAMILIA, provided an additional 38,000 years of contra-

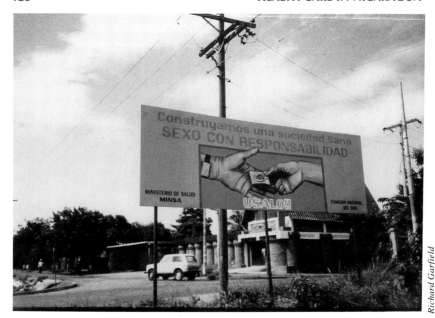

Richard Garfield

Billboard about using condoms: "To construct a healthy society, SEX WITH RE-SPONSIBILITY. Use it!"

ceptive protection, mainly through its community-based distribution program. Together with private-sector care, they provided effective contraception to 15 to 20 percent of the country's fertile women.

WOMEN IN SOCIETY

While infant mortality receives widespread attention around the world, childbirth-related deaths among mothers are scandalously high and often neglected.[25] Yet women's health problems affect everyone: The health of the next generation depends primarily on the well-being of today's mothers. It is telling that a recent review of infant mortality decline in developing countries found the enfranchisement and autonomy of women to be the strongest single predictor of child health.[26] Women are the main "consumers" and "producers" of health services. While they undoubtedly benefited from Nicaragua's revolution, many continue to suffer from *machismo,* ignorance and lack of control of their own bodies, domestic violence, and dependence on dangerous and illegal abortions.

To change these conditions will require continued legal and social reform and new attitudes among both women and men. Recognition of the need for such changes—and the commitment to carry them out—has grown slowly. It has begun to reshape society, but radical changes are still beyond the horizon. In many ways, the 1990 election may put women further behind as traditional values are reasserted. A chilling expression of this was the arrest of a doctor in 1991 for performing abortions. Issues in the health field have led the push toward empowering women in Nicaragua. Even new Minister Salmeron, a devout Catholic with a large family, has modified his views under the pressure of the HIV epidemic. According to former Minister Tellez, "Women have to define their own needs, their own sexuality. But these are not the problems of women alone. They are questions for the whole of society."

8

Child Survival

It used to be a crime to be young in Nicaragua. Punishment
was by death from the National Guard if you were over five or
death by "natural causes" if you were under five.

DR. OSCAR FLORES,
former director of women's health,
Maternal-Child Health Division

In August 1988, MINSA launched a national program to cut infant mortality by half within three years. For a country at war and in the midst of a severe economic crisis, it was a remarkable initiative. To skeptics it seemed unrealistic, even foolhardy. Many health workers and community leaders, however, welcomed the initiative as a means of giving the health system a much-needed sense of direction and focus.

The first four years of the Sandinista administration were marked by unprecedented gains in child health. The Literacy Crusade of 1980 reached tens of thousands of mothers, helping them to understand the causes of disease and its prevention.[1] More food was also available. Basic goods such as maize, beans, flour, milk powder, cooking oil, soap, eggs, and kerosene were available at subsidized prices from a growing network of local shops.[2] Many people gained access to improved water supplies, electricity, roads, and sanitation facilities.[3]

Infant mortality—one of the best indicators of a nation's health—fell rapidly. Prior to 1979, there were approximately 90 to 100 deaths per 1,000 live births.[4] The rate rivaled that of Haiti, Honduras, and Bolivia as the worst in the hemisphere. By 1983, infant mortality fell to a rate more typical of middle-income developing countries, about 70 per 1,000. This chapter examines how that decline occurred, why progress seemed to slow in the mid-eighties, and what has since been done to restore the momentum.

DIARRHEA

> The parade of small coffins tells me that the rains have come.
> DR, FERNANDO SILVA, Director
> of "La Mascota" Children's Hospital, Managua[5]

Diarrhea remains the number one killer of young children in the developing world.[6-11] During the seventies, it accounted for almost 40 percent of all hospital deaths in Nicaragua among under-five-year-olds.[12-14] The frustrations of treating children with diarrhea helped turn some young doctors into revolutionaries.

"Diarrhea has to do with water, food, nutrition, and people's education," according to one FSLN activist. "At the hospital, we would treat a malnourished child for diarrhea and send him home to the same conditions. Soon he would be back in the hospital. It would go on like that until he died. This was obviously not a medical problem but a social one. Doctors were part of the problem, because we taught the people that hospitals and dangerous medicines were the answers to their problems."

During the late seventies, consultants from USAID helped promote the use of oral rehydration solution (ORS)* through trained community volunteers.[15] The volunteers, however, lacked credibility since they were not linked to the formal health system. Nor were they encouraged to educate mothers in the prevention and treatment of diarrhea within the home. Their attempts to sell ORS packets on a commercial basis were a failure: The average volunteer sold only nine packets of ORS per year—enough for four or five days of treatment for one child.

In hospitals, children admitted for diarrheal dehydration were routinely treated with intravenous therapy, which was costly and often unnecessary. Food was withheld as a matter of course, a practice now recognized as harmful.

Two months after the Sandinistas came to power, a national program to combat diarrhea was launched. The program encouraged treatment and prevention of diarrhea through improved hygiene, sanitation, clean water supplies, and the promotion of breast-feeding. The main emphasis, however, was on the use of oral rehydration therapy (ORT) to prevent or treat diarrhea-caused dehydration. The program began by training auxiliary nurses to administer ORT.

The curative emphasis of the program was reflected in the rapid spread of oral rehydration centers *(unidades de rehidratación oral),* or UROs,

---

*A combination of sodium, potassium, bicarbonate, and sugar mixed in a water-based solution. The solution is used to treat children with diarrhea by replacing essential electrolytes and improving the retention of necessary fluids.

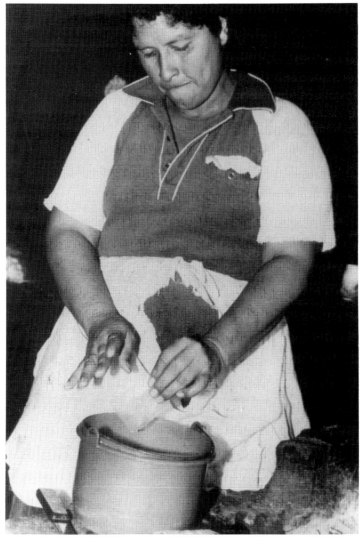

Marixa Arbizu prepares an oral rehydration solution in her home in León.

throughout the country. The original objective of 225 UROs was reached before the end of 1980. Many were set up in community centers established for the National Literacy Crusade. Others, particularly in isolated areas, were started in private homes. Most, however, were set up in health posts and health centers. Little equipment was needed: a few benches and chairs, a cot, a weighing scale, a saucepan (for preparing the ORS solution), cups and spoons, and a supply of ORS packets. By 1986, over 400 UROs were in operation around the country. Surveys in that year indicated that use of ORS for diarrhea among young children varied from about 20 percent in some urban areas to up to 56 percent in rural areas.

"Our Babies Are Like Flowers: They Need Water to Survive"

Many communication methods were used to educate the public about the dangers and treatment of diarrhea. In 1980, a half-hour radio program on diarrhea was incorporated into the regular broadcasts of the National Literacy Crusade. A forty-second radio announcement repeatedly broadcast the message: "A child with diarrhea can die. Take yours immediately to the nearest oral rehydration center." The same message was shown on colorful posters and roadside billboards.

An eight-minute television program demonstrating ORT and the facilities available at UROs was shown repeatedly at peak viewing times. Newspapers published 200,000 copies of special four-page inserts, in comic-strip form, on the causes and treatment of diarrhea. These were distributed through outpatient waiting rooms, neighborhood groups, churches, trade unions, adult literacy classes, and schools. A flip chart and slide show were also produced for health workers to use in training volunteers and teaching patients.

Meanwhile, pediatric wards in hospitals were undergoing a major transformation. No longer were children admitted for diarrheal dehydration routinely put onto an IV drip and starvation diet. ORT became the standard therapy, combined with continued feeding. Intravenous therapy was used only for severely dehydrated children unable to take fluids by mouth.

Initial results of this national effort were most encouraging. In 1980, 72,000 children were treated at UROs, helping to relieve pressure on the hospitals. At the height of the rainy season in 1980, Dr. Ivan Tercero, then director of Maternal and Child Health, remarked: "During the Somoza era, the Velez Pais Hospital would be completely filled with children with diarrhea. This is the first year in which there has been a decrease in severe diarrhea in this hospital. As a result, we are now able to deal with children who have other problems, such as respiratory infections."

Diarrhea deaths in hospitals were halved between 1980 and 1982 despite a rise in the number of cases treated. Between 1980 and 1984, diarrhea fell from the first to the sixth most common cause of infant and child deaths in hospitals. But since only about a quarter of all infant deaths occur in hospitals, this drop had only a limited effect on the country's mortality profile. Diarrhea remained the most common cause of death among infants nationally, although many health leaders and foreign observers believed otherwise.[16]

Many doctors had initially been skeptical about the benefits of ORT. They continued to use antidiarrheal drugs, antibiotics, and IV therapy for hospital admissions. But evidence from the ORT program seemed convincing: The therapy protected against dehydration at low cost and could take pressure off hospitals and clinics.[17]

In 1983, URO nurses were encouraged to give greater priority to teaching mothers how to prepare and administer oral rehydration fluids at home.[18] The health worker was to become more of a teacher than a care-giver. The new slogan was "Make every home a URO." Most families, however, continued visiting UROs and clinics for supplies of ORS as well as to seek antibiotics. A review of 161 cases of diarrhea treated in Estelí showed that while a quarter had used ORS prior to hospitalization, 53 percent had used antibiotics. It was not until 1986 that ORS packets became widely available at a modest price through commercial outlets, thanks to a subsidy from UNICEF. In rural areas where packets are unavailable, health workers promote a home mix of sugar and salt solution.

Education, sanitation, and nutritional improvements could prevent most of the diarrhea cases but could not be implemented quickly. Instead, the health system emphasized treatment via UROs. Between 1979 and 1987, the number of children with diarrhea seen by the health system more than doubled (see Figure 8–1). In 1987, 264,000 children were treated at UROs—nearly a fourfold increase over 1980 (see Figure 8–2). Only 2 percent received IV therapy.[19] Surveys carried out in sentinel sites throughout the country showed that children treated for diarrhea who were treated at UROs increased from 25 percent in 1980 to 39 percent in 1986.[20] Most of these were infants suffering from mild dehydration (see Figures 8–3 and 8–4). It is widely believed that the URO program is responsible for most of the decline in diarrhea mortality and much of the decline in overall child mortality.[16,21–24] Limited and inappropriate utilization of ORS treatment at UROs put this assumption into question.

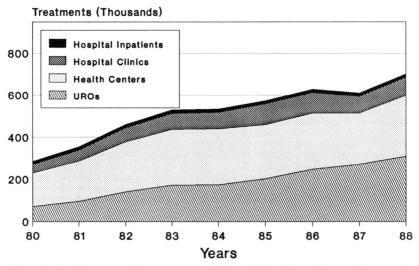

Figure 8–1 Gastroenteritis treatments, all sites, 1980–1988. Although the number of children seen at oral rehydration centers (UROs) rose rapidly during the 1980s, even more children with diarrhea continued to be seen via the primary and secondary health system.

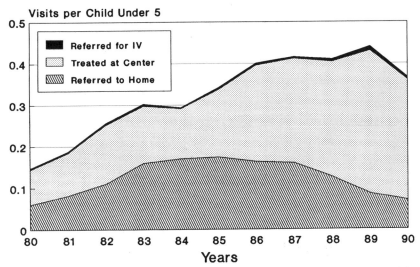

Figure 8–2   Treatments at oral rehydration centers, 1980–1990. Contraction of the health system after the 1990 change in government resulted in a reduction in the number of visits to oral rehydration centers.

Inappropriate Care

Contrary to expectations, UROs did not lead to a reduced demand for doctors' services. Diarrhea was the main reason for 16 percent of visits to a doctor in 1986.[18,25] At least 90 percent of these children could have been treated more efficiently by auxiliary nurses at an URO. The lure of doctors

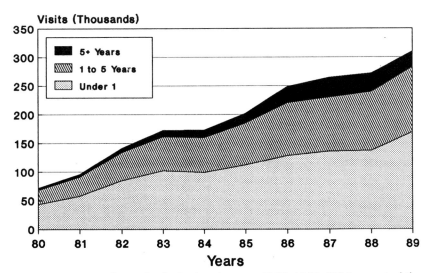

Figure 8–3   Visits for oral rehydration, by age, 1980–1989. While most of the children seen at UROs are under one year of age, a growing proportion of the total are above age one.

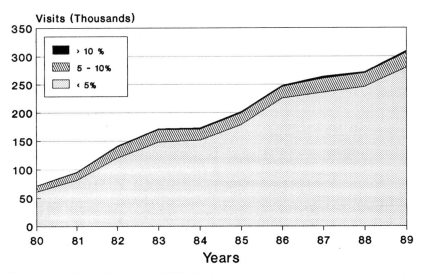

Figure 8–4   Expanding use of UROs in the 1980s is associated with growth in the proportion of children with only mild dehydration.

and hospital-based medicine remains stronger for many people than the convenience and immediate attention at an URO.

Even more disturbing are the large numbers of children who receive inadequate treatment from doctors and UROs. A review of 316 diarrhea deaths in 1985 revealed that 34 percent had received medical treatment on three or more occasions in the recent past, and 30 percent had recently been hospitalized.[26,27] New treatment norms were implemented to reduce such deaths.[28] Under-five-year-old children with severe malnutrition or persistent diarrhea are now admitted to a hospital. In addition, if dehydration brings a patient back within twenty-four hours of initial treatment, it is assumed that the mother is not using ORS correctly, and the child is hospitalized.

Because of the war and the health system's reduced capacity to provide services in the late eighties, a growing number of children in or near the war zones with diarrhea received too little care. The number of visits for oral rehydration in war-affected areas fell by more than 20 percent between 1985 and 1988. Because of the dangers and difficulties of travel, children in these areas were brought for treatment later, when dehydration was more severe, malnutrition was worse, and there was less chance to save the child's life.

Poorer access to health facilities and deteriorating living conditions led to a sharp decline in the number of children hospitalized for diarrhea and an alarming rise in the death rate among those hospitalized.

Between 1983 and 1986, admissions to a hospital for diarrhea declined 29 percent nationally, while the case fatality rate rose 79 percent (see Appendix E). From 1983 to 1986, the reported number of deaths due to diarrhea rose by 20 percent in hospitals and 10 percent outside hospitals. While the 1986 data is affected by improved reporting, and the reported number of deaths was still lower than in 1980, it suggests that diarrhea-related mortality was on the rise. With better control over the education of doctors and tighter treatment protocols for diarrhea, mortality from diarrhea in hospitals began to drop again in 1989. During July and August of that year, deaths due to diarrhea dropped by 25 percent, to 337, compared with the same months in 1988.

Reduced access to doctors and medicines since 1990 will likely have an important impact on child health. Remarkably, the number of visits to doctors for diarrhea remained stable that year. Nonetheless, there is likely to be a shift to private care and/or UROs when people believe that medicines are unavailable or at market prices through the public system. Such a shift appears to be occurring for diarrhea, as the number of visits to UROs continued to rise in 1990. If this shift is not accompanied by a decrease in access to hospitalization for potentially fatal diarrhea cases, it can lead to a more efficient system of care.

ORS packets as the mainstay of treatment have been heavily debated. Critics argue that parents should be encouraged to use a homemade solution of salt and sugar since these ingredients are more widely available than packets of ORS. Such home solutions already were the mainstay of treatment in isolated areas and war zones, where the ubiquitous Coca-Cola bottle is used for mixing. Home mixes made with rice water or coconut milk are also becoming popular in some UROs, where mothers and clinicians report a more rapid resolution of diarrhea.

The use of ORS packets, it is argued, perpetuates dependency on the health service and imported goods and encourages a focus on treatment rather than prevention. Defenders of ORS packets argue that their use has helped to give UROs the status of providers of medicine rather than "merely" educational centers. In addition, health volunteers in rural areas gain additional status and credibility by having packets of ORS to distribute.

A study in several parts of Managua in 1989 showed that 87 percent of children who died of diarrhea had used ORS. According to some health educators, overemphasis on ORS packets can be "insufficient, technocratic, and lacking in creativity."[29] ORS packets have been regarded as a cure-all, making it difficult for health education to "intervene effectively to change popular values and practices." Further, the use of packets may prevent clinicians from assessing the need for more careful treatment for children with chronic diarrhea, associated respiratory infections, and serious nutritional deficiencies.

In the seventies, diarrhea accounted for about half of all deaths among children; it now accounts for about 28 percent. The government's goal is to halve diarrhea mortality. It hopes to do this through improved treatment norms and more education on diarrhea for health professionals and mothers. The goal confronts a serious decline in living standards since the mid-eighties.[30] This decline perpetuates the conditions under which diarrhea is most common and serious: lack of sanitation and clean water supplies, poor hygiene, substandard housing, poverty, and poor nutrition. Fernando Silva, former director of "La Mascota" Children's Hospital in Managua, reflected:[31] "We've carried out massive immunization programs in the community. There you have an action followed by an immediate reaction: an immunization, which gives protection. So you have less measles, less whooping cough, less polio. But the only 'immunization' against diarrhea is for us to find a way out of poverty and underdevelopment."

BREAST IS BEST

> Your milk is irreplaceable, and comes with love.
>   Roadside billboard

Bottle-feeding is a leading contributor to infection, malnutrition, and death among infants and young children in developing countries. Whereas the educational level of the mother is widely considered the most important risk factor for malnutrition and death, a 1988 study in urban and rural Managua showed that breast-feeding could protect infants from many of the unhealthy effects of being born to poor, illiterate mothers. Children of illiterate mothers who were breast-fed had a rate of moderate or severe malnutrition (5 percent), which was similar to that of children of literate mothers. By contrast, children of illiterate mothers who were bottle-fed had a rate of moderate and severe malnutrition that was more than three times higher.

A large study in 1975 found that 58 percent of urban mothers and 69 percent of rural mothers breast-fed for at least six months.[32] The practice, however, was declining rapidly. Formula manufacturers were aggressively marketing their products along with their image of the "modern" woman. By 1978, a quarter of all mothers and a third of the mothers in Managua reported having never breast-fed their last child.[33] In 1980, MINSA launched a national campaign to promote breast-feeding and discourage bottle-feeding. Messages stressing the unique contribution that breast milk can make to a child's health and well-being appeared on thousands of posters, billboards, and T-shirts.

Hospital staff were instructed to encourage mothers to breast-feed, and "rooming-in" of newborns with mothers was instituted to enable breast-feeding on demand.[34] Bottles were banned from maternity wards, and milk

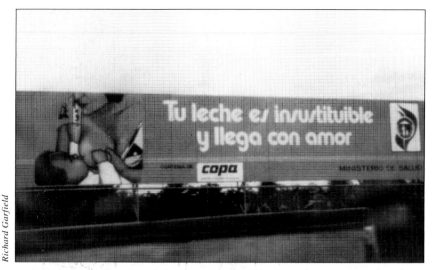

Roadside billboard: "Your milk is irreplaceable and comes with love." The message was correct, but largely ignored.

banks set up for babies who were unable to breast-feed.[35,36] In 1981 a law was adopted based on the International Code of Marketing of Breast Milk Substitutes in order to curb the marketing practices of infant formula manufacturers. The Labor Code was also amended to allow women workers twelve weeks' maternity leave and to give mothers two half-hour breast-feeding breaks at the workplace.

The campaign tread a thin line between openness and modesty. In 1980 the government banned advertising that used women's bodies to promote the sales of commercial products. At the same time, the breast-feeding campaign showed images of plump, well-filled breasts, usually attached to the mouths of contented babies, on roadside billboards, T-shirts, and posters.

The campaign seemed to have an impact in Managua, where a survey in 1982 found that the percentage of mothers giving breast milk exclusively for the first four months rose from 26 to 50 percent.[37] This progress was short-lived. Other modernizing forces related to the revolution—urbanization, increased employment among women, greater exposure to mass media—led many women to turn to the bottle. A survey in 1988 showed that more than half the mothers stopped giving the breast by the child's third month and only a quarter were still breast-feeding at six months.[38,39] One nurse observed, "They leave the hospital breast-feeding but have a bottle in their hand before they get home."

The problem is cultural, social, and economic. About a third of all households are headed by women. Most of these women work where breast-feeding is impractical. Women employed as domestic servants or in factories, hospitals, or offices have the legal right to maternity leave and breast-feeding breaks at work, but without day-care facilities, and in the present harsh economic climate, these rights are often forgotten.

Many women who intend to breast-feed for months start bottle-feeding after just a few weeks. Why do so many stop? "I didn't have enough milk," "The baby wasn't satisfied," "The baby didn't want it," and "My doctor advised against it" are common responses. They are partly the result of pervasive media images of the "modern" woman, and the difficulty of maintaining mixed breast- and bottle-feeding. They are also due to the failure of health workers to back up the breast-feeding campaign with appropriate counseling and advice.

The government itself has not acted consistently. Until 1986, the National Institute for Social Security and Social Welfare (INSSBI) provided infant formula to all new mothers at subsidized prices. MINSA has distributed bottles and infant formula to mothers through health posts and centers. In 1986, when baby bottles were so scarce they reached a black market price equal to a woman's weekly salary, the government appealed to the international community for 50,000 new bottles. These were rushed from Italy and put onto the market in record time. Former Minister Tellez explained the dilemma: "We have a culture of medicine-taking and milk supplementation. We have tried to eliminate imports of infant formula for economic reasons, but this created political problems. Working people want powdered milk, but we are working with half the dollars we had in 1983, and they must be prioritized for truly urgent imports, such as those for surgery."

This dilemma highlights an issue in the role of government. A populist state might try to meet the demands of the population without serious critique. A socialist state might try to modify or restrict the role of such popular demands, preferring to define them in its own terms.[40] The Nicaraguan state's response to the demand for imported milk shows elements of both populist and socialist approaches.

"If You Had Only One Egg . . ."

"If you had only one egg in the house, who would you give it to?" asked nutritionist Rosario Sandino, speaking to a group of expectant mothers at Velez Pais Hospital in 1986. "Would you give it to your child, who is growing and needs it to build strong bones and muscle? To your husband, who works long hours and always comes home tired and hungry? Or would you eat it yourself to provide the nutrition you need to breast-feed your new baby?"

Every member of her audience agreed that the man should get the egg. After all, he was the one who brought home most of the money. If he fell ill or left the family, there would be even more days with only one egg.

Sandino argued in favor of giving the egg to a child, or to the mother herself, but the women refused to budge. Each had faced this dilemma at some time. They were already used to having children who were small for their age; loss of a male partner seemed worse.

Before 1979, more than half of the under-five population suffered from some degree of malnutrition. During the first year of the revolution, INSSBI distributed emergency rations via health and social welfare facilities.

In 1981, the government stopped distributing rations routinely and began distributing food to families in need. INSSBI also distributed food via an expanding network of children's day-care centers. By 1988 about 38,000 children were attending 190 centers on cooperatives and state farms, and also in urban areas[38] (see Figure 8–5). In rural areas, the centers often consist of a wooden shelter with a thatch roof, a dirt floor, and no walls. Food is cooked in great iron pots and served on plastic plates. If there is no cutlery, fingers are used. Despite poor physical conditions and a chronic shortage of staff and supplies, the centers are a great advance over the nine nurseries (eight of which were private) that existed before 1979. They are extremely popular with working mothers: "If there was no day-care center in our cooperative," said one mother, "I'd have to take my two young children with me into the fields. The only shelter there is under the trees or bushes. If it rains they get wet. They play in the soil and get dirty. But in the center they get food and clothes, and books to read. They draw pictures. They're happy there, and I'm happy too."

The day-care centers have helped protect tens of thousands of young children of low-income families. Despite a tenfold increase in the number

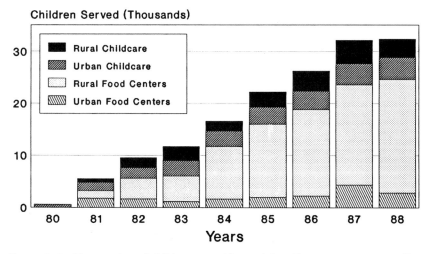

Figure 8–5   The number of children served by social welfare centers rose steadily through the 1980s.

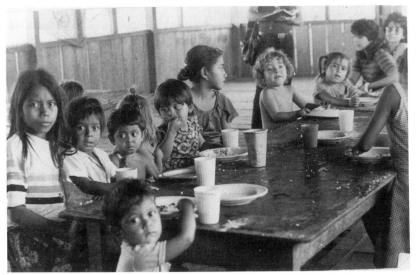

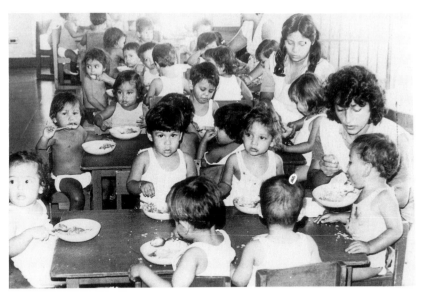

Rural and urban day care centers. Although material conditions differ for rural and urban children, both received better care and nutrition in such centers.

of children served, they still care only for a small proportion of preschool children. Many children in need of nutritional assistance, especially in towns and cities, have no local day-care center to attend. Social worker Patricia Alfonso helped to organize a door-to-door survey by community volunteers in Ciudad Sandino in July 1988. The survey identified 539 malnourished children: "These are the kids who at one year of age only weigh ten pounds. They are kept hidden, out of sight. The children's feeding cen-

Table 8–1 Prevalence of undernourishment among children under five years old, various studies, 1966–1988

Year	Location	Coordinating agency	Number of children studied	Percent malnourished[a]	
				Moderate (1– standard deviations below normal weight for age)	Severe (more than standard deviations below normal weight for age)
1966	National	INCAP	723	42	15
1969	Managua	Ministry of Health	1,500	45	11
1974	South Zelaya	CARE	156	46	38
1975	Region 2 (rural)	Ministry of Health	1,102	46	23
1975	South Zelaya	UMAN	2,400	36	27
1977	National	Ministry of Health	—	47	21
	Urban		—	45	18
	Rural		—	49	24
1981	Ocotal	MINSA	363	51	17
1988	Region 1	MINSA	8,848	33	22
	Region 3	CIES	2,800	38	11
	Rural	MINSA	450	46	16
	Region 6	MINSA	3,833	27	17

Sources:

MINSA Analisis preliminar de la situation de salud en Nicaragua.

Unidad de analisis del sector salud, 1979.

Materia Para Fines Docente, Biblioteca de Salud Luis Felipe Moncada, Area de Nutricion, 1980.

MINSA/CIES Enfoque de riesgo y estado nutricional de Los ninos menores de 5 anos en la region 3. Managua, CIES, 1988.

MINSA. Boletin del Sistema de Vigilancia Epidemilogica Nutricional No. 1, January 1989, p. 5.

[a]Weight for age is used as an indicator of chronic malnourishment, representing the child's previous nutritional and socioeconomic status.

ter is an initial effort to do something, but we know that this doesn't reach much of the population who need help."

With economic crisis and the war, malnutrition among under-fives has again become widespread and nutritional rehabilitation units in hospitals are again full. Overall, there has been a modest decline in the proportion of moderately or severely malnourished children since the sixties (see Table 8–1), but 10 to 15 percent of babies born in hospitals still weigh less than 2,500 grams[41–45] and 18.5 percent of children under five years attending day-care centers were seriously underweight.

The "glass of milk" program in Managua was designed to address the needs of school-aged children. Between 1986 and 1990, the daily provision of a glass of milk at school each day provided nutritional supplementation and encouraged many more children to attend. (For further discussion of nutrition issues, see Chapter 12.)

Malnutrition is beyond the control of the curative health system. It is determined largely by factors such as the parents' education and income, the physical environment, the availability of food in sufficient quantity and quality, and overall economic conditions[46,47] (see Chapter 12). The escalating Contra war and the country's economic decline since the mid-eighties combined to perpetuate widespread malnutrition among children.[48]

Prenatal care appears to be an important factor to prevent infants from malnutrition. Those mothers who received prenatal care in 1988 had a rate of infants with low birth weight that was 23 percent lower than those who didn't receive prenatal care. But while nutrition-related programs have

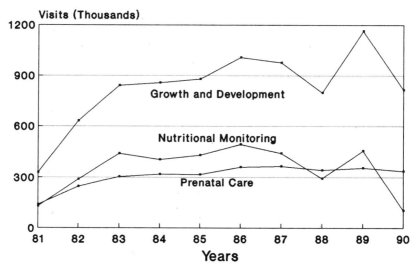

Figure 8–6 The campaign to defend the lives of children yielded a marked increase in the use of preventive health services; following the 1990 change in government the use of these services declined.

grown in recent years, the number of prenatal visits has not (see Figure 8–6).

IMMUNIZATION

Immunization against the six major vaccine-preventable diseases of infancy and childhood increased dramatically since 1980 (see Figure 8–7). While mass campaigns (see Chapter 4) helped boost polio and measles coverage, routine immunization at health clinics also increased from year to year.

BCG coverage is now almost universal. It is carried out as part of the medical checkup that almost all babies receive (whether born at home or in the hospital) during their first year. Unfortunately, the vaccine provides only limited protection from tuberculosis.

Other vaccines have to be given when a child is older and therefore are no longer easy to bring to the health post. They are, however, far more important, as they provide excellent protection against deadly diseases. Diphtheria-pertussis-tetanus (DPT) coverage increased to 57 percent of the infant population. Immunization against polio has been over 80 percent each year since 1983. Measles coverage, after reaching almost 60 percent in 1985, fell to just over 40 percent in 1987. Immunization of pregnant women against tetanus (which protects newborn babies against infection) reached 40 percent in 1986.

The impact of improved immunization coverage on child health has been considerable. Reported cases of measles fell from about 1,000 a year during the seventies to only 80 in 1984, when the quality of reporting had greatly improved. Reported tetanus deaths (the great majority among newborns) fell from an average of 240 annually before 1979 to around 50 in the mid-eighties. No cases of polio were reported between 1982 and 1990, while pertussis and measles epidemics began in 1990 (see Chapter 4).

THE WAR

Among those under fifteen years of age, there were 455 war-related deaths, 691 kidnappings, and 1,542 war-induced injuries. Some 1,200 children have suffered long-term disabilities as a result of the war.[48] These include 200 spinal cord injuries, 100 burn victims, and 290 amputations.[49] More than 10,000 children lost a father or mother, and 600 children have lost both parents in the war. An estimated 180,000 children have been forced to leave their homes to seek safety (see Table 8–2).

Child health programs were seriously disrupted in the war zones. In the community of Patastillal, near Jinotega, for example, immunization

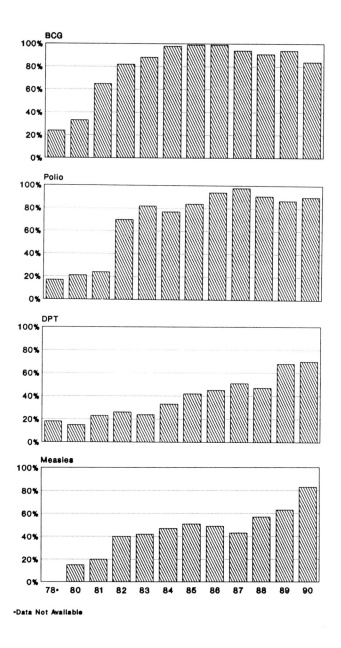

BCG

Polio

DPT

Measles

78• 80 81 82 83 84 85 86 87 88 89 90

•Data Not Available

Figure 8–7 Vaccine coverage among under-one-year-olds improved in the 1980s but is still inadequate for measles and diphtheria-pertussis-tetanus vaccine. These MINSA estimates are calculated at the beginning of each year, prior to that year's vaccination campaigns.

146

Table 8–2 Number of Nicaraguans under age seventeen affected by the war, 1988

	Nicaragua	Honduras	Cost Rica
Living in the war zone	130,000		
Living in the periphery of the war zone	225,000		
Displaced from war zone, living in Nicaragua	175,000		
Refugees outside of Nicaragua			
In camps		13,000	4,000
Out of camps		14,000	24,000
Returned refugees	12,000		

Source: CARE Children's survival assistance program needs assessment team field report: Nicaragua. New York, CARE, 1988.

stopped completely after Contra troops murdered one of two local health volunteers in late 1986. It was not until April 1988, during a cease-fire, that a health team was able to vaccinate children and pregnant women. Local residents also took the opportunity to rebuild the school and health clinic, both of which had been destroyed by the Contras. A new health volunteer also came forward for training. Tim Takaro, a U.S. doctor working in the area, reflected: "Just think how much could be done if peace broke out. . . ."

WHY DID INFANT MORTALITY FALL?

Despite the Contra war and declining living standards, a Nicaraguan child's chance of survival improved dramatically in recent decades. Infant mortality declined by about two deaths per 1,000 births per year during the sixties and early seventies. The accelerated decline during the seventies and eighties, averaging about four per 1,000 per year, was striking (see Figure 8–8). Estimates of the actual decline depend on the quality of mortality data and assumptions about mortality levels during the seventies. National mortality rate estimates for 1978 vary from a low of 90 to a high of 120 per 1,000 live births. A superb review of demographic studies by Behm suggests that the lower figure is more accurate.[4]

Infant mortality declined 47 percent, from 120 to 64 per 1,000 live births during the twelve-year period 1974–1986. It is still not clear why the accelerated decline began in the seventies. Sandiford et al. note that social welfare programs, the reduction of female illiteracy, malaria control, protection from vaccine-preventable illnesses, and breast-feeding promotion were so limited as to contribute little if any to the decline in the seventies.[50] They suggest that nutritional improvements were a contributing cause. But

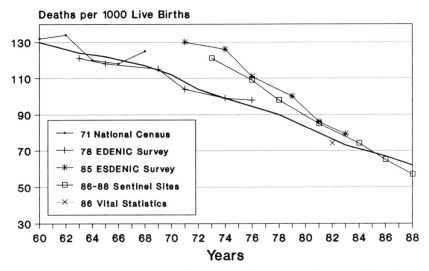

Figure 8–8 Data from a variety of surveys and censuses show a rapid and sustained decline in infant mortality which began in the 1960s and continued through the 1980s.

food amount and quality declined during those years. The supplemental food distribution programs they mention reached only a small portion of the population and were not targeted to those at high risk, and access to food-producing land declined during the seventies.

They also argue that primary care developed in the seventies because of a decrease in access to hospital-based care and an increase in the number of health workers. Indeed, the bed-to-population ratio declined steadily during the seventies and eighties. This does not imply, however, that the hospital sector had less impact or that primary care developed by default. Modernization and intensification of the hospital sector meant that a declining number of beds yielded a rising rate of hospitalizations. Only in recent years have a notable portion of these hospitalizations occurred in primary care sites.

While Sandiford et al. note that income growth was much faster in the sixties than in the seventies, this does not necessarily imply that increased income had little impact on infant mortality decline in the seventies, as they argue. Comparative cross-national studies show that income and income changes sometimes have ambiguous or delayed impacts on health status. Although latrine and water system expansion did not accompany the country's growing agricultural affluence, growing access to radios, television, and mechanized transport did. The indirect impact of these factors may be considerable. A retrospective national study carried out in 1977 showed the presence of a refrigerator in or near the homestead to be the strongest predictor of improved child survival.[51]

Other aspects of modernization in the country's export-agriculture econ-

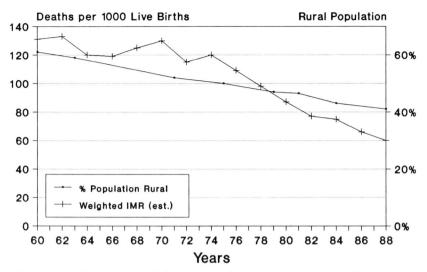

Figure 8–9   The accelerated decline in infant mortality during the last three decades is closely associated with an increase in urbanization.

omy in the seventies might have had a strong indirect impact on health. Roads, electricity, and other infrastructure reached much of the country for the first time. Urbanization and paid employment for women increased rapidly. Although these changes resulted from unpopular policies forced upon the populace, they may have improved the health of young children. Increased female employment and the information revolution presented by broadcast media may have led to improved utilization of existing food and other resources. Although rapid urbanization led to crowding, it meant that existing limited water and sanitation facilities in urban areas may have been used more intensively by the population (see Figure 8–9). Slowly improving literacy probably accentuated the cumulative effects of these modernizing processes in the seventies.

Why Did Infant Mortality Continue to Fall Rapidly in the Eighties?

The Nicaraguan experience in the eighties suggests, remarkably, that health outcomes can improve during extended periods of economic disaster. During the eighties, per capita GNP declined by a third, breast-feeding declined in popularity, and social disruptions became commonplace. Yet despite these profoundly adverse conditions, infant mortality continued to decline rapidly. The following factors may have contributed to the decline during the eighties:

1. Popularization of early treatment of diarrhea among young children
2. Increased application of vaccinations against measles, pertussis, and tetanus

3. Equalization of salaries
4. Rapid expansion of social welfare programs, including those for food supplementation
5. Rapid expansion in effective resources, geographic access, and utilization of primary care services, including pharmaceuticals
6. Land reform, transferring 20 percent of the country's arable land to about half of the country's peasant families.
7. Legal empowerment and accelerated integration of women into the work force
8. Improved literacy, especially among women

It is difficult to determine which of these variables contributed to protecting the infant population from the unhealthy effects of the social and natural disasters of the eighties. The single most important factor may be improved maternal literacy. Among children born to illiterate mothers in 1982/83, 95 of every 1,000 newborns died before reaching twelve months of age. Among mothers who were literate but had not attended school, only 75 per 1,000 died (see Figure 8–10). In 1980, 78 percent of illiterate mothers-to-be without schooling became literate; this could account for a decline of about 16 percent in infant mortality, representing more than a third of the total decline during the period from 1980 to 1986.

Unlike the seventies, it is possible in the eighties that curative medical services provided a critical safety net to protect infants from the unhealthy effects of the social and economic disruptions of the eighties. A comparison

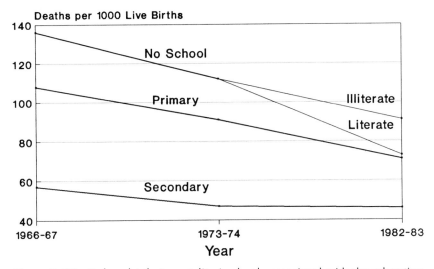

Figure 8–10 Reduced infant mortality is closely associated with the education level of the mother. Literacy alone may be responsible for much of the reduction in the risk of infant death in the 1980s.

of mortality rates among reported deaths for children aged one to four in 1975/76 and 1985/86 is suggestive (see Figure 8–11). Deaths from vaccine-preventable diseases and diarrhea declined markedly. This period included 1980–1984, when community health campaigns brought vaccines and oral rehydration to homes throughout the country. Most of the expansion in the early eighties was, indeed, via primary care. The relatively poor quality of this care and a lack of coordination between primary and secondary care services in the early eighties may explain the relatively modest decline in infant deaths due to respiratory diseases during these years.

Nicaragua and Honduras have long had similar population, economic, and mortality dynamics. A comparison of infant deaths registered by cause during 1985/86 reveals the near-disappearance of deaths from vaccine-preventable diseases in Nicaragua (see Figure 8–12). Deaths from diarrhea and respiratory disease were also lower. In both countries, respiratory and diarrheal diseases remain the main preventable causes of infant deaths. It is likely that the rate of perinatal deaths in Nicaragua and Honduras is similar; data in Figure 8–12 probably differ because of the higher rate of hospitalization (and therefore greater likelihood of registration) of infants in Nicaragua.

The affluent experienced infant mortality rates that were one-fourth those of the poor during the seventies. While the magnitude of this difference has narrowed by half in Nicaragua, it remains broad in most of the rest of Central America. This narrowing appears to result both from improved liv-

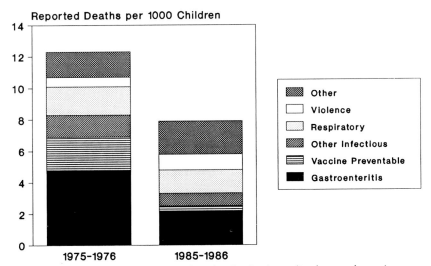

Figure 8–11   Over the span of a decade, deaths from diarrhea and vaccine-preventable diseases among one- to four-year-old children were considerably reduced. Deaths from violent causes, however, increased.

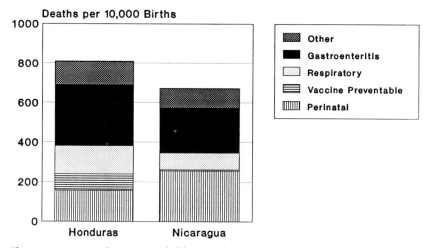

Figure 8–12 Deaths among children under age 1 in Nicaragua and Honduras, 1985–1986. Infant mortality rates in Nicaragua are notably lower than those for Honduras for causes that respond to the major child health programs in Nicaragua. These include vaccination for vaccine-preventable diseases, oral rehydration for diarrhea, and antibiotic treatment for respiratory infections.

ing conditions for the poor (at least through 1985) and deteriorating conditions for the affluent.

Mortality among children aged one to four declined more slowly, dropping about 25 percent from 1978 to 1987.[52] This decline is only half as great as the decline among infants. This is probably because infant mortality responds well to targeted medical and social interventions, while mortality among one- to four-year-olds responds more to the overall living conditions. About 100 of each 1,000 one-year-olds die before reaching age five.

These improvements still left a great deal to be done. Of the more than 100,000 children born in Nicaragua each year, approximately 10,000 die before the age of five; about 6,000 in their first year and 4,000 during years one to four. Only one in every five Nicaraguans is under five years of age, but 42 percent of all estimated deaths in the country occur in this age group.[4] Late fetal deaths also remain high. Stillbirths occur at a rate of about fifteen per 1,000 live births. Many of the same measures that will reduce infant mortality will reduce these late fetal deaths.

Large geographic disparities also still exist. Infant mortality has fallen faster in rural than in urban areas. This may be due to the government's efforts to target social and economic development programs toward the rural poor as well as to increase maternal literacy. However, mortality is still about 50 percent greater in rural areas.

In the poorest regions, infant mortality is about twice as high as the most affluent regions.[53] Although the level of the mother's education is closely

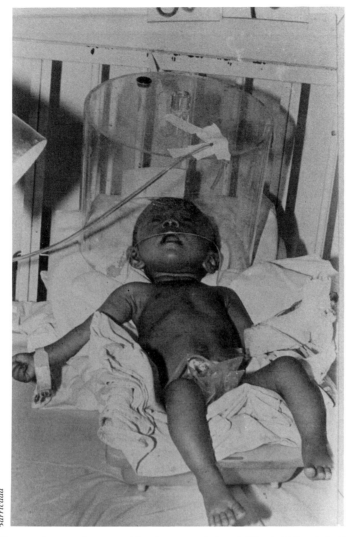

Barricada

Attacking respiratory diseases with a homemade humidifier in Velez Pais Hospital, Managua.

associated with risk of death during the first five years, even children of illiterate mothers in the department of Managua had a better chance of surviving than the children of mothers who graduated from secondary school in outlying regions.

Even more disturbing was the fear that, since the mid-eighties, the downward curve in infant deaths stopped. In 1987 the infant mortality rate in Nicaragua was estimated at about sixty-five per 1,000 births. This rate was similar to that for El Salvador, Guatemala, and Honduras, and much higher than that of Costa Rica.[54] There were good indications that infant mortality in urban areas was actually on the rise.

Yet such high rates of infant and child death are not inevitable, even in a country with a long legacy of war and a severe economic crisis. Most infant and child deaths are still due to several preventable diseases. The Latin American Demographic Center (CELADE) projects that at least two-thirds of the deaths among under-five-year-olds could be prevented through improved nutrition, diarrhea control, and the prompt treatment of respiratory infections.[40]

Seemingly a miracle, data from the late eighties show that infant mortality continued to decline rapidly. This decline may result primarily from improvements in clinical services for respiratory illnesses and perinatal conditions that accompanied the Campaign to Defend the Lives of Children, detailed below.

DEFENDING THE LIVES OF CHILDREN

MINSA launched the Campaign to Defend the Lives of Children in 1988, in a speech expressing the government's intention to make the campaign a major national priority. Then-President Ortega called on "all political parties, churches, and people's organizations to join together to combat infant mortality."

The campaign aimed to cut infant deaths by promoting diarrhea control, immunization, breast-feeding, birth spacing, maternal care, treatment of respiratory infections, and improved nutrition.[55] The campaign had a strong intersectorial approach. Other government ministries, including Education, Transport, and Social Welfare, were prominently involved. At the community level, organizations such as the Sandinista Defense Committees, trade unions, and youth, student, and women's organizations were to play leading roles. But the government also sought support from sections of the community that had been hostile to the revolution, such as business leaders and the Roman Catholic church.

The campaign was the major planned program to be undertaken by MINSA during the last years of the eighties. It was launched with few new resources and was implemented as the health budget and staff were reduced by 30 percent.

Local government was thus key. Plans to improve water and waste disposal were to be developed locally under each mayor's direction. Community organizations were called upon to help identify malnourished children and provide them with supplementary food, depending on local resources. Cooperatives and state farms, for example, set aside a cow or chickens in order to provide a secure supply of milk or eggs to children in need. At a national meeting of the agricultural workers' union (UNAG), male delegates were skeptical of this provision. Female leaders pushed through a resolution supporting this MINSA request.

The campaign's main focus was to educate parents on promoting children's health. Unlike past health programs, which targeted whole sectors of the population, the Campaign to Defend the Lives of Children focused its limited resources on those groups in greatest need. Nutritional programs in the workplace, for example, targeted pregnant women. Special efforts were made by health workers and community groups to reach mothers-to-be who are illiterate (15 percent of the total), geographically isolated (5 percent), or at high risk because they are either under twenty (21 percent) or over forty years old (2 percent).[38,56,57]

The potential to improve the health of children appeared to be great. Hospitals and health centers were directed to review their records and identify patterns associated with high infant death rates when the campaign began. It was found in Berta Calderon Hospital, for example, that most deaths among newborns occurred late at night or in early morning, when no pediatric specialists were present. Neonatalogists were put on duty at regional and national pediatric hospitals at all times late in 1988. As a result, the mortality rate among newborns in hospitals fell by 40 percent in the first eight months of 1990 compared with the same period of 1988.

Much of the potential for health promotion still went unexplored. Nutritional education, growth monitoring, and rooming-in for breast-feeding, for example, are only occasionally carried out. These preventive actions would bring enormous benefit to vulnerable children, but their appeal to doctors with a curative orientation is limited.

Despite the importance of improved medical outcomes, the main focus of the campaign was to be on education. According to campaign leader Dr. Ivan Tercero, "We need to do three things for child health: Improve water and sanitation, provide better nutrition, and carry out more education. We hardly have the funds even to start doing the first two, but improved health education and use of resources is within our reach."

For immunization, the goal was to reach at least 80 percent of the target population for each of the six main vaccine-preventable childhood diseases. One-hundred-percent coverage was reached in some parts of the country. Ironically, Managua is one of the regions plagued by low coverage. While polio vaccine coverage was estimated at 82 percent nationally for 1988, it was only 74 percent in Managua.

For a country beset by war, a ruined economy, and natural disasters, the campaign was extremely ambitious. There were no precedents in the developing world for such a dramatic reduction in infant mortality under similar conditions. Many believed that the campaign would be a success if it simply prevented infant mortality from rising. Some data suggest that it did indeed drop, although not at the rate envisioned. During the first eight months of 1989, the total number of registered infant deaths in the country dropped 11 percent, to 2,535, compared with the same period in 1988. The decline was mainly in the Managua region, primarily due to a decrease in perinatal deaths through improved treatment norms in hospitals. Registered infant deaths remained stable through 1991. These deaths are estimated to be about 40 percent of the total in the country, and include those from the new "active case-finding" system employed for a wider search for deaths.

The campaign also was designed for a wider impact. As Program Director Carolina Siu said: "The war has left us a divided society. We hope this campaign can be a point of departure from which to rebuild our society, to strengthen the social fabric. If effective, this campaign will help unite all of Nicaragua, like the Literacy Crusade did in 1980."

This was a goal the campaign failed to achieve. The country was, by 1990, too poor and too divided to mobilize and unite efforts. The new Chamorro government assumed the campaign as part of its health policy, and the original director of maternal and child health in MINSA remained in charge. In fact, though, the campaign lost momentum and direction following the change in government. In the context of further cutbacks and privatization, intersectoral coordination between government ministries, mayors, and agricultural co-ops became impossible. During 1990, local meetings and MINSA encouragement to regional offices fell off. By 1991, the campaign had de facto been absorbed into the routine activities of the Maternal-Child Health office. A unique, identifiable campaign in most areas was no longer seen.

Further, campaign supports from other ministries of the government disappeared. Despite large donations of milk from Japan, the Ministry of Education lost interest in the "glass of milk" program, which atrophied. INSSBI stopped using its social welfare centers for campaign education and outreach. The army was called upon to assist other health campaigns in 1990 when the usual supports failed; it could do nothing to promote the ongoing, informal activity that improved child survival. The Nicaraguan experience shows that well-designed health programs, targeted toward specific groups and implemented with the participation of a wide cross section of the community, can achieve impressive results. Immunization and malaria programs are the most obvious examples. It seemed that the new campaign focused on educating and involving the community rather than perpetuating dependency on doctors, hospitals, and medicines. Ironically, the major apparent result of the campaign was improved medical norms. At this time, health education seems to make its major contribution by encouraging the parents of more children in need to seek medical care.

Throughout 1990, leftist newspapers attacked the new Chamorro government with articles that infant mortality was rising rapidly. Even the respected *CEPAD Reports* stated that "hospitals reported record numbers of children's deaths from measles, diarrhea, and other preventable diseases."[58] Yet these reports simply were not true. With the exception of the serious measles epidemic, reported deaths from each of the major causes were stable or still dropping.

Koch-Weser and Yankauer, in an editorial about Nicaragua, note that governmental leadership will make or break these opportunities.[59-63] The above analysis of causes for mortality decline in the later 1980s may encourage health and political leaders by documenting that their efforts have had a major impact. Changes outside the direct reach of MINSA, such as major improvements in the nutritional and sanitary environments of young children, will be of critical importance in the years ahead. Nonetheless, changes in the application of existing resources and educational opportunities need not await affluence; they can be done now.

The primary care strategy as defined as Alma Ata a decade ago focused both on the need for political commitment and for intersectoral coordination. The political commitment to promote child health exists in the central government and MINSA of the new Chamorro government. Yet this commitment is severely constrained by the weakened relations with community groups and the Ministries of Education and Social Welfare. Such coordination and shared commitment is difficult to mobilize in a political environment that is mainly focused on privatization; this first post-Sandinista wave will have to run its course before it becomes possible to return to the campaign for children. It is up to MINSA to shorten the course of the privatization wave and seize new opportunities for intersectoral coordination as soon as they appear.

9
Health Professionals

The state will establish mechanisms to involve health professionals in the formulation and implementation of the health
plan.   *Proclamation of the Government*
of National Reconstruction, 18 July 1979

We have the power to decide who lives and who dies. We have
to adopt that omniscient position.
FREDDY RUIZ, director of surgery at Jinotepe Hospital

From the moment they came to power, the Sandinistas were haunted by the
fear of a mass exodus of doctors. Recent precedents in other Latin American countries were hardly reassuring. In Cuba, the emigration of about half
of the country's doctors within three years of the revolution of 1959 destabilized the health and political systems.[1] In Chile, medical opposition frustrated reforms initiated by Salvador Allende's socialist government, helping
to create favorable conditions for the right-wing coup of 1973.[2-6] Sandinista
leaders feared a similar "fight or flight" reaction in their country. The issue
was as much political as medical. Doctors were prominent members of the
middle class. They would need to be won over for the Sandinistas to succeed in their stated intention of developing a "pluralist" society and a
"mixed" economy. This chapter analyzes the effects of the government's
attempt to retain the doctors while training many more new health technicians and professionals.

Doctors did begin leaving the country, but in a trickle rather than a flood.
There were three main reasons why the much-feared mass exodus failed to
occur. First, opportunities to work in the United States were far more restricted in 1979 than they had been in 1959.[7] Second, as one of the inher-
itances of the Somoza era, many doctors trained in Nicaragua did not meet
the technical standards required by other countries. And third, the revolutionary government made herculean efforts to satisfy the doctors. First
among these efforts was the appointment of a nonpolitical neurosurgeon,
widely respected in medical circles, as the first minister of health. Doctors

believed, with good reason, that the government would respect their professional integrity.

The early trickle of doctors out of the country was largely offset by an influx of foreign health professionals, who numbered about 800 in the peak year of 1982. Dozens of Nicaraguan doctors who favored the overthrow of Somoza also returned to the country immediately after the dictator was overthrown.[8] Most of the *internacionalistas* came from Western Europe and Latin America, especially Mexico and Cuba; some also came from the United States. Most provided services to populations in rural areas never reached by the physicians who had migrated to North America.

The absence of Nicaraguan doctors was most notable in the specialties, including anesthesia, ophthalmology, and internal medicine. Later, when the Contra war became more widespread, rehabilitation and neurosurgery were the specialties in greatest shortage. In a small country, where there are normally only two or three specialists in many fields, the loss of even one can be serious. The lack of specialists was felt most acutely in the medical school in León, where teaching in some subject areas had to be suspended for lack of qualified staff.

Opposition political groups quickly seized upon the issue of foreign health workers. *La Prensa* published inflammatory stories suggesting that foreign doctors were unqualified to practice medicine in their own countries, were covert military personnel rather than health professionals, and spread venereal diseases due to their poor health and immoral behavior.[9] Cuban doctors were a particular target of rumor, innuendo, and defamation. None of the accusations appear justified. On the contrary, many Cuban doctors have served where national physicians preferred not to venture in isolated rural and war zones.

A big surge in the numbers of departing doctors occurred in 1983, when the Contra war began to escalate and a military draft was initiated. In the first half of 1983, about 200 doctors (including eighty-eight specialists) left the country.[10] Consequently, some urban neighborhoods and rural communities that had grown used to having a doctor suddenly found themselves without one. By the end of 1986, 646 doctors, close to half of all those working in the country before 1979, had left.[11] Their departure deprived the health system of valuable medical expertise. Others saw a great success in the retention of about half the doctors. American doctor Anthony Dajer observed: "Medical personnel are easy migrants, for their skills find a ready market. The fact that they remain at their posts, trying to improvise in a steadily deteriorating setting, speaks volumes. . . ."[12]

Moderate Sandinista policies had minimized the impact of this brain drain. The loss had been gradual and its destabilized effect was limited. In the meantime, hundreds of newly trained doctors and many more technical and administrative staff had begun to work (see Figures 9–1 and 9–2).

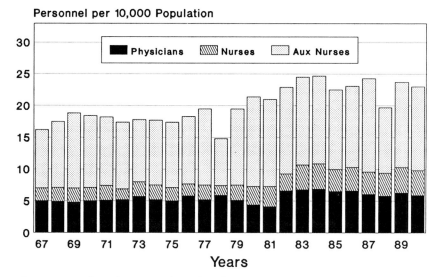

Figure 9–1 Clinical personnel employed, 1967–1990. A rapid rise in the number of health workers employed in the 1980s only moderately exceeded the rate of population growth.

The continued emigration of physicians was nonetheless a cause for deep concern. Especially alarming was the realization that many specialists trained after 1979 were also leaving. Of the twenty-nine obstetrics-gynecology residents working in the country in 1985, twenty-two had left by 1988. The pro-Sandinista newspaper *El Nuevo Diario* appealed to the

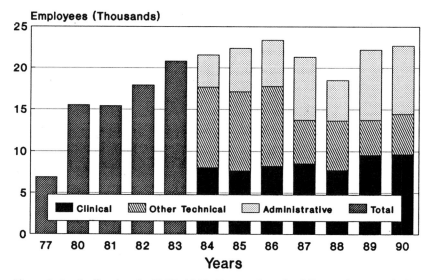

Figure 9–2 Staffing levels, 1977–1990. Contraction of public employment during the economic crisis of the late 1980s only slightly reduced the number of personnel directly providing health services. Most of the administrative personnel lost in 1987 and 1988 were replaced by 1989.

government to try to reduce medical emigration:[13] "A policy of encouragement would include sufficient salaries and technical facilities to carry out
their work efficiently, and other actions that the health authorities can well
determine. This would not be creating a privileged sector of professionals,
but would respond to the objective reality of a country which has a grave
and chronic shortage of doctors, and which cannot afford the luxury of
sitting by passively while doctors continue to leave."

Nubia Herrera, a prominent nursing leader, took a different view: "If
half the doctors leave but the ones who stay are with the revolution, we'll
be OK. The problem now is that half the doctors are dragging their feet and
weakening the health programs."

THE WHITE COAT EMPIRE

A dramatic fall in real income and the economic chaos caused by rampant
inflation have been key factors in the brain drain. Many doctors also resent
government attempts at regulation and a loss of status in the revolution's
more egalitarian society.

Regulation of medical practice was sorely needed. During the Somoza
regime, there was no system even for registering physicians. Nor were there
any criteria for official recognition of specialists: Doctors would simply
advertise themselves in the press as "pediatric hematologists" or "renal
surgeons" without any specific qualifications. In addition, many doctors
exploited the public health service by drawing government salaries while
spending most of their time in private practice. Some doctors worked only
a few hours a day in public clinics but were paid for as many as twenty
hours of work. The total number of reimbursed medical hours even surpassed the physical capacities of some of the most notorious clinics.

Such administrative disorganization was key to the system of privileges,
which favored leading physicians but kept the medical profession as a
whole politically weak. This sense of impotence was clear in a plea from
one physician published in the *Lancet* following the 1972 earthquake. Fearing that the piecemeal approach of the government after the disaster would
lead to epidemics, Camilo Vigil wrote, "There is increasing evidence that
the voice of the medical profession is seldom heard. . . . If preventive medicine in this situation is to be more than a myth, prompt action is vital. We
wait and hope."[14]

In 1980, the government proposed a bill to regulate medical practice.
This was fiercely opposed by the medical establishment, which organized
a one-day walk-out of hospitals in protest at what was called government
interference in their professional affairs.[9] The heavily political character of
the medical opposition, including threats of mass emigration to Miami, had
a chilling effect on relations between doctors' leaders and the government.

A MINSA official said angrily: "These people live in a dream world. They say that if we pressure them they will go to the U.S., where they can pursue their profession freely. But in the U.S. there is far more regulation and control over medical practice than has been proposed here."

Representatives of the *Colegio de Medicos* took part in redrafting the bill, and some of its provisions were watered down. Only in 1983 did it finally become law.[15] For the first time, the medical establishment was obliged to accept the right of the government to regulate professional practice. As a result, doctors receiving a salary were required to increase their scheduled public practice to at least six hours a day and to fulfill their contracted time. Salaries for public service at each professional level were standardized and a maximum salary level established. The one-year social service requirement for medical graduates was extended to two years, increasing the number of doctors working in rural areas.

These changes were not well received. An anonymous letter writer to *La Prensa* on 12 June 1985 complained:[16]

> Today the doctor has a lower social rank. Doctors come mainly from the middle class and aspire to a better standard of living. Today doctors feel limited or even worse, pushed down the social ladder. It is not uncommon to hear doctors complain that in hospitals they are treated as though they were plumbers or air-conditioner repairmen. This style of egalitarianism is a fallacy, because in all industrialized countries of the East and West, doctors have certain social privileges.

Yet the influence and prestige of the medical profession remains enormous. One group of doctors has concentrated on strengthening the formal organs of professional influence, the powerful *Colegio de Medicos* and *Federacion de Sociedades Medicas*. These associations are now better organized and more influential than before 1979. A second, smaller group of pro-Sandinista doctors is active in the health workers' union, FETSALUD. A third group has avoided all forms of organization, any of which they view as open to government manipulation. In their various ways, these three groups are well placed to influence the political process. In 1985, for example, when the government formed a commission to try to standardize the anarchic system of doctors' fees in private practice, the organized opposition of the medical profession led to abandonment of the idea.[17] There were, however, important new limits to the political power of organized medicine. When doctors in Managua went on strike in August 1988, the health minister soon got them back to work by threatening to replace them with Cubans.

Many aspects of medical practice remain lax. When the nurse in charge of the health post in San Lorenzo, Boaco department, moved to Managua in 1987, she was replaced by a social service doctor straight out of medical school. Within weeks, what had been an exemplary rural health service began to disintegrate. The young doctor spent only three days per week in San Lorenzo, devoting the rest of his time to establishing a private practice three hours away in Managua. Worse still, he charged for medical consultations in the health post.

Since his was the only service available, the local people had little choice but to pay him or go without care. When they finally complained to the regional health authorities and asked for another doctor to be sent in his place, visits to the post had so declined that San Lorenzo could no longer be considered a high demand area. The people would have to wait until more new doctors graduated. Meanwhile, someone scrawled a common sentiment on the wall of the health post: "Too bad doctors do social service rather than compulsory army service on the war front. . . ."

PRIVATE MEDICINE

In 1979 it was thought that all medical practice would eventually be completely socialized, as in Cuba. According to Dr. Antonio Jarquin, one of the early architects of the system, "It was impossible to do this with the resources we had. [For the time being] private medicine would be like a safety valve."[18]

Yet in 1990, most doctors still had private practices. Only in isolated areas, where foreign volunteers and recent Nicaraguan medical graduates work, is private medicine absent. Following two years of social service, doctors are free to go private. This issue was raised during debates in the National Assembly on a new constitution during 1986. Sandinista delegates, including several doctors, denounced private medicine as an exploitation of the people, while representatives of other parties defended the right of doctors to exercise their professional skills outside the state health system.

The constitution, as finally approved, was a compromise, referring only to the area upon which most delegates agreed, namely, that it is the responsibility of the government to ensure that the health needs of the population are provided. The right of medical professionals to practice privately is not explicitly recognized, but neither is it denied.

As the Contra war and the economic crisis worsened, as many as 90 percent of doctors depended on private practice. According to Leonel Arguello:

> Attitudes toward private medicine have changed a lot. We thought that if health could be considered a right, private care would have to be eliminated. At first it was regarded as being only for the ethically weak or politically

uncommitted. But theory and practice weren't the same. Progressive doctors started leaving MINSA in order to make ends meet. Now, many revolutionaries have gone into private practice on a part-time basis, and no one accuses them of backsliding. It is, in fact, the only realistic option available.

In a few hours of private medical practice, a doctor can earn the equivalent of a month's salary in the public health system. This combination of public service and private enterprise is also carried out by many nurses and other health professionals, albeit at lower levels of remuneration.

In Managua, typically, private medicine is practiced at an office in a clinic or attached to the home. In small towns it may be an office, complete with an elaborate sign, off the town square. Those who use private care the most are middle-class patients, market traders, and government employees. Some of the best care available is private, as well as some of the worst.

Dr. Antonio Dajer worked with a typical small-town doctor: "He had trained in Mexico, and insisted that penicillin, in high enough doses, could overcome any infection. He even produced an *Annals of Pediatrics* article from 1956 to 'prove' it. He was notorious for dumping sick kids on the hospital when they were close to death. If they survived, he claimed credit and charged them half a year's income."

Work in the public system has some important advantages. It offers far greater opportunities to utilize modern medical equipment and interact with other professionals. Another benefit is easier access to basic commodities such as rice and soap, and imported goods such as cars. Most physicians, including those trained since the revolution, work six hours a day in public medicine and two to four hours a day in their private practices.

The widespread role of private medicine leaves a fundamental inequality in the health system. Private patients routinely receive better care and have more of the limited resources of the health system available to them. On the other hand, more of the limited human and material resources are in the country precisely because private medicine exists.

Private practice is nonetheless growing stronger. Since 1988, new health centers built by MINSA had public and private offices under the same roof. In 1989 a private ward was established in a public hospital in Jinotepe and one in Rivas.[19] These experiments in privatization were tried because these hospitals had relatively low utilization and served relatively affluent populations. In this way, MINSA hoped to generate additional operating funds and persuade newly trained physicians to remain in the country. Nonetheless, the government was nervous about the uncontrolled growth in private medicine. A *La Prensa* editorial mocked this concern by suggesting that MINSA believed "there are more clinics in Managua than food shops in the *barrios*."[20]

Whatever its drawbacks, private care does help meet the social aspirations of doctors and provide treatment that is preferred by affluent patients. It also absorbs surplus money that is difficult to spend because of the lack of luxury goods for sale. In this way, both doctors and their better-off patients are able to maintain a semblance of middle-class life despite the rampant inflation and chronic shortages that beset the country.

In the postelection environment after 1990, private practice came back with a vengeance. Many more new graduates tried to avoid their social service obligations, left their posts early, or charged for care that was supposed to be free to the public. While Minister of Health Salmeron condemned such abuses, there was little he could do to stop them in the conservative environment fostered by the central government.

TRAINING DOCTORS

In 1979 there was one doctor for every 2,100 people, but their distribution was highly skewed. In the major cities there was an average of 1,400 people per each doctor, compared with 5,000 in the rest of the country. Admission to the one medical school, in the city of León, was tightly restricted. No more than fifty-five students were admitted each year. At this rate, a desirable doctor/patient ratio would never have been reached. The revolutionary government therefore decided to train a large cadre of new doctors, at the rate of 500 per year. Professor Fabio Salamanca, former dean of the León Medical School, explained:

> Many of us had participated in the revolution and were sympathetic to the Sandinistas. In the seventies we had tried to make changes in the curriculum, to accept students from rural and poor backgrounds, and to make practical experience and independent thinking a priority. But our efforts were stopped by the directors of the school. When the Sandinistas came to power, we saw our opportunity to make important changes in the curriculum. But more importantly, we felt that it was necessary to produce more, to turn out more physicians as our contribution to the revolution.

A second medical school, in Managua, was started in 1981.[21] Five years later, 400 newly graduated doctors took up their social service posts. Eighty-two of these young physicians sat in the small auditorium of the surgical hospital in the northern town of La Trinidad, which only six months earlier had been attacked by contra troops. They listened anxiously as health officials briefed them on the local situation. Their arrival would, at one stroke, double the number of doctors in the region. Their medical education, however, differed in many important ways from that of their older colleagues.

What Doctors Learn

The plan for medical education underwent extensive revision in the early eighties.[22,23] The number of doctors in training rose tenfold, while classroom and laboratory supplies and spaces hardly changed. Most students only got to see real textbooks in the library; they studied and worked from mimeographed notes that they bound into homemade texts. The clinical and teaching expertise of many teachers prior to 1979 was limited. Following 1979, many of the best teachers either left the country or took leadership positions in MINSA. Gaps in clinical training became painfully apparent. The rightist "León Document" a decade later blamed this situation on "the entrance of new teachers with mediocre medical training, no teaching ability, . . . and educated in Eastern socialist countries in a way which doesn't correspond to Western medicine."

The revised medical curriculum emphasized disease prevention, participation in a health team, the role of the community in promoting good health, and the social roots of disease.[24] Social science courses were added, along with courses in epidemiology, health administration, and environmental health.

The major innovation of the new curriculum was the work-study program. From their first week in medical school, students spent one day every week working in the community with patients and local organizations. Together with health volunteers, first-year students conducted community health surveys, including evaluations of the health status of families. They also administered vaccines, gave educational talks, and helped link the community with local centers. This sort of hands-on experience can have a strong effect on students. As one student said, "When I first arrived in the community, people began to ask me questions and I had no idea of the answers. So I came back to medical school and studied more."

In their second year, students worked with children in primary schools, learning about growth monitoring, immunization, health education, and diarrheal disease control. During their third year, they studied nutrition, collected stool samples, and inspected work sites. In the fourth year, their course work focused on occupational health, and they worked in factories and health centers. In their fifth and final year, they worked in health centers and hospitals and learned about maternal and child care.

In addition to their work-study program, most students spent two months a year working in special work brigades. Many staff and students helped with the coffee or cotton harvest or assisted during emergencies such as the aftermath of Hurricane Joan. Some also served as medical orderlies in militia and army units.[25] These "mobilizations" were enormously time-consuming. Denis Silva Torres, who in 1983 became the first medical student killed in the Contra war, had spent more time off campus than on during his four years of training.

The loss of course time through mobilizations contributed to a decline in the quality of clinical training. In 1985, a majority of all third-year students failed one or more clinical courses, and one-third had to repeat the entire academic year. A reassessment in 1986 led to important changes. Students are no longer permitted to volunteer for health campaigns, harvests, or service in the militia or army, except as part of a program sponsored by the medical school. Although male students can perform military service, they are kept for only one academic year. The work-study program has also been cut from 20 percent to 10 percent of course time, and basic sciences have been reintroduced in the first year of medical studies.

Efforts were made to bring students from less-affluent families into medicine. These efforts include a scholarship program, a residential premedicine high school course organized at the medical school for rural students, and on-campus housing for medical students from outlying regions. Regional quotas also gave students from outside Managua (60 percent of all students) a better chance to matriculate. According to Nubia Herrera, former director of the Medical School Department of Preventive Medicine: "These students are middle class by local standards, but would be considered poor by Managua standards. Some of them do better than students from Managua, because many didn't suffer as much disruption in their secondary education as those from the city."

The proportion of female medical students rose steadily from 1980, and in 1984 passed the 50 percent mark.

Contrary to comments by some foreign observers,[21,26] it seems that preventive medicine and community health training were weakened by aspects of the Sandinista medical education. There are several reasons for this. First, the schools were not run by MINSA but by the National Higher Education Council,[27] a group more interested in the development of expertise than its application. Second, the best teachers of preventive medicine were no longer at the schools; they had become MINSA leaders. Finally, the work-study program often exploited students for their labor, encouraging little motivation for the field.

Training remains heavily oriented toward hospitals, and little classroom time is devoted to ambulatory or primary care. As a result, many new graduates are more prepared to prescribe medicines than to encourage breast-feeding, growth monitoring, rooming-in, home-mixed oral rehydration therapy, or to work with traditional birth attendants. According to Ennio Cufino, formerly of the Managua office of UNICEF, "The only aspects of preventive medicine to gain respect among medical students are programs like immunizations and malaria treatment, which don't intrude upon the hospital-based, curative care system."

This situation may soon change. With the electoral defeat of the Sandinistas in 1990, many progressive health leaders have returned to the university. Autonomy and independence of the national university has been reestablished, and leftists have been elected to leading posts. It appears that in the nineties, like in the seventies, the university may become a focal point for social reforms.

NURSING IN CRISIS

Like medicine, nursing in Nicaragua was organized on a model "made in the U.S.A."[28] Military and other nurses who accompanied the U.S. Marines to Nicaragua early in this century introduced high standards of clinical education that were poorly suited to the needs of a developing country. Most Nicaraguan nurses were in fact auxiliaries, or aides, trained in courses of six to twelve months. Others known as "empiricals" had no formal training at all.[29]

The Somoza regime feared that nurses would exert a progressive influence through social agitation in politics, labor, and health care issues. The regime tried hard to keep nurses divided. Professional responsibilities and salaries varied widely: The salaries of nurses in hospitals and clinics in Managua were about three times higher than those working in outlying areas. Responsibility for the training of nurses was something of a merry-go-round. When the North American director of the nursing school left in 1950, control was assumed in turn by a religious order, the Ministry of Health, the university, and then the Ministry of Health once more.

The revolution's new health programs created an enormous need for more and better-trained nurses.[30] They would be key personnel for primary care and the needed link to more sophisticated hospital-based care. The government trained large numbers of nursing auxiliaries: Between 1980 and 1987, the number increased tenfold. At the same time the number trained in a basic, three-year course increased fivefold (see Figure 9–3). This is still far from adequate, as about 8 percent of nurses leave the profession every year: Some emigrate to the United States, but most find other work in the country due to dissatisfaction with pay and working conditions.

The growth in training of allied health staff has been hailed as a great advance,[21] but the shortage of nurses is now more serious than that of doctors. In 1976, Nicaragua had 39 professional nurses per 100 doctors; by 1984 this had improved to 55 per hundred, but still lagged behind the rate for Central America of 68 per hundred (see Figure 9–4). In industrialized countries, by contrast, nurses almost invariably outnumber doctors: In the United States, for example, there are four professional nurses for every doctor.

New Graduates per 10,000 Population

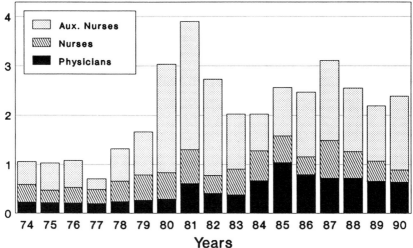

Figure 9–3 Health personnel graduated, 1974–1990. New auxiliary nurses trained in the first years of the revolution soon came into the work force, while new physicians only began to practice in 1984.

The shortage of nurses is acutely felt in primary health care, but it is even more serious in hospitals. In 1985, 43 percent of the nursing posts in primary care were filled, while only 31 percent of the hospital nursing positions were filled.[31] The number of nurses and nursing auxiliaries failed to keep pace with the increase in hospital beds. Between 1980 and 1983, the

Nursing Personnel per Physician

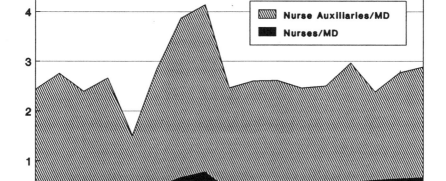

Figure 9–4 Despite a plan in the 1980s to increase the nurse-to-doctor ratio, there are still less than one professional nurse and only three auxiliary nurses for each physician.

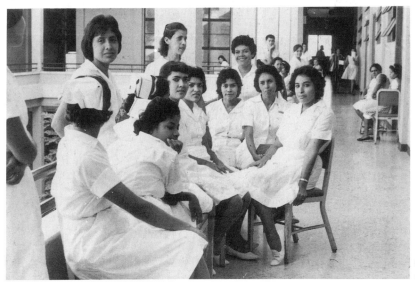

La Prensa

Nurses from a more tranquil time. Graduates of the nursing program at El Retiro Hospital in 1970. The earthquake in 1972 leveled Managua's only hospital.

number of hospital beds increased by 546, but the number of nurses working in hospitals by only 171, and the number of auxiliaries by 176. The shortage was greatest in the five new hospitals opened since 1979. Some of these institutions have been so short of nursing staff that the opening of new wards has been delayed for months or years. In the "La Mascota" Children's Hospital in Managua, for example, there are 137 nurses and 70 auxiliaries for 207 beds. This yields a staff-to-bed ratio one-third to one-fifth that expected in hospitals in the United States.

It is striking that many of the problems facing nurses in Nicaragua are similar to those found in among nurses in industrialized countries. The shortage of nurses, especially in hospitals, is due in part to MINSA's policy of investing heavily in the training of large numbers of doctors. Ironically, it is the doctors who now realize that hospital-based medicine depends largely on nursing staff and are now demanding improved conditions for nurses. Salaries are poor, training facilities are inadequate, training is frequently isolated from practice, and working conditions are often extremely difficult. Poor advancement opportunities in the nursing education system make a career in medicine relatively more attractive. Despite heavy competition for entrance to medical school, since 1984, nursing school classes have been undersubscribed. The profession has failed to attract many male trainees.

The poor quality of working relations with doctors further discourages many from becoming nurses. Many doctors assume that nurses know little and pay little attention to their views. It is common for doctors not to explain to nurses the medical orders they have written. When challenged on their diagnosis or treatment, obscure claims of *criterio medico* (medical criteria) discourage nurses and give them little motivation to coordinate with doctors. Former Health Minister Lea Guido made efforts to change this situation. She led an educational effort to develop teamwork and "treat each patient like your own mother or father." But the heart of the problem was the quality of relations among doctors and nurses, which is changing only slowly.

Unlike doctors, nurses have been able to exert little influence on the political process. The weakness of organized nursing was seen in the closure of the university-level nursing program in 1983, the elimination of the national nursing office in the Ministry of Health in 1985, and the lowering of entrance qualifications in 1986.[32] Vehement opposition to these moves by the nurses' professional association *El Colegio de Enfermeras* led to the establishment of a national advisory group on nursing in 1988.[33] This group succeeded in reestablishing the three-year basic program for nursing education, expanding the training options available, increasing some salary levels, and allowing nurses to enter a postgraduate program in epidemiology.

MINSA sought to employ two nurses and three auxiliaries for each doctor. This would require twice the present number of about 1,000 graduate nurses. To meet this goal, nurses were trained at six regional hospitals and auxiliaries are trained in one-year programs in each region of the country.[34] Even so, undersubscribed classes and rapid abandonment of the nursing field delayed the improvement in the doctor–nurse ratio for another decade. The new leaders of MINSA, while more doctor-oriented in their political outlook, are less burdened by the phobia of emigrating physicians than were the Sandinistas. They see that the primary care system will likely function more effectively and at lower cost if nursing is encouraged. Still, such changes are likely to be slow and will have to involve nursing leaders in a way that MINSA has never found possible.

PUBLIC HEALTH

In 1983, physicians were recruited to the first postgraduate public health training program in the country. The Centro de Investigaciones y Estudios de la Salud (CIES) was developed because the new national health system needed trained leaders at all levels. Until that time, only a handful of people had received formal public health training in other countries. During the eighties, about 100 doctors (and a few nurses) were prepared for regional and national posts as administrators and epidemiologists. The CIES was jointly administered by the university and MINSA.

Following the 1990 election, CIES moved to become a direct dependency of the university. It also absorbed some of the leftist ex-MINSA officials. Many view the CIES today as the key institution for preserving and transmitting the Left's view of health to the next generation of medical reformers. To do so, the institute must also become successful in selling itself financially and politically. Like the other progressive health group formed after the 1990 election (see Chapter 13), it is coordinating some community health research projects. It also provides leadership to the preventive medicine departments in the country's two medical schools, develops local courses for hospital administrators, and runs international programs. It is a unique and important resource as the only postgraduate public health program in Central America.

New Priorities

In 1987, there were 1,955 physicians in Nicaragua (see Table 9–1). The specialists include among them 46 epidemiologists and 160 health administrators. About 1,300 doctors, 1,300 professional nurses, and 3,800 nurse auxiliaries were trained since 1979.

A rapid increase in the number of doctors trained was a political necessity in the first years of the revolution. It was a long-held dream of social reformers and responded to the felt need of both organized medicine and the population. It also enabled MINSA to cope with the gradual emigration of almost half the doctors.

Some observers viewed an excessive focus on medicine as little danger in a country with a primary health orientation.[35] Yet training and employment of physicians is many times more costly than it is for paramedic personnel. A large group of nurses or *brigadistas* could be trained more rapidly, would cost less to employ, and would probably have been more willing to live and work in isolated rural communities, outlying regions, and poor neighborhoods. In fact, it is still mainly nurses and *brigadistas* who provide care in isolated rural areas.

Table 9–1   Doctors, by level of training, 1987

Level of training	Number
Interns	283
First year of social service	214
Second year of social service	241
Generalists	300
Residents	280
Specialists	637
Foreign specialists	103

Source: Direccion de Docencia, MINSA.

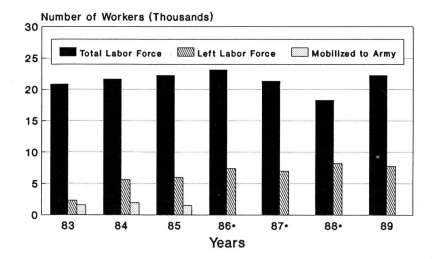

*Data Not Available on Those Mobilized

Figure 9–5 Labor force changes, 1983–1990. Despite a rapid turnover in personnel employed by the health system, high levels of employment were maintained throughout the 1980s.

Given the relatively small number of students qualified to enter the university, it is also questionable whether admitting 500 students every year into medicine was the most effective employment of scarce human resources. These students might well serve the country more effectively in fields such as engineering, agriculture, or public administration. And although newly graduated doctors may be able to bring health care to people who have never had it before, they also generate more demand for expensive medicines and supplies.[36] With these concerns in mind, MINSA in 1989 began to restrict the size of new medical school classes to 150 per year.

Despite MINSA's best efforts to retain the country's doctors, at least half of those trained before 1979 and a third of those trained since 1979 left the country during the eighties (see Figure 9–5). Most have found work in the United States, Mexico, Panama, and Venezuela. Some miss the status and respect they enjoyed in Nicaragua and return to their old posts after some months abroad.*

If there were no shortage of doctors, the political pressure they exert might be lessened. Most worrisome is the emigration of specialists trained since 1979. An end to the war and an upturn in the economy might make the prospect of staying in the country more attractive. This was only to

---

*In 1979 there were about 400 Nicaraguan physicians in Florida.[7] When efforts to waive the registration exam for foreign medical graduates failed, a few chose to return to their posts in Managua. "It is better to be a respected doctor here and earn twenty dollars a month, than to be a faceless cab driver in Miami for a hundred dollars a day," said one.

begin after the FSLN lost the election in 1990, but funds and coherent personnel policies for health were slow to come. Lack of funds in the health system and a lack of cohesion in health policy made day-to-day operations even more difficult than under the Sandinistas. Doctors staged a six-week strike in early 1991 to demand materials with which to work and their salaries, which had not been paid in months. The strike resulted from the refusal by Minister Salmeron and President Chamorro to renegotiate wage scales. Many doctors felt betrayed by the irony of ministerial intransigence, now that there was finally a physician in the minister's post.

10

Medicines and Medical Equipment

> MINSA announces that beginning March 15, there will be a
> charge for medicines that are dispensed at health centers
> throughout the country. With this measure, MINSA hopes to
> control the indiscriminate use of medicines.
>
> Radio Sandino broadcast, 7 March 1986

Under the Somozas, the provision of pharmaceuticals was left to the invisible hand of the free market. Predictably, the Somoza family managed the invisible hand via ownership of SOLKA, the country's second largest pharmaceutical company. Drugs were promoted like cigarettes or Coca-Cola through advertisements on billboards and radio and in newspapers and magazines. Doctors and pharmacists earned special premiums for promoting the products of particular drug companies. In addition, the political domination of the U.S.-allied elite created a strong image of the American "good life," which dominated the media and popular culture. The result was what is now referred to as the "culture of medicines." In the minds of medical leaders and the public, the more drugs they took and the higher the doses given, the better. This commercialism reached absurd proportions. A popular B-vitamin complex, Neurobion, sold for thirty-eight cordobas a vial. An identical formula marketed under the name Vitalgia sold for fourteen cordobas but was much less popular. Almost no one taking either formula could derive a health benefit from it.

But there was another side to the story. While affluent Nicaraguans and Social Security beneficiaries consumed too many drugs, most other people remained dependent on home remedies and traditional medicines using plants, powders, and the secret potions of folk healers. Especially in rural areas, there was almost no access to modern drugs. This chapter describes how these imbalances were addressed both when the health system expanded rapidly after 1979 and when it pulled back, starting in 1984.

With the advent of the revolution, everyone wanted to fill their medicine chests. Doctors often responded by providing unnecessary injections and drugs on demand for simple ailments that required little or no medication. For a child with influenza, doctors commonly prescribed two antibiotics, an analgesic, multivitamins, and a tonic. None of this was needed and much of it was harmful. The revolution's health system had to respond to the people's felt needs, but at what cost? If the people wanted too many expensive, ineffective, or dangerous medicines, should the government provide them? Breaking the grip of the "drug mentality" would prove to be a singularly daunting task.

FREE DRUGS FOR ALL?

In July 1979, within days of taking power, the new government decreed that all drugs dispensed in public hospitals and health centers would be free of charge. More than any other act, this decree convinced the population that the health services were theirs. The full financial implications of this policy were not yet clear, however, and the government soon found itself retreating from this promise.

The top priority was to provide essential drugs to those who previously had little access. The rapid expansion of the primary care system between 1979 and 1983 (see Chapter 2) meant that drugs could be provided at health centers and posts. As MINSA concentrated on opening new health centers and getting doctors and nurses to staff them, lack of organization was the rule in the pharmaceutical system. Millions of dollars worth of drugs were imported on credit. Many of these medicines, as well as products from the country's twenty private drug firms and countless petty importers, found their way onto the black market. It was not unusual to see a private pharmacy run by a conservative opponent of the Sandinistas whose shelves were stocked with donated Cuban products.

Although supplying the rural areas was sometimes a problem, the real nightmare was in the cities. Lines into hospital pharmacies backed up to the street. Doctors filled a sheet full of prescriptions, only about 60 percent of which could be found in any given hospital. Patients began to migrate from one hospital to another in search of their prescriptions. This meant that the public health system—above all, the hospitals—were distributing so many medicines that supplies were usually short. Middle-class patients complained vigorously about the empty pharmacy shelves.

Byron Molina is a landowner in Jinotega. He visited a foreign doctor at the local health center, complaining of indigestion and asking for an American antacid, Mylanta. Since this brand was not available, the doctor wrote a prescription for aluminum and magnesium hydroxide, the generic name for the same product. He flatly refused to accept the prescription. Since the available medicine was from Cuba, he presumed it to be of poor quality and waited until relatives sent him the bulky medicine from the United States.

A wide variety of medicines are available from private pharmacies. From 1980 to 1982, private pharmacies increased their share of the burgeoning drug market from 59 percent to 85 percent. To decongest hospital pharmacies and to provide a source of over-the-counter medicines for the urban poor, thirty public pharmacies were opened in 1983. Thirty-one more were opened in the following five years. About 60 percent of the people responding to a 1984 survey in and around Managua said that they obtained medicines from either these pharmacies or primary care facilities.[1] These sites were preferred because the supply was similar to the private pharmacies but prices were subsidized. Another 20 percent reported buying medicines on the open market, while a similar proportion reported buying from *curanderos* (folk healers).

In a somewhat chaotic fashion, basic drugs (as well as other medicines) became much more widely available after 1979. In 1981, for example, more than 10 million prescriptions were filled, representing a near doubling from 1978.[2] The number of prescriptions peaked in 1985 at more than 15 million (see Figure 10–1). Yet demand was rising even faster than supply, and widespread complaints were heard about the growing unavailability of medicines!

Despite excessive use of medicines, the reduced prices and wide availability of pharmaceuticals since 1979 have helped many. This is most apparent in rural areas. Bosco Liviana is a peasant farmer in Matagalpa. He started becoming thin, weak, and had a persistent cough in 1985. He did

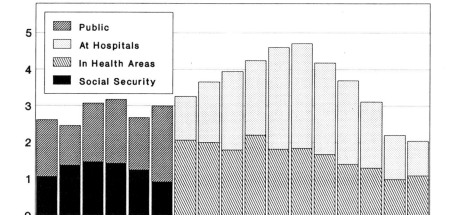

Figure 10–1 The number of prescriptions filled per capita nearly doubled from 1978 to 1985 and then declined to levels below 1978. A decreasing proportion of all prescriptions were filled at hospitals in the late 1980s.

not need a doctor to know what was happening—he had tuberculosis. His father and brother had died from tuberculosis in the seventies when they could only occasionally afford to purchase antibiotics to treat it. (Interruptions in treatment promote resistant strains of the tubercular bacillus like the one Bosco contracted.) He started to visit a health post, as he could get a fairly steady supply of appropriate antibiotics there at no cost. Visiting a pharmacy would have taken most of his income. He has had no symptoms since 1987 and is now considered cured.[3,4]

Public pharmacies in 1982 started taking turns to provide twenty-four-hour service, something the health centers would offer only four years later. Yet the government soon found that providing free drugs sapped the health system of needed funds and encouraged the overconsumption of unneeded or dangerous medicines. The value of one month's imported pharmaceuticals in 1982 equaled that of a whole year's imports during the late seventies.

In March 1982, the Ministry of Health imposed a "registration fee" for prescriptions; the drugs themselves were still free. In 1986, a more radical shift occurred: There would be a charge for prescription medicines, albeit heavily subsidized. Moreover, not all drugs would be charged for. Those needed in special programs, such as tuberculosis, venereal disease control, and immunization, would still be free. Drugs for hospital inpatients would also be free.

Some people stopped visiting the clinics and health centers; any prescription fee was prohibitive for them. The new policy still left a huge gap between drugs sold at "official" prices through government health facilities and drugs sold "commercially" by private pharmacies. Between March 1982 and June 1987, for example, the cost to patients of essential drugs sold at government health facilities was only about 25 percent of their commercial value. This glaring discrepancy led to two serious problems.

First, some popular drugs sold out rapidly each month. For weeks at a time there were none to be bought. Hospitals and health centers had in stock an average of 60 to 70 percent of all programmed medicines.[5] Second, "professional" patients made a business of obtaining drugs at official rates and selling them on the black market for much higher prices. Calling this the "war against the ants," health leaders tried to identify and educate those who abused the health system in this way.[6] It turned out that many of the culprits were health workers themselves, popularly labeled "white-coat bandits."

Subsidized prices and good supply stimulated many forms of black market activity. Near the northern and southern borders, people opened lively resale trades with Honduran and Costa Rican traders. The most widely black-marketed medicines were contraceptives. Since supply from government sources was irregular, doctors providing family planning services in clinics around the country sometimes had to buy pills on the black market, in order to provide them to clinic patients.[7] The pills usually were originally purchased at public pharmacies and sold to traders in the market.

To deal with these interrelated problems, the government resorted to a measure that, only a few years earlier, would have been regarded as political hersey. In 1987, subsidies were slashed to abolish the difference between essential drugs sold through official and commercial channels. Essential drugs, however, still received an indirect subsidy through a favorable foreign-exchange pricing policy. The elimination of direct subsidies meant that except for several special disease control programs, the prices of essential drugs at government health facilities and private pharmacies were similar. Private pharmacies continued to sell more nonessential, or "popular," drugs, which provided them with the bulk of their profits.

The policy took another spin when a single rate of foreign exchange was established in the national monetary reform of February 1988. Meant as an emergency measure to attack inflation and improve the business environment, it also eliminated the indirect subsidy for medicines. The effect was a fivefold increase in the price paid by the consumer. The public's reaction was immediate. After ever-rising consumption of medicines for the last nine years, sales of medicines plummeted. "There is a drastic reduction in demand," said Byron Ramirez of the Ministry of Internal Commerce. "If someone needs ten pills, at best he'll be able to buy only five now." Medicine sales fell so drastically that prices had to be cut by 35 to 50 percent to avoid letting the products become outdated prior to sale. Children under six years of age, pregnant women, the disabled, and the retired, as well as anyone receiving treatment for tuberculosis, syphilis, or malaria, still receive medicines without charge.

The High Cost of Drugs

Nicaragua's drug bill is much too high. The per capita annual cost of medicines in Nicaragua is about twenty dollars. This is at least five times higher than in Bangladesh,[8] a much poorer country that has made great strides in improving access and reducing the cost of drugs. In 1985, Nicaragua spent $31 million to import drugs or the products to manufacture them.* This was equivalent to the value of the country's cotton crop (its second biggest export).[9] The reasons for excessive costs were identified as early as 1981.[10] First, over 90 percent of all products used to fabricate finished medicines are imported. At least 80 percent come only from capitalist countries,

---

*This figure does not include donations, which could be worth another $10–$15 million per year.

where the terms of trade were unfavorable. Nicaragua routinely pays two to five times more for its drug imports than necessary. Improved purchasing mechanisms could reduce the bill by at least $3 million a year.

In 1986, PAHO established a program to enable all Central American countries to purchase essential drugs in bulk at competitive prices on the world market.[11,12] With a grant of $4 million from the Dutch government, PAHO set up FORMED—a revolving loan fund through which each country can obtain sixteen essential drugs of value up to $650,000. PAHO procures the drugs in bulk, paying only one-quarter to one-third of the average price paid by the Central American governments. The governments then reimburse PAHO, making two rounds of bulk purchases annually.

ESSENTIAL DRUGS

Reducing the vast number of medicines on sale would save at least $5 million a year. In the late seventies about 3,500 pharmaceutical products were registered. These included fifty-two different types of ampicillin preparations. Many unregistered products—the so-called popular drugs—were also readily available. Apart from narcotics, any drug could be purchased without a doctor's prescription. There was some logic in this, since most of the people never saw a doctor. But with a multiplicity of drugs on sale in shops, supermarkets, market stalls, and pharmacies, the inevitable result was widespread self-medication using drugs that were either useless (such as vitamin B_{12} injections) or harmful (such as chloramphenicol).

In 1977, an Export Committee of the World Health Organization published the *Model List of Essential Drugs,* which recommended 220 drugs and vaccines as essential in good medical practice. All were of proven safety and efficacy and possessed well-understood therapeutic properties. Most were no longer protected by patent.

In 1981, MINSA began to develop a list of essential drugs for the country. The project met with immediate hostility from many doctors. Physicians saw the formulary as a threat to their freedom to prescribe. Domestic and foreign pharmaceutical companies feared for their profits. Even patients were mobilized to resist the plan. Many people had a trusted brand name; consumers at all levels were encouraged to accept no substitutes for their tried-and-true product. Only in rural areas, where preferences for particular brand names had not yet developed, were generic Cuban and Eastern European pharmaceutical products readily accepted.

Finally, after widespread and painstaking consultations, a National Pharmaceutical Formulary was published in 1984 with 667 products.[13] It designated the number and types of drugs to be supplied at each level of the health system, based on the training of health workers at that level. In 1985 the Formulary was reduced to 475 products, of which only 65 were listed as indispensable for general use. Another 343 were reserved for specialists with access to diagnostic facilities, and a further 76 were designated as "high-risk" drugs to be used only under strict protocols. In 1988 a revised Formulary was prepared, consisting of 392 products, of which 253 items were designated for distribution only by prescription.

At each step, organized medicine opposed the implementation of the various formularies. As a result, the lists have been observed mainly in the breach. Importers continue to sell any medicine without official sanction. At the end of 1988, for example, both public and private pharmacies had ample supplies of useless products such as injectable vitamin B_{12}. At the same time, pharmacies ran out of birth control pills and were unable to obtain further supplies. The formulary has had its major impact on the urban and rural health posts, where at least half of the sixty-five "indispensable" medicines were usually available.

"People widely see the formulary as just a way to try to reduce MINSA's medicine bill," according to Jaime Orozco, one of the authors of the current formulary. "We have to change this conception, and even that's not enough. . . . If we are not careful, we can still abuse our patients with the improper use of medicines on the formulary."

Local Production and Distribution

Local production of some pharmaceuticals may reduce the drug bill. Production costs are relatively high because of Nicaragua's limited domestic market and lack of export opportunities. Heavy investment in technically sophisticated equipment is also needed to ensure good quality control. On the other hand, the promotion of self-reliance in medicines creates employment, helps to establish an industrial base, and reduces dependence on unpredictable outside markets. Reducing the percentage of medicines that are imported as finished products from 60 to 40 percent would reduce costs by about $5 million a year.[14]

In 1984, a COFARMA, a pharmaceutical distributing company, was formed to manage the importation and distribution of all drugs and raw materials for local production. COFARMA supplies fourteen privately owned drug manufacturers and two state-owned firms. Since the trade embargo imposed by the United States in May 1985, Nicaragua imported raw materials for its pharmaceutical industry mainly from Spain, Holland, socialist countries, and Mexico.

Local drug production is concentrated among 100 of the 350 products listed in Nicaragua's National Formulary of Essential Drugs. State-owned SOLKA produces only essential drugs; the private companies produce nonessential, or "popular," drugs as well.

SOLKA receives foreign aid in the form of equipment, technical expertise, money, and basic materials from Holland, Argentina, Italy, and Spain. Nevertheless, SOLKA works at only 40 percent of its capacity and has never provided more than 20 percent of the country's essential drug needs. There are continuous shortages of basic materials and spare parts to repair old machinery. In addition, low salaries make it difficult to recruit the highly specialized staff needed to manage a drug company. While private drug firms can offer higher salaries, they also suffer from a lack of basic materials and spare parts, and their production levels are well below capacity.

Although state-controlled, COFARMA has considerable independence and pays salaries comparable to those in the private sector. COFARMA distributes about 80 percent of the drugs imported to government health facilities and 20 percent to private pharmacies. Its budget reached about $12 million in 1989. All drugs, whether purchased or donated, are first stored in Managua for distribution to stores in each of the regions. COFARMA's warehouse, bookkeeping, and inventory practices have put an end to large-scale medicine thefts. Production and distribution, however, still lack the efficiency needed. Then-Vice-minister of Health Pablo Coca observed in 1987 that 2.5 percent of funds for medicines were wasted by deterioration, lack of attention to the expiration dates, or theft. About $3 million could be saved by improving administrative efficiency. According to Byron Ramirez, "Sometimes emergency importation is necessary, such as when dengue fever broke out in 1986. Medicines were bought quickly, in dollars, on the open market. By the time our factories could produce the required medicines, the market was already flooded with imports."

Local supply, particularly in war zones and other rural areas, is also a problem. On 14 July 1988, for example, contras attacked a convoy of trucks carrying medicines and other supplies to the small town of Mancotal, in Jinotega near the Honduras border. No one, including the local priest, risked a resupply operation for fear of another attack. It was two months before a *brigadista* from a neighboring area was convinced to take on the task.

OVERCONSUMPTION

Despite improved coordination of distribution and the elimination of subsidized prices, Nicaraguans still often consume medicines that are ineffective or harmful. Sixty percent of all imported medicines are antibiotics. Enough antibiotics are consumed to provide each person with five full courses of treatment a year—more than is used in Europe or the United States. But people often take antibiotics for only one or two days at a time,

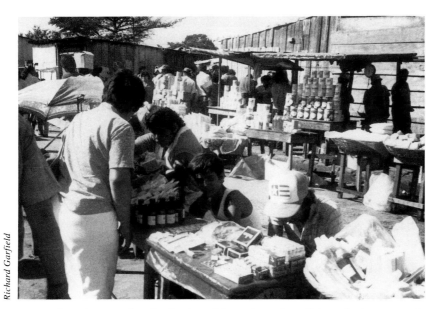

Richard Garfield

Despite laws limiting the distribution of formula and medicines, both are openly sold in stalls at Managua's Eastern market.

making each dose ineffective and promoting resistant bacterial strains. With the recent elimination of pharmaceutical subsidies, the tendency to take less than a full course of treatment is even greater.

Part of the problem of overconsumption has been the easy availability of a wide variety of drugs on the open market. It was not until June 1987 that the government issued a regulation making a doctor's prescription necessary for essential drugs. The large private sector and black market in medicines make it difficult to ensure enforcement of this regulation. The government still has no control over nonessential drugs, which remain on the open market. In February 1988, a researcher from the Central American University in Managua found a wide range of potentially dangerous drugs on sale:[15]

> In supermarkets, aspirin, high-powered antibiotics, and all kinds of other medicines have been sold—and are still being sold—on the same shelves as buttons and crackers. Ampicillin and vitamin B complex are everyone's favorite self-prescribed medicines for whatever disorder, no matter how light or serious. For mental exhaustion or migraine, vitamin B injections; for indigestion of whatever cause, milk of magnesia; for any degree of flu, ampicillin by the dozens and for nervous tension, Valium.

The drug mentality affects both doctors and the public. In a 1984 survey, more than half of those responding believed that colored pills were more effective than white pills. The pressure on medical practitioners to overprescribe drugs is intense: A doctor who advises bed rest and plenty of fluids instead of prescribing several drugs for a common cold may be called a quack. Worse, patients might have labeled him a counterrevolutionary for denying them the right to what they believed were essential services.

Efforts to improve doctors' prescribing practices have had only limited success. Most doctors receive little training in pharmacology and are unprepared to make optimal choices. Large numbers of patients and poor diagnostic facilities leave overprescribing the most expedient solution for a harried clinician. This also avoids confrontations with patients, many of whom are convinced of the need for a particular injection and seem unwilling to accept "no" for an answer. "I had a usual morning treating outpatients and supervising medical students," said U.S. doctor Tom Freiden. "I had already seen three patients with colds who demanded antibiotics, which of course I wouldn't give. When a medical student spoke up, I thought she would say that they needed injections. Instead, she said, 'Where I come from, people use the eucalyptus plant for colds—why not suggest that to them?' She was right. There were ten more colds that day, and we recommended it to them all."

Such examples are rare. Staff at the pharmacy of the Granada hospital are now protected from the public by an iron grille. "The people receive medicines prepacked and complain that they don't get enough. They shout at the girls," according to pharmacy director Fidelia Arguello. "Not long ago one of the patients beat up one of our pharmacy staff—that's how ag-

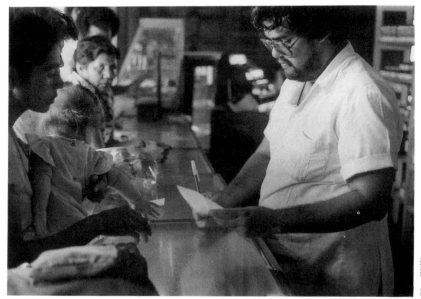

Glen Williams

Many Nicaraguans still suffer from a "drug mentality," which creates unnecessary demands on the health services. Pharmacists are often at the receiving end of complaints from patients when drugs are unavailable.

itated they get." One specialist invariably prescribes eighty-four capsules of ampicillin. The hospital pharmacy, however, follows a policy of giving only sixteen capsules at a time to avoid overprescribing. "This leads to conflicts with both patients and doctors. Every month we discuss with the hospital staff the problems of drugs and prescription, but they don't listen. On the other hand, patients are seldom satisfied either."

Traditional Medicine

Former Health Minister Tellez's prescription was to "replace the culture of antibiotics with our older culture of herbs. We need to remember camomile, bitter orange, saliva, and pasote." Traditional health care in Nicaragua is less well developed than in countries such as Guatemala, where the large indigenous population has maintained a long pharmaceutical tradition. Since 1986, health educators have nonetheless led an effort to recover and systematize information on herbal medicines in rural Nicaragua. Much of this knowledge resides with traditional birth attendants and has only recently been researched systematically.

There are widely varying views on the value of traditional medicine. Decentralization, the economic crisis, and an inability to meet the demand for modern medicines have encouraged experimentation in this area. In 1985, a botanical pharmacy was started in Estelí. Among its activities was a national meeting in which 850 school students and teachers presented the results of 3,000 interviews with people about herbal medicine.[16] The pharmacy has also drawn up an inventory of herbal resources and has classified about a thousand medical plants. Thirty-three of these were identified as priority products for cultivation and biochemical analysis in Germany. Three cooperative gardens outside of Estelí grow, package, and sell about a dozen of the most popular herbal remedies. The most important of these are camomile, eucalyptus, lemon grass, and guava. Many applications in the field of mental health have been made. Additional stores were set up in Matagalpa and Juigalpa. New surveys were carried out in these areas to uncover differences in the use and marketability of herbal medicines. Infusions and ointments are being developed to supplement the more typical teas.

In August 1987, the ministers of health of the seven Central American countries, meeting in Managua, issued a declaration stating that the time was ripe for the integration of traditional and local health systems. In November 1987, the first Central American meeting for the "rescue of traditional medicine" was held in Estelí.[17] These initiatives, together with the formal training of traditional *parteras* (see Chapter 7), reflect increased official awareness of the potential contribution of traditional medicine to health. "We don't want to overdo it. We can't try to use these medications to treat every kind of pathology or illness," said former Minister Tellez. Investigation into the utility of several herbal preparations and commercialization of these products has progressed rapidly. "We've had good results. Once the study is finished and the war is over, we plan not just to keep it at this level but to cultivate more of these plants commercially."

EQUIPMENT AND SUPPLIES

Laboratory equipment is an essential component of modern health care.[18,19] In hospitals and clinics, over 1,000 products are used in diagnosis and treatment. Unlike pharmaceuticals, most of these can be purchased locally. Given the strong public demand for medicines, however, this area has received less priority. While 90 percent of the drug purchases planned for 1987 were made, only 60 percent of materials (such as sheets, bandages, and cleaning supplies), 50 percent of lab reagents, and 60 percent of the small instruments in the plan were purchased.[5] By 1990, drug purchases dropped to 56 percent of planned levels.

For months at a time none of the five blood gas machines in Managua works. The only way to get an indication of the oxygen perfusion of the blood at such times is to look at it in a syringe and judge its brightness. The hemodialysis unit in Managua has been out of commission most of the time since 1980 for lack of parts. Old X-ray machines produce pictures so dim as to be of questionable utility: Twins have been delivered on several occasions following an X-ray that showed only one faint fetal skull. A similar situation is found with the one cobalt-based cancer treatment unit. A waiting list of six months for therapy is in effect, partly because the cobalt bomb is so old that patients must lie under it for an hour or more to receive an effective dose.

The most serious bottlenecks in the health system stem from the slow repair of equipment.[20] This was a problem before the war; the severing of credit and commercial relations by the United States made repair of most of the country's medical equipment even more difficult. It is estimated that 70 percent of the medical equipment in the country is from the United States. Of the four hospitals in the north-central region of the country, sterilizers for surgical equipment are usually out of service in two. This results in delays in surgery, higher infection rates, and higher transportation costs in taking equipment from one hospital to another for sterilization. It also contributes to poor job satisfaction among health workers. Gustavo Jerez Talavera, a hospital administrator, summed it up: "We cannot disconnect one child to hook up another."[21] Sometimes trucks must be hired to take materials to a distant hospital for resterilization. Laboratory equipment in health centers may take up to a year to repair.

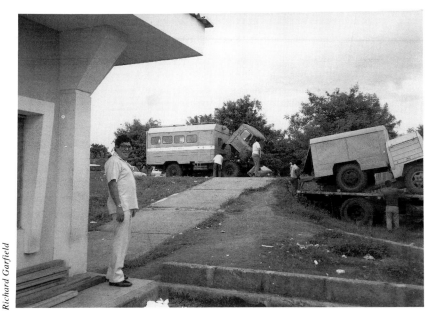

Richard Garfield

Like monuments to the past, these gifts, portable laboratories, sat unused in the back of the national MINSA office for years. Outdated when built, these heavy trucks were almost impossible to move. The wide variety of brands and styles of medical equipment donated to poor countries makes medical care administration all the more difficult.

In 1987, MINSA took its first complete inventory. It found that there were about 4,000 pieces of electronic equipment for direct patient care and diagnosis.[5] Twenty to thirty percent of the equipment was out of service. Hospitals and health centers depended on 257 pieces of major electromechanical equipment, of which 40 to 50 percent were out of service.

The inventory also showed that MINSA ran 83 operating rooms, 12 of which were out of service; 63 X-ray machines, more than a third of which were not functioning; and 112 clinical laboratories, most of which had some nonfunctional equipment. MINSA has thirty warehouses and twenty administrative buildings.

Transportation is also problematic. In 1987, MINSA owned 87 ambulances, 369 pickup trucks and jeeps, 63 large trucks, 26 vans, 12 small buses, 38 cars, 4 trailer trucks, 1 tractor, 5 river boats, 22 motor boats, and 23 bicycles. About 35 percent of these vehicles were out of service at any given time. Repair is made more difficult by the wide variety of donations and purchases received. MINSA's vehicles come from 28 manufacturers and include 188 different models. Poor skill among drivers is another problem. In 1986, MINSA vehicles were involved in 114 accidents. The situation continued to deteriorate; by 1990, half of all equipment was not working, including 60 percent of the country's ambulances.

The training and social service practice of local doctors prepares them for some of these limitations. Dr. Rodolfo Correa is doing his social service at the health center in Matiguas, Matagalpa. "A Nicaraguan doctor is a clinical doctor. To diagnose amebiasis, we don't need a test. We check to see if the stool has some mucus, is bloody, watery, green, or yellow. . . . To diagnose diabetes, we will ask a patient, 'How have you been feeling? Are you thirsty?' It's guerrilla medicine. We sometimes make mistakes, and sometimes we do well. Everything is a fight. We improvise."

BALANCING PRIORITIES

Misuse of medicines weakens the health system. It robs the system of needed funds to repair and maintain transportation, supplies, and essential medicines. A comment by Julio Briceno, then vice-minister for medical care, was illuminating in this regard. Explaining in 1983 why MINSA had for two years spent its foreign exchange on antibiotics and other medicines rather than replacement parts for hospital equipment, he said, "It's more logical to invest the few dollars we have in preventive medicine."[22] This expense, in fact, had little impact on preventive medicine. It went into the arena of progressive doctors, albeit ineffectively, for primary health care. This meant that funds were less available for secondary care in hospitals (the domain of more conservative doctors) and preventive care (the domain of nurses and community volunteers). As in other aspects of the health system, the pivotal role of physicians as leaders and legitimizers of the political system, with greater commitment to medicine than health, emerges.

Elimination of misuse and overconsumption will require a great deal of education and better organization. Both professionals and consumers need to better understand the uses and limitations of antibiotics, pain relievers, and vitamins. This will require both cultural evolution and technical education over an extended period of time.

Despite misuse and high cost, Nicaragua during the eighties was one of the few Latin American countries where essential pharmaceuticals were available most of the time at urban and rural primary care facilities. Nicaragua spent less than half as much for imported pharmaceuticals in 1989 ($14 million) as it did in 1985 ($31 million). The massive effort and repeated organizational and administrative changes made to keep medicines flowing were a key expression of the country's high commitment to meeting basic needs.

It is also in the area of pharmaceuticals that the weaknesses of post-Sandinista MINSA become most apparent. The first new director of COFARMA lived in Miami and ran a medicine-exporting firm. Charges of misappropriated funds and absentee positions of authority, while unproven, were reminiscent of regimes prior to the Sandinistas.

The medicine policy got caught up in the wave of privatization sweeping Nicaragua and Eastern Europe in 1990. Even orders already paid for were not shipped, as private firms in Eastern Europe refused to honor commercial commitments made months earlier when they were still state-run companies. As a result, remaining subsidies and free medicine programs disappeared in Nicaragua. Medicines went to market value just as hyperinflation returned to destroy the buying power of salaries.

In addition, tight central controls imposed by MINSA on distributing medicines were lost. In their place, health units were to order medicines of choice through fixed budget allocations. This budgetary decentralization might have worked in a different political environment and under careful supervision. Lacking careful norms and supervision and under new leadership, pharmaceutical distribution deteriorated. Health centers and hospitals complained of shortages worse than any experienced under the Sandinistas, and many health posts reported no medicine deliveries at all for months. Many viewed this approach as an attempt to bankrupt and privatize COFARMA itself.

Minister of Health Salmeron reiterated MINSA's policy of free medicines for high priority groups and asked for public assistance in policing the pharmacies. In the environment of radical privatization, though, this became increasingly difficult. State pharmacies were de facto privatized, eighty new profit-oriented pharmaceutical importing firms sprang up,* and free or subsidized medicines became a thing of the past.†

The picture of access to medicines had a few bright spots. One was access to new sources of donations for medicines. The largest of these was USAID, which provided several million dollars' worth of pharmaceuticals in 1990. Even more important was the attitude of many poor communities, which were losing access to modern medicines after the election. They organized self-reliant approaches to protect themselves. This included development of local revolving funds for families needing to purchase medicines, seeking direct donations from foreign groups, and an explosion in the cultivation of medicinal plants.

These bright spots do not make up for the losses of recent years. The double blows of increasing impoverishment and privatization have robbed the poor of one of the most important advances they experienced during the eighties. It can only be hoped that improved administration and the clarification of health priorities in the months ahead can reestablish good supplies and effective distribution of basic medicines.

*There had been 380 registered pharmacies in the country prior to 1990.

†Except for vaccines and tuberculosis medicines. For the latter, supplies were guaranteed by the International Union for the Prevention of Respiratory Diseases.

11

Stretching the Shrinking Cordoba

> If you want to invest $100 million in a private hospital with
> 100 beds and modern, scientific technology, welcome . . .
> But please! Get it out of your head that there might be
> any government resources to finance private investments in
> medicine.
>
> Minister of Health ERNESTO SALMERON

Health systems in developing countries are difficult to scrutinize with economic analysis.[1,2] Few health leaders have a complete overview of monetary issues, and key information is often unavailable. The mixed public/private character of the Nicaraguan health system, however, gives us a view of the bottom line.

HOW MUCH SHOULD HEALTH CARE COST?

This question confronted MINSA when a budget was to be developed in 1979. Since no reliable data on the Somoza period were available, officials guessed at the budget of the prerevolutionary agencies dealing with health and then doubled that amount. Contrary to what many investigators have assumed, Nicaragua was already investing heavily in health prior to the revolution. During most of the seventies, the health sector absorbed about 8 percent of the government's budget (see Figure 11-1). This was double the average size of health budgets in developing countries. The public health sector represented 1 to 2 percent of the national Gross Domestic Product (GDP). The role of health in the GDP was greater than in any other Central American country except Costa Rica.

With the revolution, health investments rose rapidly. By 1981 the health sector represented 13 percent of the government's budget and 4.7 percent of the GDP. Despite rising inflation, the value of public funds invested in health rose far more rapidly. Furthermore, MINSA represented only about 40 percent of all health-related expenses in the country. Private physicians and dentists, private medicine purchases, and health investments by other

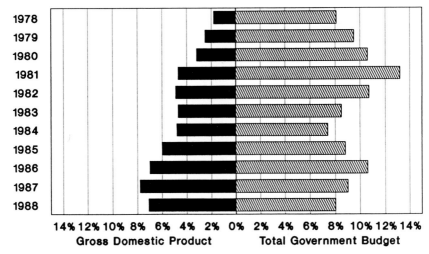

| | 14% 12% 10% 8% 6% 4% 2% 0% 2% 4% 6% 8% 10% 12% 14% |
| Gross Domestic Product | Total Government Budget |

Figure 11–1   The health ministry comprised a large component of the government's budget from the late 1970s. As the government budget represented an increasing proportion of the country's economy in the 1980s, the proportional role of health in the national economy has similarly grown.

Table 11–1   Estimated expenditures for health in Nicaragua, 1986

Source	Cordobas (billions)
Government	
Ministry of Health (MINSA)	23.8
Water and waste (INAA)	2.4
Armed forces (EPS and MINT)	2.0
Social welfare (INSSBI)	0.5
University health training (UCA, UPOLI, UNAN)	0.5
Total government	29.2
Private individual payments	
Private physicians	14.1
Private dental care	1.8
Water supply payments	5.3
Private pharmaceuticals	3.4
Charges for public pharmaceuticals	0.4
Private hospitals	1.2
Lab tests and eyeglasses	0.5
Folk practitioners	0.5
Total private	27.2
Charities and health industries	
Red Cross	1.4
PROVADENIC	0.3
Popular organizations	0.2
Health industries	0.6
Total charity and industries	2.5
Estimated total health expenditures	58.9

Source: Roemer, MI. The Health System of Nicaragua—Under Fire. Los Angeles, Mimeo, 1986.

Table 11–2 Economic recession and changes in
health spending

Country	Percent per capita GDP, 1980–1984	Percent per capita health spending, 1980–1985
Guatemala	− 15	− 58
El Salvador	− 26	− 32
Costa Rica	− 12	− 17
Honduras	− 12	− 15
Nicaragua[a]	− 65	− 2

Sources:
Direccion de Finanza, MINSA.
Ministerio de Finanza, JGN.
Cornia, GA, Jolly, R, and Stewart, F. Adjustment with a human face. Oxford,
Clarendon, 1987.
[a]Calculated with official inflation index.

ministries surpassed the expenses made by MINSA (see Table 11–1).
Health spending thus constituted a whopping 10 to 15 percent of the GDP
during the mid-eighties.

After 1984, further increases in the number of cordobas devoted to the
health system were eaten up by inflation. By 1986, MINSA had only
slightly more inflation-adjusted cordobas to spend than it did in 1980. Compared to the other Central American countries, where economic problems
have been less severe, the Nicaraguan health sector has nonetheless fared
very well. Nicaragua throughout the eighties maintained most of its health
funding, while in the other countries it was severely cut back (see Table
11–2).

BUDGETARY CHANGES

Despite rising military spending throughout the eighties, the health sector
maintained its prominent position in the national budget. In 1982, 19 percent of public expenditures went to the military (see Figure 11–2). This
rose to 46 percent of the budget in 1987. Despite a serious reduction in
availability of funds to other sectors, the social sector in general and the
health sector in particular were largely spared from cuts prior to 1988. "It
may seem contradictory," said a government planner, "that although the
war costs us more, we need to invest in the health system to reduce the
war's impact on the general population." The maintenance of high investments in health, in the context of a shrinking national economy, increased
MINSA's relative share of the GDP from between 1 and 1.5 percent in the
seventies to an amazing 7.8 percent in 1987 (see Figure 11–1). It did not,
however, ever reach 14 percent of the government budget, as has been
reported.[3]

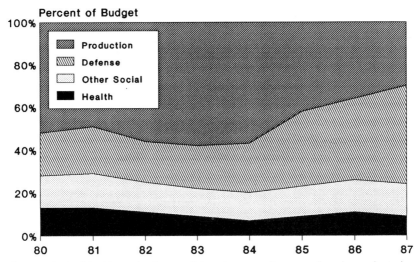

Figure 11–2 Health and other social sector spending was largely neglected as defense took an increasing proportion of the national budget in the 1980s.

Sources of Operating Funds

Prior to the revolution, the largest pool of health funds was generated by the Social Security system (see Figure 11–3). Following the revolution, these payroll deductions continued to fund health services that were administered by MINSA and opened to the whole population. A unique arrange-

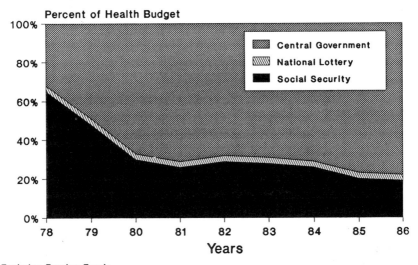

•Excludes Foreign Funds

Figure 11–3 Public health funds from domestic sources only, 1978–1986. The central government provided an increasing proportion of funds used by MINSA as the value of social security contributions declined.

ment was made to transfer 9 percent of all Social Security deductions to MINSA for its general operating budget in what came to be known as the "solidarity fund." Social Security health funds in 1978 represented 65 percent of all health expenditure. Increasing investments from other sources reduced the relative value of this pool to 30 percent of MINSA's budget in 1980, 28 percent in 1983, and 19 percent in 1986.

National lotteries are used to fund health systems in many Latin American countries.[1] In Nicaragua it is estimated that 3 to 6 percent of the health budget is provided by funds generated by the lottery. Domestic charitable donations were an important informal source of operating funds prior to the revolution, making up as much as 10 percent of the budget. The size and variety of programs since 1979 have dwarfed this source.

International moneys were an important source of funds for routine program operations in the early eighties. Most of these funds were part of an Interamerican Development Bank loan to construct or refurbish health facilities. Such funds equaled up to 20 percent of MINSA's budget in 1981, but diminished to 6 percent in 1984. U.S. government efforts to block any further grants or loans have been largely successful: Direct dollar donations to the government for health were an insignificant portion of MINSA's budget from 1985 to 1989.

Following the Chamorro election in 1990 and the end of the U.S. economic blockade, new moneys started to flow. USAID spent about $14 million for health-related services for contras returning from Honduras, provided over $4 million directly to MINSA for emergency pharmaceutical purchases, and provided several more million for health to U.S. organizations such as Project HOPE. European governments pledged even more in a $70-million package. These funds would nearly double the effective budget of MINSA, but were not made available until old loans in arrears were renegotiated. As a result, MINSA, like the rest of Nicaragua, was still starved for development funds a year after Chamorro took over.

A decrease in the value of international loans, domestic charity, and Social Security funds left the central government to provide an increasing proportion of the health sector budget. In 1987, the government provided about 80 percent of all funds for the MINSA budget. Even after being cut by 30 percent in January 1989, health continued to receive more than 10 percent of the total government budget. Such high dependence on regular government funds again highlights the remarkable strength of the government's commitment to the health sector.[4] When the National Assembly debated next year's budget in November 1990, Minister of Health Salmeron had almost daily press conferences on AIDS, the measles epidemic, and other major issues. His strategy seemed to work. Health received a stable allocation of funds from the central government at $83 million (see Figure 11–4).

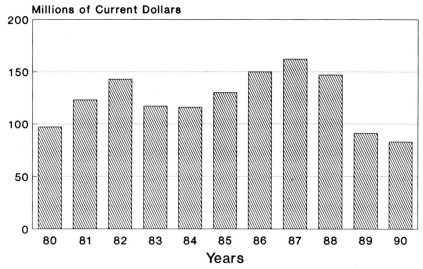

Figure 11–4   The size of the MINSA budget has varied greatly from year to year.

Destination of Health Funds

The destinations of various components of the health budget have changed little since 1980. The largest single component has always been the hospitals, utilizing close to half of the entire budget. On average, each of the thirty-one hospitals utilizes about little over 1 percent of the national health budget. In 1983, MINSA began to shift funds toward primary care. This trend slowed in 1984, when falling quality of care in hospitals and war-related demands dictated a return to traditional funding patterns. Nonetheless, funding for primary health care expanded from 14 percent in 1981 to 26 percent in 1987 and to 33 percent in 1989. Funding for hospitals rose dramatically from 46 percent to 50 percent of the health budget in the first year of the Chamorro regime. The main component of the health budget cuts in the latter eighties was administration. Decentralization helped reduce the cost of administration from 25 percent in 1981 to 14 percent in 1986 and to 6 percent in 1990. Preventive components of the MINSA budget receive smaller funding allotments. Health education and malaria control together account for about 8 percent of the total budget. International funding of the health budget has been concentrated in these latter components and in primary health care.

More than half of all local currency funds are destined for salaries. Most of the rest goes to equipment and supplies. Because of the preferential rates of exchange applied through 1988 and the availability of donations to reduce overall costs, medicines distributed by the health system appear to cost relatively little. Their cordoba value was only about as much as food consumed by patients and less than other medical supplies. Investments in construction and repair of facilities consume the rest of the budget. Expenditure on construction peaked at 14 percent of the budget in 1982 and declined to 1 percent in 1986. By the late eighties, national funds went almost exclusively to salaries. Foreign funds were needed for almost all other program costs. In 1990 the situation had become more extreme. Minister Salmeron stated that his 23,000 employees would absorb virtually all MINSA funds for nonfixed expenditures. There were no funds left in the budget for maintenance, let alone construction or improvement of facilities or initiation of new programs.

IMPORTS

The economic crisis is reflected in a scarcity of dollars and imported goods. Health, more than other social sectors, depends on imported goods such as pharmaceuticals, spare parts and equipment, books and journals, reagents, expert consultation, and medical care for patients treated outside the country.

By far the largest foreign exchange purchase is pharmaceuticals. More than half of the $40–60 million in value imported by MINSA in most years is destined for medicines. In 1986, $18 million was spent on finished medical products and $12 million went for medicines that would be finished in Nicaraguan processing plants. By contrast, $800,000 was used to purchase equipment, and $300,000 to purchase vehicles. It was estimated that an additional $1.5 million would have been sufficient to repair most of the broken medical equipment in the country. By contrast, double that amount was being spent to import powdered milk, which could actually harm the health of young children.

International Donations

While the country received $100–150 million in donations each year during the eighties, few international donations were designated to supply dollars for imports. Registered donations (mainly from UN-related agencies), totaling about $10–$15 million, probably cover less than half of all imports for health. Donations of goods-in-kind considerably exceed donated currency. In 1986, MINSA programs received $10 million in cash donations while UN-related organizations provided $13.5 million in health assistance,[5,6] Western European countries gave about $1 million in medical aid, and medical solidarity groups in North America and Europe provided about $3 million. Some 40 percent of all materials donated to MINSA were unsolicited.[7]

Donations in kind via medical scholarships provided a further estimated $800,000 in value. Medical teams and supplies provided for foreign-run hospitals by the Soviet Union, the German Democratic Republic, and Cuba were estimated to be worth $2.5 million in 1986.

Although these sums are small by the standards of some countries, they represent an enormous amount in the context of a small, impoverished

Table 11–3   Partial list of foreign assistance for health in Nicaragua, 1990[a]

Sweden	Malaria control	0.3
Norway	Various projects, especially for the Atlantic coast	1[b]
The Netherlands	Rotating medicine fund	0.4
	Various projects in region 5	2[b]
Denmark	Atlantic coast facilities	0.9
Finland	Rehabilitation services	1
	Malaria control	0.4
	Equipment maintenance	1
Japan	Ambulances	2
	Milk	9
Italy	Health facilities in region 4	4[b]
	Child survival activities	0.9
	Facilities and water in Bluefields	3
Germany	Operation of Karl Marx Hospital	–[c]
Canada	Water systems in major cities	1.2[b]
	Water and health education in region 6	0.8
Spain	Training health workers	–[c]
Soviet Union	Building a hospital in Chinandega	–[c]
PAHO	Various programs	1.3
UNFPA	Family planning	2[b]
UNICEF	Child health and training	–[c]
USAID	Contra repatriation	12[b]
	Running four hospitals	1[b]
	Water system improvement	5[b]
	Pharmaceuticals	4[b]

[a]In millions of U.S. dollars.
[b]Estimated value per year.
[c]No information on value of program available.

country. A danger thus exists for the loss of national decision making, subverting national plans and developing some sectors of the health system at the expense of others on the whim of international organizations. Donahue discounts this dynamic by showing that foreign moneys supported much of the primary care system that was developed during the eighties.[8,9] In fact, foreign moneys supported most of the health system; primary care would likely have proceeded more rationally if foreign support didn't simultaneously subsidize inefficient pharmaceutical, food supplementation, and health personnel policies.

This danger became greater following the electoral defeat of the Sandinista government and the collapse of Eastern European socialism in 1990. The Eastern bloc had provided the second largest pool of international resources for health prior to 1990, exceeded only by UN agencies. Suddenly, this source seemed to disappear. At the same time, declining financial support from solidarity groups was increasingly disbursed directly to community groups and nongovernmental organizations, bypassing MINSA.

Western European governments and the United States nominally supported the government that their war had brought into power and partially made up for lost sources of funds and materials. By 1991, however, with attention turned to Eastern Europe and the Persian Gulf, these funds fell far short of needs. Only the Scandinavian countries provided continuity in high levels of support for health during the eighties and nineties (see Table 11–3).

A SHORTAGE OF DOLLARS

As the national currency weakened with rampant inflation since 1985, the relative value of imported goods has grown and the importance of donations has skyrocketed. In 1987 the value of donations (about $20 million U.S., detailed above) exceeded the value of the total national health budget at black market rates of exchange. Of course, the goods and services produced by the health system far exceed the real value of donations, but rampant inflation has made such comparisons meaningless. The economic embargo, the war, and the declining economy have left the government, and its health system, increasingly dependent on outside assistance.

The health system imports expensive goods for which it must pay in hard currency from central government funds. In 1987, more than two-thirds of all MINSA dollar purchases were paid for with central government funds. The commercial debt of MINSA, begun in 1982, grew to about $20 million by 1987 (see Figure 11–5) and fell to $17 million in 1990.

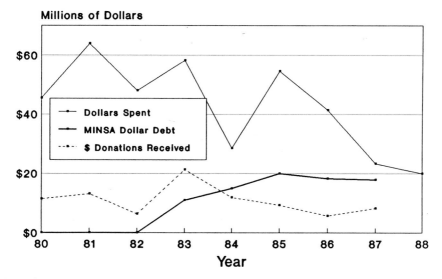

Millions of Dollars

*Some Data Not Available for 1988

Figure 11–5   MINSA has spent considerably more U.S. dollars for imports than it has received from international sources; thus, MINSA incurred a growing debt during the mid-1980s.

Reducing Dollar Dependence

Notable advances have been made by the health system in five areas of import substitution. First, an increasing proportion of medicines are being finished within the country: Nearly all intravenous fluids, for example, are now fabricated nationally. Second, centralized purchasing and restriction in brands has helped rationalize supply. Together, these changes save the country about $5 million a year.

Third, pesticide purchases have been reduced by more than half through revising the strategy for control of malaria, saving the country $1–$2 million a year. Fourth, innovations in the repair, reuse, or fabrication of spare parts may save the country $500,000 a year. Finally, the expanded use of herbal medicines makes an intangible but important contribution to reducing the demand for imported pharmaceuticals.

Value Destroyed in the War

The health system was hit hard by the Contra war. Great as the destruction has been, this represents only a small portion of the total destruction wrought by the war. As in previous natural and manmade disasters in Nicaragua, most of the damage was sustained by the agricultural and industrial sectors. About 3 percent of all direct destruction in the contra war was sustained by the health system. This included $2 million for the destruction of twenty-nine health posts and 3 health centers, $2.8 million for destruction of ambulances and infrastructural facilities, and $1.2 million for medicines lost or stolen.[10]

While large stocks of medicines were destroyed in attacks on several health centers in 1984 and 1985, the greatest single loss occurred in the October 1983 bombing of the Pacific coast town of Corinto. In destroying the country's main oil depot, large warehouses with medicines, clothes, pesticides, and food worth several million dollars were lost.

MINSA estimated in January 1988 that reconstruction of destroyed facilities would cost 200 billion cordobas. This total was more than twice the cordoba value of the country's annual health budget at that time. Perhaps as much as 50 percent more value was lost in destroyed or stolen equipment and supplies.

THE COST OF REBUILDING

In 1990 it was estimated that MINSA needed $1 million on average to repair each of ten hospitals, as well as $1 million to operate all of the thirty-one public hospitals each month. Looked at another way, the country needed $17 million to provide pharmaceuticals, $9 million for other medical materials, and $74,000 for laboratory supplies to maintain services at their already-inadequate levels. Yet most of these funds were not readily forthcoming.

Put in the context of war-related destruction and the economic crisis gripping the country, the strong commitment of the government to maintain its investment in health seems remarkable. International donations are essential in making that commitment effective. It appears, however, that such donations distorted health funding in the eighties, making inefficient use of scarce resources for pharmaceutical purchases. These inefficiencies were increasingly corrected as the deepening economic crisis tested the ingenuity of health leaders. Yet as Minister Salmeron reflected, "Even if we doubled the health budget, it would be inadequate . . . the demand for care is still not being satisfied."

12

Health in a Survival Economy

> Good food, housing, money, and employment contribute to
> maintaining health. . . . A garden, however small it may be,
> is better than a doctor.
>
> ALEJANDRO DAVILA BOLANOS, circa 1960

Health services may improve the length or quality of people's lives, but
their impact depends on the opportunities afforded by the underlying economic and social environment. Before 1979, the chance to live a long,
healthy life in Nicaragua was reserved for a privileged few. Among this
group, life expectancy was nearly as high as in the United States and other
industrialized countries.

The poor majority, by contrast, were deprived not only of health care but
also of the other factors that play a role in health—food, land, income, safe
water, sanitation, housing, education, and other basic services.

The goal of "health for all" could not be achieved simply by expanding
the outreach of the health services. Fundamental changes in society were
needed to narrow the health gap between the privileged few and the poor
majority. These changes would entail, above all, a radical transformation
of the country's economy.

But the economy was shattered in the eighteen-month insurrection: Factories, homes, hospitals, schools, and public buildings had been destroyed
or damaged by Somoza's National Guard. The total cost of the damage
during the insurrection was estimated at $1.3 billion.[1] When the Sandinistas
came to power, they found only $3.5 million in the national treasury and
faced a national debt of $1.6 billion.

The new government decided to embark on a two-track policy of economic and social development. On the one hand, the economy would
undergo a process of *restructuring* in order to distribute resources and opportunities more evenly. At the same time, large-scale *reconstruction* would
be encouraged to repair and rebuild infrastructure needed for growth.[2-4]
This chapter traces changes in economic policy, exports and imports, and
food production that have influenced health during the last decade.

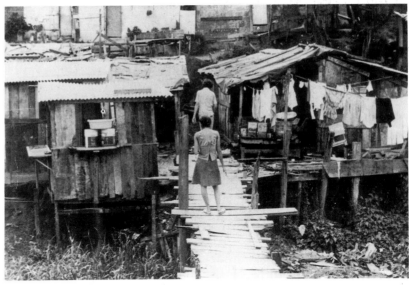

A typical neighborhood in the Atlantic coast town of Bluefields. A semitropical environment and poor infrastructure make good hygiene and sanitation almost impossible.

THE "MIXED" ECONOMY

The Sandinistas stressed their commitment to a "mixed" economy, in which the private sector would continue to play a role. Most business leaders and large landowners, however, deeply distrusted the Sandinistas and resented the government's intervention in the economy. One of the government's first steps was to nationalize all property belonging to Somoza and his associates. This included one-fifth of all farmland, half the agroprocessing industry, one-third of manufacturing capacity, and nearly all the fishing, forestry, mass transport, and construction industries.[5] Foreign-owned assets in the mining and banana industries were also nationalized. In addition, the government took control of banking and foreign trade, but limited expropriations of businesses and land outside the Somoza group.

Despite opposition from much of the business community, the early years of the Sandinista revolution were marked by social progress and economic growth:

Between 1979 and 1984, expenditure on education increased fourfold, the number of children attending primary school increased by 70 percent, and the number of school teachers doubled[6,7]

The population covered by social security rose from 200,000 to more than 1 million[8]

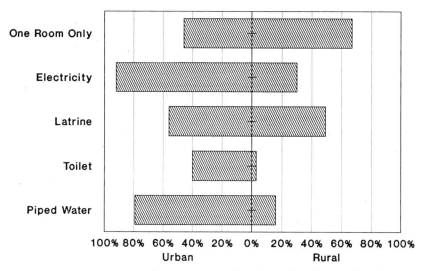

Figure 12–1 Housing conditions in 1985, by place of residence. Despite poor urban living conditions, people living in rural areas generally fared worse.

300 new health posts and five hospitals were constructed[9]

800 kilometers of new roads were built, including the first land route between the Pacific and the Atlantic coasts[10]

Electricity was brought to 14,000 new users in rural areas[10]

50,000 new telephone lines were installed, and direct telephone communication was established with the Atlantic coast for the first time[10]

Light industry grew rapidly, including food processing (milk, vegetables, cooking oil, seafood, sugar), clothing, pharmaceuticals, and leather goods[11]

New housing was built for 20,000 families[9]

New water supply systems reached 280,000 people in 450 communities; sanitary waste disposal reached 100,000 new users[9] (see Figure 12–1)

These developments were fueled by large public expenditures made possible by loans from international banks, grants from UN-related organizations and Eastern European governments, and credit lines from Western European and Latin American governments during 1979–83. The introduction of a progressive tax system also pressed wealthy Nicaraguans to contribute to the country's social development.

THE QUEST FOR FOOD SECURITY

The health of poor families depends, above all, on being able to grow enough food on their own land, or having the income to buy it. Before 1979, hunger was a daily fact of life for thousands of families. For the poorest half of the population, average calorie availability was only about 80 percent of what the body requires.[12] In the poorest regions, only a third of the people had enough income to supply an adequate diet.[13] The richest 5 percent, by contrast, consumed nearly double the calories they needed.

One of the new government's basic aims was to ensure that all social groups had enough food. Such a system of "food security" would require radical changes in land ownership, agricultural production, food pricing, and distribution. It would also have to pay special attention to the needs of the most vulnerable groups, especially low-income families.

When the Sandinistas came to power, the country faced a major food deficit. The final months of the insurrection had severely disrupted the planting season in many parts of the country, resulting in sharp falls in the maize, beans, and rice harvests. The Ministry of Agriculture moved fast to help small and medium-sized farms. Before the revolution, 90 percent of credit for farmers had been used for export crops grown by large landowners.[14,15] Now, for the first time, credit was made available to small- and medium-scale farmers to grow food for the national market.

Between 1978 and 1981, the number of small and medium-sized farmers receiving credit rose from 23,158 to 80,455.[16] Another popular measure was a drastic reduction in rents on land used to grow food crops. New institutions were created to provide small- and medium-scale farmers with technical assistance and a regular supply of seed and fertilizers.

To meet the food deficit, the government imported large quantities of maize and beans. Grain, milk, oil, and sugar were distributed as emergency rations. Food was sold at subsidized prices through community stores, supermarkets, and workplace commissaries and canteens. Schools provided milk and health clinics distributed food to pregnant and lactating women and to families with malnourished children. The Ministry of Social Welfare started nurseries where the children of working parents were fed every day (see Chapter 8).

Emergency rations were phased out in 1980 and replaced by a system providing food supplements to families in need. By 1981, food availability was generally above prerevolutionary levels (see Table 12–1).

Malnutrition was declining and it seemed that the nutritional rehabilitation units of hospitals could soon close. A physician working in one of these units commented, "These cases are leftovers of the past. Soon they will be no more."

The new agricultural policies had mixed results. In 1981 the bean crop was up, rice production was stagnant, and maize was down by 45 percent.[17] Most rural residents began eating much better, but at the cost of large food imports. This was a cost the government could not afford indefinitely.

An already difficult situation was exacerbated when, in early 1981, the United States abruptly suspended a wheat loan worth $9.6 million. This

Table 12–1   Annual per capita food availability, 1966–1989

Food								Quantity				
	Years:	66	76/78[a]	81	82	83	84	85	86	87	88	89
Eggs	Dozens	14	10	11	14	13	13	14	10	10	8	5
Milk	Liters	163	90	61	74	85	88	85	81	67	54	48
Oil	Liters	17	9	12	10	15	11	9	11	10	9	9
Meat	Pounds	72	39	39	41	42	42	42	35	34	32	22
Beans	Pounds	40	35	31	28	38	40	33	28	26	24	30
Rice	Pounds	64	37	81	64	70	73	76	71	63	45	54
Sugar	Pounds	51	97	90	102	104	100	119	102	90	67	62
Maize	Pounds	—	158	123	124	149	129	135	123	123	112	117

Sources:
INCAP. Evaluacion nutricional de la poblacion de Centroamerica y Panama. Guatemala, 1969.
Programa Alimentaria Nicarageunse (PAN), unpublished.
[a]Average.

was the first of a series of economic sanctions aimed at crippling the economy and destabilizing the government.

In response, the government launched the National Food Program (PAN) in April 1981. PAN's central task was to ensure the supply of basic foods to the whole population by promoting the production of food crops by small and medium-sized farmers.[17] In the heady optimism of the days before the contra war, government planners expected PAN to achieve national self-sufficiency in maize, rice, and beans within three years. (Ironically, the Spanish word *pan* means bread, which could not be made without using imported wheat.)

The new program concentrated mainly on helping peasant farmers through price incentives, credit, seed, technical assistance, mechanized services, training, improved crop storage facilities, and transport. To overcome dependence on imported wheat, the government promoted the use of maize. Festivals were organized involving recipe competition, song, and dance, all based on the theme *el maiz, nuestra raiz* ("maize, our roots").

Self-sufficiency in basic foods, however, proved elusive. Torrential ruins on the Pacific coast washed away the first maize crop of 1982. Those farmers who managed to replant were then ruined by a prolonged drought. Meanwhile, public demand for maize rose rapidly due to the growing population, heavily subsidized food prices, and the use of maize as a substitute for sorghum in animal feed. In 1983, the country faced a massive shortfall in maize, which was covered by record imports (see Figure 12–2). Drastic measures were needed to boost production of the country's major food grain.

The government responded by making large investments in maize production on state land.[14,18] Irrigated lands in the fertile Pacific region, nor-

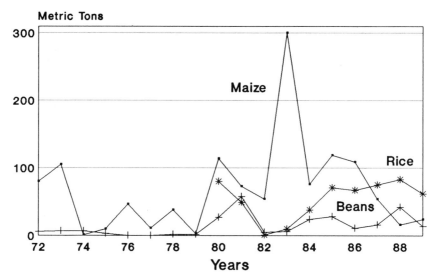

Figure 12–2 Food imports were used to make up for production shortfalls in the early 1980s. This policy was too expensive to maintain, and imports declined in the latter 1980s.

mally used to grow cotton, were dedicated instead to maize for part of the year. As a result, maize grown on state farms almost doubled between 1982/83 and 1983/84. Yet it still accounted for only 14 percent of total maize production. And because it relied on imported equipment, state-produced maize was much more expensive than maize grown by peasants. The National Farmers' Union (UNAG) condemned the policy because it absorbed finance, equipment, and expertise that otherwise could have been used to boost peasant food production.

Land to the Tiller

The inauguration of PAN was followed in late 1981 by the government's long-promised Agrarian Reform Law. This was potentially the single most important step toward boosting food production. Nicaragua has relatively abundant agricultural land, with an average of 23.7 hectares per rural family. (In nearby El Salvador, by contrast, the average is only 3.5 hectares per family.) Before the revolution, however, this land was divided very unevenly. In 1978, about 3,000 large farms accounted for nearly half the total agricultural land. Situated on the fertile plains of the Pacific region and using modern agricultural technology, these farms mainly produced export crops such as cotton, sugar, and tobacco. Their owners (2 percent of the agricultural work force) also dominated bank credit and technical assistance.

The other half of the country's farmland was owned by small and me-dium-sized producers, who accounted for one-third of the rural work force. These farmers produced 70 percent of the country's main staple foods—maize and beans—yet received little government credit or other assistance. Another third of rural families were poor farmers owning only 2 percent of the land, receiving no government assistance, and unable to grow enough food for their needs. The other third were either salaried or seasonal work-ers owning no land at all, most living in conditions of abject poverty.[16]

The new agrarian law was moderate in scope. Properties of over 300 hectares in the Pacific region and over 700 hectares elsewhere could be expropriated. Below this level, expropriation could be applied only to in-efficient farmers, or those who maintained unusually exploitative land ten-ure and labor relations. The law allowed for land to be distributed to peasant cooperatives, individual families, and indigenous communities. In practice, the Ministry of Agrarian Reform (MIDINRA) favored cooperative owner-ship rather than individual land titles where peasants could be encouraged to form them.

Disincentives to Production

While MIDINRA tried to boost food production, other government policies had the unintended effect of *discouraging* farmers from producing food crops. One disincentive to farmers was the lack of consumer goods and farming tools at government-controlled shops in rural areas. Through their trade unions, farmers and farm workers complained bitterly that there were insufficient shops and that those in existence did not stock the machetes, rubber boots, kerosene, clothes, shoes, and household goods they wanted. Said one farmers' leader: "What's the point of working all year only to sell our products at low prices, and then not be able to find or buy what we need to clothe, feed, and look after our families?"

Food subsidies were another disincentive to grain production. In order to provide enough basic foods to the urban poor and landless farm workers, the government "froze" prices in 1981. This was achieved through massive consumer subsidies. Television commercials explained how ENABAS pur-chased maize at the relatively low rate of 1.8 cordobas a pound and sold it to the consumer for only one cordoba a pound—the difference, plus the cost of transport, packaging, drying, and storage, being paid by the gov-ernment. A similar system applied to items such as beans, milk, flour, cooking oil, and even lettuces imported from Costa Rica.

It became cheaper for many farmers to buy food from the government than to grow it themselves.[18] Many small-scale farmers stopped growing maize and beans and sought work in the cities instead. Large cotton and sugar estates stopped planting maize and beans for their workers. Instead, even on some state farms they bought these items at subsidized prices.

The Bubble Bursts

Total per capita production of basic grains during 1980–83 rose to 74 percent of the levels during 1974–76.[19] Despite price and marketing problems, the production of basic foods continued to increase. The 1983/84 rice and bean crops reached record levels and maize production exceeded 500,000 metric tons for the first time since 1978/79.[17] Available calories were 40 percent higher than prerevolutionary levels. Eating habits also changed. People ate less beef but more rice, maize, chicken, and eggs than before the revolution (see Table 12–1).

The overall economic outlook was still hopeful. In contrast to the other four Central American nations, the economy was still expanding: In 1983, the economy grew by 5 percent.[20–22] The cost of living was also lower in Nicaragua than anywhere else in the region, due largely to heavy government subsidies on common items such as food, kerosene, soap, and cooking oil. About 24,000 families received land through the Agrarian Reform Law. Although government expenditure had increased enormously since 1979, inflation was still modest.

Most people seemed to approve of the policies of the government. In November 1984, the FSLN won 68 percent of the popular vote in the country's first general election since the end of the Somoza era.

But the bubble was about to burst. Nicaragua could no longer escape the consequences of the world economic recession, mounting external debts, and falling prices for its agricultural products. A massive trade deficit placed the economy under intolerable strain. In 1984, Nicaragua imported goods worth $826 million, while the value of the country's exports was only $386 million.

Nicaragua also faced special problems because of the war. In 1984, about 120,000 people left their farms to seek safety in cities or special settlements, resulting in a sharp fall in the area planted with maize and beans.

The coffee harvest—which provided 60 percent of export revenue—was also severely hit because pickers could not move safely in many of the mountainous areas where the Contras operated. In the 1984/85 coffee harvest, more than 200 pickers were killed by Contra forces and production valued at $69 million (one-fifth of total exports) was lost.

At the same time, intense lobbying by the U.S. government led to the denial of access to important regional and international sources of finance and development aid.[23] The governments of the United Kingdom and the Federal Republic of Germany also eliminated their aid. In May 1985, the

United States, which for decades had been Nicaragua's main trading partner, placed an embargo on most trade and commerce.

A "SURVIVAL" ECONOMY

By 1985, the Nicaraguan economy was in deep trouble. Production of food and cash crops fell, export income declined, and rampant inflation eroded the value of wages. The people complained bitterly about shortages of food and consumer goods.

The Sandinistas responded by abandoning some of the policies they had pursued so wholeheartedly since coming to power. Proclaiming the need for a "survival economy," they first set about reducing government expenditure, which was a prime contributing factor to inflation.[24] Development projects, including roads, bridges, housing, sewerage, and water supplies, were suspended. The budgets of nearly all government ministries were frozen or cut. The only exceptions were Health and Defense, both of which increased.

The government also took steps to boost the production of food and cash crops. Food subsidies were reduced.[17] This step was popular with farmers, but brought hardship to many urban poor and landless rural families who had to buy all or most of their food.

The government also ended the monopoly of ENABAS, allowing grain and bean producers to sell their crops to other buyers. Private cooperatives began to replace state enterprises in the sale of agricultural tools, basic foods, and consumer goods in rural areas. In the department of Estelí, for example, the local branch of the farmers' organization UNAG established a network of shops selling items such as boots, shirts, seeds, kerosene, tools, and clothing. The larger shops also served as storage and marketing centers, helping small farmers and cooperatives to market their crops more efficiently.[15]

The government decided to accelerate the pace of agrarian reform and to reduce the emphasis on collective agriculture. Between 1984 and 1986, about 74,000 rural families received land—60 percent individually and the remainder via cooperatives. In early 1986, the Agrarian Reform Law was amended to permit the expropriation of underutilized private farms without regard to size.

By the end of 1986, Nicaragua's agrarian structure had changed profoundly. Two million hectares of farmland (40 percent of all arable land) had been distributed to 98,000 families, either individually or through cooperatives.[12] Large-scale farmers owned only one-fifth of all farmland, compared with half in 1978 (see Table 12–2). About 40 percent of the rural

Table 12–2   Land tenure: Percentage of all agricultural land by type of ownership

Type of ownership	1978	1986
State farms	0	13
Cooperatives	0	13
Private land		
<35 hectares	18	22
35–141 hectares	30	30
>141 hectares	52	22

Source: Solon, L, Barraclough, S and Scott, MF. The Rich Have Already Eaten.
London, Transnational Institute, 1987.

population had received land through the agrarian reform. Landless laborers were still 25 percent of the rural work force, but many more had year-round employment and the benefits of membership in the agricultural worker's union.

Economic and military attacks focused the attention of Sandinista leaders on economic and political survival. Ironically, the result was increased *privatization* of agricultural production and services via individual holdings and cooperatives, rather than greater control by the central government. The effects on production were soon evident: In 1986/87, the maize harvest was well above the prerevolutionary levels, rice production doubled, and bean production reached a new record (see Figure 12–3).

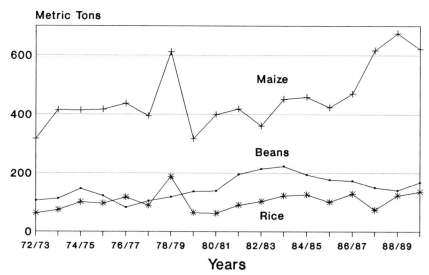

Figure 12–3   Between 1972 and 1990, increased maize production did not keep pace with population growth. Bean and rice production fared even more poorly.

Protecting the Poor

Agrarian reform was an essential step in reaching food security, but it was not enough. Special measures were needed to ensure that the most vulnerable—especially the urban poor and landless farm workers—also had enough food. This was the purpose of the "guarantee card" system introduced in 1982. Intended originally to distribute sugar more evenly, the system was later extended to cover rice, beans, cooking oil, and soap, which were sold at subsidized rates through community shops.[15] The system made these items more available and helped hundreds of thousands of poor families meet basic living expenses.

But with the escalation of the contra war and the deterioration of the economy, the guarantee card system was gradually whittled away. By early 1988, the government could guarantee only one kilo of sugar, a half-kilo of rice, and one bar of soap per household every month.

1988—"The Worst Year"

As the Nicaraguan revolution approached its tenth anniversary, the country coped with a crippling economic crisis compounded by eight years of war. At the start of 1988, the government declared a state of food emergency after a severe drought wiped out 75 percent of the bean crop, 45 percent of sorghum production, and 25 percent of the maize harvest. Said Henry Ruiz, minister of economic cooperation:[25] "Food security is not a question of balancing proteins and calories. It's a question of having enough rice and beans to last out the war."

The economy was now in desperate shape. Export revenues plummeted to about $200 million annually, a 30 percent decline from prerevolution levels (see Figure 12–4). The national debt reached $7 billion. This is the highest per capita debt in Latin America, representing an amount similar to the entire country's GDP for two years. Foreign aid and credits reached a high of $1.2 billion in 1985; they fell to $385 million in 1987. Galloping inflation reduced economic planning to guesswork. Real wages in 1988 had lost 94 percent of their value compared with 1980[26] (see Figure 12–5).

The impact of the war on the economy was devastating. Between 1984 and 1987, the country lost the equivalent of 40 percent of its export earnings through destroyed infrastructure and lost agricultural and industrial output. Direct destruction was valued at $222 million, while total losses (including lost production and the value of secondary industries) were estimated at $2.6 billion.

The war also had more insidious effects on the economy and health. With defense spending absorbing half of the budget, all other sectors suffered. Routine maintenance was neglected due to the chronic lack of foreign cur-

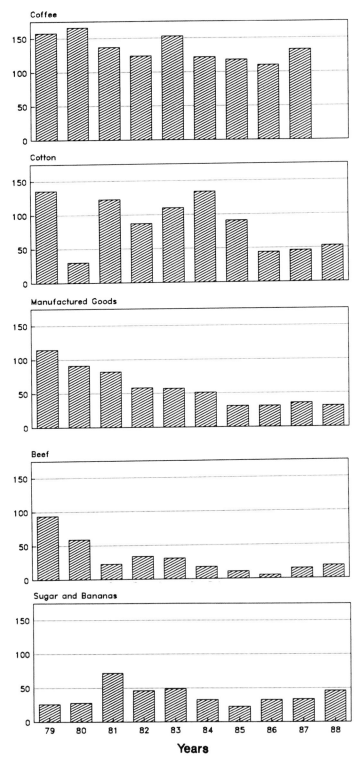

Figure 12–4 The economic disaster of the 1980s is reflected in stagnant or falling production of all major exports.

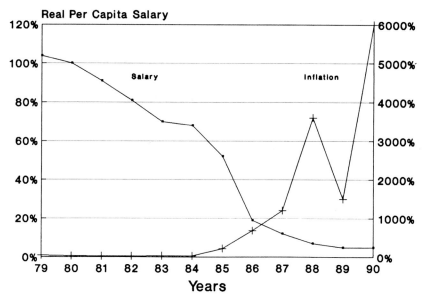

Figure 12–5 Economic indicators, 1979–1990. Inflation destroyed the buying power of wages, especially after 1984.

rency to purchase supplies and spare parts. A survey in Boaco, for example, found that only a quarter of the rural water systems built after 1979 were still providing water of acceptable quality.[27] The collection of urban refuse was irregular or nonexistent because of a lack of vehicles, tires, and spare parts. In Managua's slum neighborhoods, the combination of unsafe water, inadequate sanitation, and heaps of fly-infested refuse produced favorable conditions for the spread of infections, especially diarrhea. Illiteracy is estimated to have risen from 12 percent in 1980 to 20 percent in 1988.

In February 1988, the government announced a series of measures designed to check the downward slide of the economy. The cordoba was devalued by 3,000 percent. Twenty other devaluations were carried out through August 1989.[28] In June, a package of economic measures was implemented that shocked many of the government's own supporters by its severity. Aimed at reducing the trade deficit and boosting exports, the measures were described by one economist as "a conventional International Monetary Fund package without the financing that accompanies IMF reforms." Price controls were lifted on most goods and services, and most subsidies were abolished. Rice and bean prices tripled, meat and fish prices doubled, gasoline rose twelvefold, cooking gas rose tenfold, and electricity rose sevenfold.

Those least affected were food producers, who continued to receive government credit and could sell their rice, maize, and beans on the free market. In the first half of 1988, a cease-fire and early rains also enabled farm-

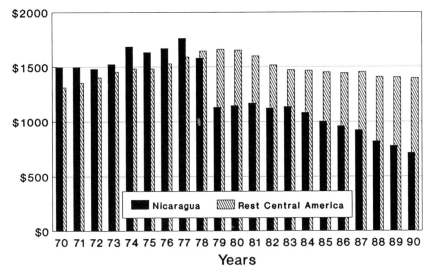

In 1988 Dollars

Figure 12–6 Nicaragua's per capita national product rose rapidly during the 1960s and 1970s. It declined sharply in the revolutionary insurrection of 1978 and 1979 and recovered only slightly in the early 1980s. It declined again and more seriously during the Contra war of the late 1980s. By contrast, the recession in the rest of Central America during the early 1980s was followed by stabilization during the late 1980s.

ers to plant 16,000 more hectares of maize and beans. The first rice, maize, and bean crops of 1988 were well up on the previous year.

These harvests were followed by Hurricane Joan, which destroyed food and export crops, roads, electricity supplies, food-processing plants, schools, health facilities, and 30,000 homes.[29,30] Total damage was estimated at $840 million—four times the country's current annual export earnings. The hurricane's effect on inflation was immediate and profound.

According to government economist Mario Arana, 1988 was "the worst of the revolution. In one year we lost all the achievements of the eight previous years." Inflation reached the unbelievable annual rate of 2,000 percent. Although all of the Central American countries suffered recession throughout the eighties, Nicaragua was by far the hardest hit[31,32] (see Figure 12–6). Production fell by about 8 percent in 1988 and by lesser amounts in 1989. Per capita GDP fell to about $300—lower even than that of Haiti, long the poorest country in the Western Hemisphere.

REESTABLISHING THE "SAFETY NET"

Austerity measures slashed the purchasing power of wage earners. Government employees and some others received some protection through the monthly distribution of five kilos of rice, five kilos of beans, and three kilos of sugar. This program reached 34 percent of the nation's homes. Low-income urban and rural workers received salary increases, but these increases only permitted a family of four with an average salary to purchase 64 percent of a theoretical "basket" of basic foods each month. As a result, consumption of all forms of animal protein (milk, eggs, and meat) went down and consumption of corn, rice, and beans went up. In 1989, calorie and protein consumption were, on average, 14 and 25 percent below minimum recommended levels (see Figure 12–7). Remarkably, the economy in many rural areas began to stabilize.

To further ameliorate the effects of the economic adjustment on children, the "glass of milk" program was launched in April 1989 in Managua and Matagalpa among preschool, first-, and second-grade students. This popular program expanded rapidly, involving each region and reaching 249,000 children each day by August 1990. The program exhibited some of the best characteristics found in other successful Nicaraguan programs. First, it was decentralized, with municipal and regional governments in charge. Community organization was important to pressure local governments to participate and to generate the volunteer labor and materials to make it run. Finally, close intersectoral coordination among the Ministries of Finance, Transport, Health, and Education was needed. As an added benefit, leaders report that school attendance and learning ability seemed to improve dramatically in many areas.

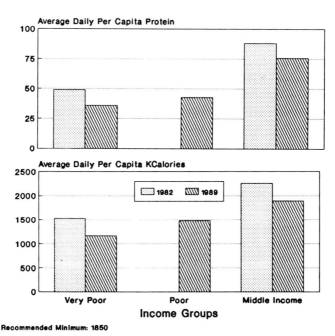

Figure 12–7   Although middle-income groups had far superior nutrition than the poor, both groups experienced worsening nutrition during the 1980s.

The weaknesses were also characteristically Nicaraguan. It was based on a relatively expensive foreign product (powdered milk) for which continuing donations had to be sought. Since the program was an entitlement for all children from preschool to second grade, it left out older children regardless of need and failed to target those younger children or those schools that had the greatest needs. It was estimated that universal distribution limited the impact to a 7 to 10 percent protein and calorie supplement, which was still inadequate for those in greatest need.

A 30 percent cut in the government's budget and a 117 percent devaluation in January 1989 reflected bold, perhaps desperate, attempts to control hyperinflation and stimulate the economy. Guaranteed food prices for consumers and most subsidies for producers were eliminated. The effects of these measures were mixed. Inflation dropped from about 90 percent a month in late 1988 to about 10 to 15 percent during spring of 1989, only to return to intolerably high levels in June.[26] But the social costs of this process were great. Public credits fell from 29 to 11 percent of the GDP from 1987 to 1989. Lacking credit, many ENABAS outlets closed, reducing access to foods and medicine in rural areas.

Agricultural investment by the government fell from 12.5 to 2.4 percent of GDP from 1987 to 1989. This meant that production for export fell further, replaced in part by small-scale production for consumption in the national market. There seemed to be no way out.

Many believe that the electoral defeat of the Sandinistas in February 1990 was born of this desperate situation. While the FSLN campaigned with the slogan "everything will be better," the Chamorro coalition promised more concretely to revive the economy with U.S. assistance within 100 days. This, too, was not to be.

Despite as many as two devaluations a week and the elimination of virtually all remaining credits and subsidies following the change of government in 1990, inflation ate up half of the value of the currency each month. The economy continued to decline through 1991, when it was estimated that 75 percent of the population was poor and 17 percent lived in desperate conditions. Half of the working population was unemployed, while the average salary of an employed person covered only 60 percent of the food purchases for a family of four.

Sizable credits from the United States and the World Bank were unavailable during the Chamorro government's first year. They began to flow in 1991 only after the new government dropped the World Court decision against the United States, which had demanded financial reparations for its military interventions. Such credits will have to be carefully and patiently applied before the economy is likely to improve. Until they work, the safety net created in the eighties, then dismantled in turn by the FSLN and Chamorro, must be reestablished.

Key among these safety nets are nutritional programs. Overall, the nutritional status of children has changed little in recent decades (see Table 8–1). By 1991, only three nutritional programs still existed. These included the monthly food distribution to government employees and the "glass of milk" programs described above. There is also a small program for nutritional rehabilitation of seriously malnourished children under five. All are now smaller in scope and exhibited some or all of the problems that have plagued Nicaragua. These include a lack of targeting those in great need, a lack of continuity, due in part to a dependence on foreign donations, and a lack of coordination with primary health services to improve prevention and nutritional education. The Chamorro government needs to develop the resolve of the FSLN to provide a safety net at least until the economy improves. At the same time, it needs the acumen of experienced administrators and the business community to determine how to reach those in greatest need in a more efficient manner.

13

After the Sandinistas

I don't want Dona Violeta so much as I want a change.
GUILLERMINA MEDINA, street vendor

Everything is so expensive and salaries have fallen through the floor. If you eat today, you don't eat tomorrow. But now maybe we will be able to work and know the sight of meat and medicine again.　　　　XIOMARA SILVA, homemaker and mother[1]

For the first time in history, a revolutionary socialist government accepted electoral defeat on 25 February, 1990. It was a result almost no one had anticipated. For many, it seemed as if another earthquake had struck. People walked the streets in a daze, breaking into tears uncontrollably. Many of the poor felt all was now lost—they had depended on the government, and it was no longer theirs. Even the Right was thrown into disarray when their figurehead candidate won. The new government and the U.S. State Department began the first of many emergency meetings; few contingency plans existed for what had seemed an impossible outcome.

The electoral upset was another expression of the deep polarization in the country. Of the 146 voting municipalities, 93 went to the center-right UNO coalition. Yet the party with the single largest voting return was the FSLN, with 53 municipalities, including Estelí, León, Jinotepe, and Rio San Juan. A slight majority of those elected to the National Assembly were parties of the Left. The scramble for power and position in the new government began.

In health, this meant establishing a transition team. A group of twelve doctors sent from the various UNO parties started meeting with health leaders to find out what they were to inherit. Most of these individuals were unknown to current health leaders. Some were party functionaries, while others were known as prominent private-sector physicians. Most of them seemed like the "old guard" that the Sandinistas loathed.[2]

Heading the transition team was Ernesto Salmeron, a leading pediatrician without party affiliation, director of the private Hospital de Especialidades and personal physician to the Chamorro family. Dr. Salmeron was a devout Christian who believed himself to be saved from a near-fatal accident the year before for a divine mission such as leading post-Sandinista MINSA. Although many of the Left considered him a reasonable man acting in a serious and respectful manner, his manner and ideology confirmed some of their worst fears of the UNO and its transition team. After debriefing the team for twelve hours, one leader stated, "They think they are inheriting the Nicaragua of 1979—where have they been for the last ten years to be unaware and unaffected by all that has gone on?" Salmeron responded, "It looks like we came from nowhere, but we were always here, always ready to serve. But since we weren't part of their little circle, they weren't interested."

As in some other ministries, workers prepared to sack their facilities. This seemed to be in line with a pledge from lame-duck President Ortega to "govern from below"; UNO leaders, in turn, took every opportunity to denounce the outgoing administration for such tactics. But Minister of Health Tellez had imposed guidelines to inventory and leave all equipment and supplies. To the chagrin of other UNO leaders, new Minister Salmeron went on television to praise the honesty and professionalism of outgoing health leaders, and asked that Sandinista vice-ministers and regional directors stay on under the new government. "I cannot lie before God," he was quoted, "they have done a good job and left every pencil and paper clip in its place."

Despite such overtures, the FSLN retired its senior staff from MINSA. They feared being identified with what they expected would be a dismembering of the public health service. The minister hired new national leaders, regional directors, and hospital chiefs. These people were criticized in terms that would have fit the new Sandinista regime in 1979: "The new people running the health ministry are clinicians with no public health experience. Many have only recently returned from self-imposed exile and have little or no knowledge of the . . . programmes undertaken by the previous government."[3]

Problems common among new and inexperienced leaders emerged. Regional MINSA and local hospital directors sacked leftist health workers to settle personal or political scores. Some new appointees were so enamored with their rapid rise that they did little more than strut with self-importance. With little experience, even sincere vice-ministers had trouble running programs with anything like the efficiency of the former administration. Salmeron's directives against firing workers for political reasons were largely unheeded.

A staff member at the new USAID office in Managua observed that "the Minister [Salmeron] probably has the most difficult job in a country full of people with very difficult jobs." Severely strapped for funds, under great

FSLN Platform	UNO Doctors' Position
Deepen and widen the campaign to defend the life of the child to reach an infant mortality of 30 per 1,000 by 1996.	Maternal and child health have suffered the worst impact of the entire (Sandinista) health program. Immunization and oral rehydration campaigns have been the only two factors to decrease infant mortality.
Strengthen the program for pre- and postnatal care to protect the life of the mother.	Attention to pregnant women was a disaster due to the lack of trained personnel.
Continue fighting malnutrition and diarrhea.	None of these (health) programs has decreased malnutrition; if anything, it has increased.
Continue improving hygiene by way of campaigns at the initiative of the people.	Neither preventive medicine, nor doctors, nor public health committees have been able to improve the terrible lack of environmental sanitation . . .
Continue fighting childhood illness with the participation of the people, as we have done with polio, tetanus, whooping cough, diphtheria, and measles.	Mass organizations don't know nor do they have any way to know, the true importance of various illnesses. . . . They didn't develop the capacity of the community. They were demagogues. . . .
Maintain direct medical care free to all. There will be a substantial improvement in the supply of medicines and the control of their price. Children under five years old and pregnant women will continue receiving medicines free.	The supposed extension of health services has been a disaster. The number of patients seen in clinics has increased, but at the expense of these same patients who are seen more and more quickly and with less attention to detail. And what good is an increase in the number of patients seen if prescriptions cannot be filled because pharmaceutical products aren't imported?

FSLN Platform	UNO Doctors' Position
Increase the coverage and improve the quality of medical care, with an emphasis on the *barrio* doctor program and rural communities . . .	They emphasized primary care and preventive medicine because they were cheaper, but curative care is just as important.
Improve the capacity of health centers and hospitals. Health posts will be built in villages and hospitals will be repaired or rebuilt . . .	It wasn't possible to maintain standards among the graduates; Curative medicine was twenty to thirty years behind the developed countries to start with; [under the Sandinistas] it regressed another thirty years.
Give special attention to the training of medical specialists and paramedical personnel. We will continue organizing scientific conferences and continuing education for our doctors . . .	Poor standards contributed to the emigration of half the teaching staff. Other factors were the mediocre preparation of new professors, lack of teaching ability, and the use of political criteria in hiring . . . The field of medicine has been deformed and is no longer attractive. The son of a worker or *campesino* should not be forced to study medicine to change the class basis of the doctors . . . The university has always been for the middle class . . . further, the appointment of nurses, dentists, and biologists to posts as administrators and teachers was a disaster . . .

pressure to perform, and lacking the cohesion in administration that either professional training or party unity can provide, he had to lead deeply polarized groups. The Sandinista electoral platform stated their objectives;[4] a postelection document informally distributed by unnamed UNO doctors at the León Medical School presented a very different view.[5]

The situation grew more confusing yet as both the Sandinistas and UNO split internally over health policy. On the Left, some kept to the policy of "governing from below" by refusing to work with or support the government, encouraging alternative institutions and strikes. Others pursued a critical support for the government in what became known as *concertación,* or harmonization. The *concertación* faction gained steam with the reappointment of FSLN leader Humberto Ortega as minister of defense, and MINSA became the FSLN test case for the policy.

UNO centrists, led by Salmeron, supported policies favorable to doctors and the private sector, but defended the need for a public health system that responds to the needs of the poor majority. Radical rightists were determined to undo everything the Sandinistas had created, and were intent on destroying the public health system. They saw the policies of Dr. Salmeron and President Chamorro as virtual treason to their cause. The situation led the minister to cry that he was "caught between two groups of bandits."

ATTACKS FROM THE RIGHT

The attack on health from the Right came primarily from other government ministries. The new minister of social welfare touched the most vulnerable nerve by publicly stating that Social Security funds should be withheld from MINSA in order to build a 120-bed Social Security hospital. The minister of education attacked MINSA's sex education and contraception policies, saying that education about sexuality must be "in the form that [God] expects, for reproduction."[6] At first Minister Salmeron agreed, trying to replace the program for "safe sex" with the slogan "Every sheep with his mate."

Under the direction of Archbishop Obando y Bravo, the Church turned up the heat. A group of bishops went on television to describe virtually all contraception as equivalent to abortion and murder. In a homily from his pulpit, the archbishop condemned the use of condoms. Citing the importance of condoms in reducing the transmission of AIDS, Minister Salmeron shot back: "How marvelous and great is God, to have given man the wisdom and means to prevent disease." Although safe-sex posters were taken down, the government's condom distribution program continued.

ATTACKS FROM THE LEFT

The health workers' union, FETSALUD, took on a renewed importance in 1990 not seen since the anti-Somoza strikes of the seventies. It participated in the country's two general strikes of 1990 and helped organize a doctors' strike in early 1991. In the first, most of the government was shut down amid demands for wage adjustments, an end to arbitrary firings, and worker participation. Salmeron testified that their demands were just, but depended on resources and policies that could only be made by the presidency. MINSA was one of two ministries to remain partially open.

The second strike was more extensive and militant, complete with street barricades. All ministries were closed and health workers took over several clinics. One of these in a rightist Managua neighborhood suffered an armed attack by sixty UNO supporters and ex-contras to dislodge what was considered a leftist stronghold. More national strikes were threatened by the FSLN but failed to materialize. It was thus with some surprise that a spontaneous action by doctors in La Mascota children's hospital in January 1991 led to the largest strike ever to hit the health system. It began as a "partial work stoppage" to protest nonpayment of salaries and lack of supplies. By the end of the month 3 hospitals, 139 clinics, and the national MINSA offices were shut. Health workers and professionals alike were fed up. A third of all workers earned about $50 a month, which barely covered a person's minimal food costs. Many salaries had gone unpaid for months, particularly in health posts and clinics, which were de facto being closed. In February the strike spread to the regions and involved three-fourths of all staff. Minister Salmeron at first refused to negotiate, saying that his budget was exhausted and he had nothing with which to negotiate. Eventually the presidency got involved, assuring job security, wages, and supplies to end the strike in March.

Most medical educators were leftists; in 1990 they successfully reestablished legal autonomy to protect the political independence of the university (see Chapter 9). Former MINSA leaders who had been political appointees of the FSLN went further. They formed the Centro de Estudios y Promocion Social (CEPS) as a progressive group to consult on public health, support community groups, and agitate against the UNO government. Among their many goals, they quickly took a leading role in supporting community health efforts, especially in poor neighborhoods and FSLN-controlled areas to "preserve the gains of the revolution." Former Minister Tellez, for her part, was elected as a delegate to the National Assembly, where she takes part in the health commission. She was also elected later that year as party chief for the Managua section of the FSLN.

INTERNATIONAL GROUPS

Both leftist and rightist groups had important foreign supporters. CEPS, the university, and community groups continued to receive support from the many solidarity groups in the United States and Europe. Although these groups shrank following the electoral defeat, interest in Nicaragua among progressives remained strong. Aid that had formerly been provided to MINSA was rapidly shifted for distribution to nongovernmental organizations in what must be the first international campaign to privatize leftist assistance for public health. This was justified by one group with the statement that "progressive leadership . . . has come only from the FSLN or its supporters."[7] The coordinating committee of the U.S. health solidarity network even adopted a policy statement that no member group could solicit or accept funding from USAID.[8] Such efforts included insulin supplies to the Nicaraguan Red Cross, a cholera prevention campaign directed by Fetsalud and the FSLN, and HIV education and condom supply directed to the private foundation Nimehuatzin.

The Cuban government reacted to the election by immediately withdrawing most of its health and other technical staff. Though they had good reason to be concerned for their physical safety, some Cuban doctors were soon sent back. In August of 1990 there were 113 Cuban doctors, whereas there had been 175 in the beginning of the year. Fidel Castro, in a televised speech, suggested that more doctors could be sent if the new government wished to pay. This offer received serious consideration. At the time, outlying regions were critically understaffed. The withdrawal of Cuban staff had, for example, left region 1 with a total of only six physicians. While the government had to support Soviet or German doctors at a cost of $750, Cuban doctors cost them only $175 per month.

The most active foreign supporters of the Right were those groups that had formerly assisted the Contras in Honduras. The biggest of these is the "Miami Medical Team," a group of anti-Castro Cuban exile doctors deeply committed to the Contra cause. They had flown in regularly from Miami during the war to perform surgery in Contra bases; Miami Medical Team Director Dr. Alzucaray flew into Managua following the election, proclaiming, "Today Managua, tomorrow Havana." Other supporters included religious and/or political groups considered rightist and engaged in health work, including the Dooley Foundation, Freedom Medicine, and the Pan American Development Foundation. One ministerial aid commented, "Frankly, I don't have much use for either the solidarity or the rightist groups. Both arrogantly assume they know the answers and can tell us what to do."

Some of these groups were supported by USAID to do health work with the Contras in Honduras; many more such groups were among the approximately fifty that submitted health proposals to USAID for Nicaragua in 1990.

Many Nicaraguans looked to USAID to save them. It seemed the only place to find the money to "fix the economy in 100 days" as Chamorro had promised, and President Bush pushed Congress to vote a $300-million emergency package for Nicaragua. But it seemed that the hostile Reagan policies still held sway at the State Department. Disturbed by the Chamorro government's 'concertación' with the FSLN and by the absence of an effective policy to promote private-sector investment, it seemed that USAID failed to disburse the money quickly. Yet more than half of the $300 million approved by Congress in May 1990 had been disbursed by the end of the year. During 1990, USAID spent at least $12 million for emergency health programs, contra assistance, and pharmaceuticals for MINSA. Much of this disbursement had an openly political character, emanating from Washington prior to the establishment of the USAID office in Managua. USAID planned to focus funding on primary health care by 1991, but pressures to provide support for hospitals and pharmaceuticals were great. To promote primary care, USAID policy is to encourage community participation and public health-oriented health professionals. In Nicaragua, these had been Sandinista policies as well, and many of the potential activists for these efforts were FSLN-related groups and individuals. They had to find a way to encourage primary care without supporting the Sandinistas.

In the postelection period of elation, European governments pledged $70 million for the health sector. These funds, however, were held hostage to the renegotiation of loans in default from the early eighties. PAHO was the only major international organization able to expand quickly enough to respond to the new health situation. PAHO provided health services to Contras returning from Honduras (see Chapter 5), assisted in the expansion of routine services in areas where the contras went, assisted the university and CEPS, and helped coordinate the development of a new five-year plan for the health sector.

SERVICE DELIVERY

Under incredible political, organizational, and financial pressures, the health system limped along bravely in 1990. Health posts closed, then reopened, then closed again when Cuban doctors in rural areas were withdrawn after the election.

In a situation reminiscent of the time when the Sandinista government was new, mobile medical services were promised for areas lacking in doctors. In some towns, local private doctors came in to help take the place of withdrawn Cuban specialists at health centers. Health campaigns went poorly (see Figure 13–1) (see Chapter 4). Where vehicles and supplies had been lacking for campaigns right after the change in government, by 1991 organization and motivation were in short supply. In Managua only half of the expected *brigadistas* volunteered. Nationally, it was reported that only 60 percent of the expected coverage was achieved.[8a] In some areas, community health committees and *brigadistas* associated with parties of the Right were formed. Such efforts were short-lived; they could not make up for a breakdown in the already mature national primary care system.

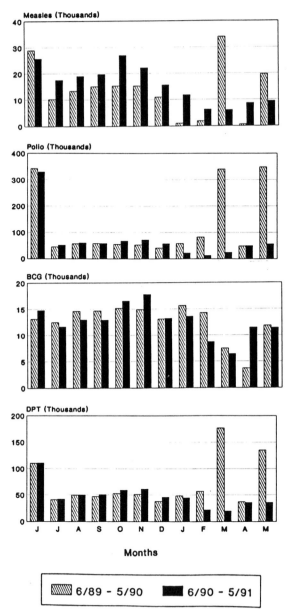

Figure 13–1 Immunization doses administered in Nicaragua, June 1989–May 1991. Following a decline in immunization doses provided during the months of transition from the Sandinista to Chamorro governments in 1990, comparable levels of immunizations were reestablished.

The greatest fear was of radical privatization. Former Minister Tellez interpreted this philosophy as "the right to health for the rich. The poor, the workers, can have as much health as they can buy."[9]

Contrary to accusations from the Left, Minister Salmeron had no intention of privatizing. Yet the decentralization of financial planning and shortfall in central government funding had a similar effect. Each unit received a fixed budgetary amount each month from which they drew to purchase supplies and medicines from COFARMA instead of the former system of monthly "care" packages of medicines. With rampant inflation and fixed budgetary allotments, health centers and posts quickly ran out of supplies and hospital directors spoke of shortages worse than any they had seen in years. To make matters worse, new leaders lacked the experience needed to face such a crisis. Some new vice-ministers worked only half a day, devoting the rest of their time to their private practices.

Some health centers were reportedly able to purchase only a quarter of the medicines they had received just months before. In 1989, 22 percent of the medicines on the national formulary were out of stock; in 1990, 39 percent were unavailable.[9a] Yet the consumption of medicine and visits to doctors declined only moderately in the first year of the Chamorro government, at 12 percent and 8 percent, respectively (see Figure 13–2). More people simply had to purchase medicines on the open market after getting a prescription through MINSA services. In this way, privatization crept uncontrollably into the public health system. With the decline in capacity of the health system, non-acute and preventive care declined. Visits for nutritional maintenance declined by 80 percent and visits for growth and development declined 30 percent.

Moreover, loss of careful administrative controls exacerbated the trend toward de facto privatization. Before, limits were imposed on the number of pills an individual could receive through the free medicine distribution program. When these regulations were abolished in 1990, a small number of people purchased large amounts. Similarly, vaccines for health campaigns fell short as they were distributed indiscriminately, without regard to previous vaccinations. Small- and large-scale robberies, last seen in 1985, reappeared. Some hospitals began to charge for X rays and some UROS even started to charge for packets of rehydration salts. Visits to UROs declined by 14 percent (see Figure 13–3).

Such deterioration was the product of the polarization and poverty that beset the country in 1990. It was estimated that 75 percent of the population was poor, 17 percent were in dire poverty, and half of the work force was unemployed. The minister of health and most of his new vice-ministers worked hard to hold the system together. Some of the former Sandinista leaders continued to work for MINSA, while others did so indirectly via PAHO and UNICEF. The new leaders sent proposals to fund health pro-

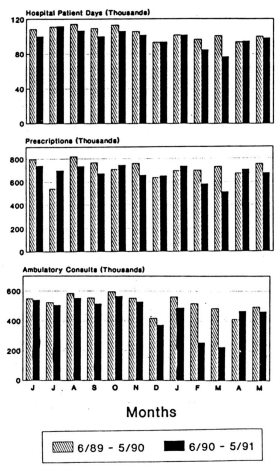

Figure 13–2 Curative medical services, June 1989–May 1991. During most months of 1990, the public health system generated only slightly fewer services than during comparable months of 1989.

grams to a meeting of government-related donors in Europe in the summer of 1990. These programs—the Campaign to Defend the Lives of Children, water and sanitation systems, and care for the disabled, among others— were nearly identical to programs promoted by the former administration.[10] A five-year health plan developed by late 1990 similarly took its priorities and programs mainly from the health plan for 1988–91 developed under Sandinista administration.[11]

The health system declined more rapidly in 1991. During the 3-month strike at the beginning of the year only emergency cases were treated at hospitals. Many health posts were so poorly staffed and supplied that patient visits plummeted. To pay for improved salaries and supplies promised to end the health worker's strike, MINSA had to reduce staff. This was

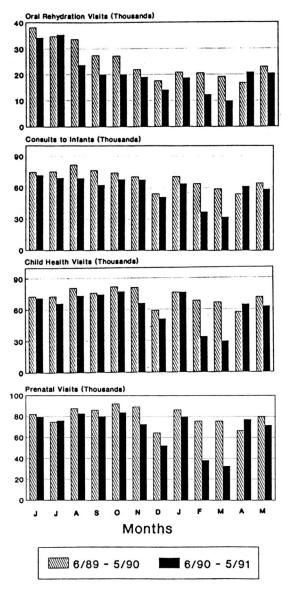

Figure 13–3   Child health services, June 1989–May 1991. Services related to preventive care for children declined much more than did curative care for adults.

achieved, starting March 1991, in the Occupational Conversion Plan. The plan provided 2 years' severance pay for workers, who could then not reapply for public employment for at least 4 years. Any and all health workers were offered the plan, 2,900 workers took it. A third of them were from Managua; 500 were nurses or doctors. Several categories of personnel, including malaria control workers and librarians, largely disappeared as most of these staff opted for the plan.[9b]

The best interests of the public's health in Nicaragua were an issue that at least the Left and the Center for the most part agreed on. Even the World Bank lent its support, stating, "It is particularly important in Nicaragua that the poor be protected from the cost of the stabilization. This is not only an electoral promise of the government, but it may be needed to form the political alliance supporting the [economic] reform program."[12] Whether these programs would succeed would depend mainly on the development of administrative skill among new leaders, the growing ability for different political groups to work together, and a reestablishment of external support.

14

The Nicaraguan Health Model

> Health is a shared responsibility of the government and people.
> Former Health Minister DORA MARÍA TELLEZ

> Eighty percent of Nicaraguans are very poor . . . this ministry
> exists to serve that 80 percent.
> Health Minister ERNESTO SALMERON

The strongest hurricane in a century hit the Atlantic coast town of Blue-fields on 22 October 1988 and cut a swath of destruction across the country. For twelve hours, the storm roared like jet engines overhead. Concrete and wood-frame buildings alike were reduced to rubble. The roof was ripped off the new Bluefields Hospital and nine clinics were destroyed. The destruction was similar in magnitude to that of the 1972 earthquake, but the reaction to it could not have been more different.[1]

Organization before, during, and after the disaster is credited with preventing many deaths. The government, working with local communities, business people, and churches, evacuated people to safe areas around the country. Energetic and efficient rebuilding efforts began the next morning, despite the U.S. embargo and only limited relief assistance from Western Europe.

There was little hopelessness, no barbed wire, and no speculation. A similar level of cooperation was noted following floods on the Pacific coast in 1982 and 1985.[1] If disasters bring out the best and the worst in people, Nicaragua had changed greatly since 1972.

In the hours before the hurricane, half a million people were evacuated to safety. As a result of this quick action, only 148 people died in the disaster. In the weeks that followed, the Bluefields sawmill worked all day, every day, even though half of its roof had collapsed. Teams of volunteers cleared the streets, piling up rubble every twenty feet. Thousands of people were given shelter in schools and other public buildings across the country. Three weeks later, only 800 people had not yet returned to rebuild their homes. Extensive health precautions were credited with preventing epidemics of diarrhea and malaria. Within two years, most people lived in new, better homes built of concrete and zinc.

Hurricane Joan was only the most recent of many natural disasters to hit Nicaragua during the past two decades (see Table 14–1). Yet despite two wars, a ruined economy, and a series of natural disasters, the Sandinistas established and maintained a health system that met the basic needs of most people. Even under revisions promulgated by the UNO government and despite all its shortcomings, the system is still eloquent testimony to the country's commitment to health for all.

A more complex social disaster hit the northern Zelaya region around Puerto Cabezas in 1990. Heavy rains were reported to cause massive flooding and loss of life. An emergency was proclaimed and international assistance was sought. A Red Cross telethon raised $70,000 nationally and more than $3 million was pledged by foreign governments and churches.[2] President Chamorro and Health Minister Salmeron surveyed the area via helicopter and Cuba sent an emergency team of twenty-three health workers.[3] But when they arrived, they found no great disaster. Flooding had been moderate, as in most years, but not severe. Pictures presented during the telethon were taken during the rains a year before, when no emergency was proclaimed.

The differences in 1990 were social, not natural. During the previous twelve months, 30,000 indigenous people returned from Honduras, an inexperienced new regional government was elected, and Cuban support in housing, health, and food supplies was withdrawn. The pretext of a natural

Table 14–1   Destruction in six disasters (millions of dollars)[a]

Disaster	Damage to health facilities	Total direct damage
Earthquake, 1972	25	5,400
Insurrection, 1978–79	8	1,300
Floods and drought, 1982	18	420
Contra war, 1981–87	6	1,050
Embargo, 1985–88	—	220
Hurricane Joan, 1988	44	840

Sources:

Espinosa, H, Murguia, W, and Perez, E La situacion de la salud en la economia Nicaraguense post-terremoto Managua, 1975. Master's thesis, UNAN.

ECLA. Nicaragua: Economic repercussions of recent political events. Santiago de Chile, United Nations, 1979.

ECLA. Nicaragua: Las inundaciones de Mayo de 1982 u sus repercusiones sobre el desarrollo economico y social del pais. Mexico, United Nations, 1982.

ECLAC. Notas para el estudio de America Latina y el Caribe 1987: Nicaragua. Mexico, UN, 1987.

INEC. Efectos socio-economicos de la guerra de agresion. Managua, INEC, 1988.

ECLAC. Report on damage caused to Nicaragua by hurricane Joan. New York, United Nations, 1988.

[a] In 1988 dollars.

disaster was used to deal with the failure of policies for social and economic development.

This chapter examines the development models of the Sandinista and UNO governments and draws lessons that may be of use for other developing countries.

THE NATIONAL AGENDA

The Nicaraguan government adopted a variety of flexible approaches in an attempt to build socialism in the eighties. These included a mixed economy and decentralized administration—characteristics more common among social democratic governments in industrialized countries. Developing countries like Nicaragua often view such policies as unaffordable luxuries because they suffer from a chronic shortage of capital for investments in social and economic development.[4,5] The U.S. decision to try to destroy the Sandinista government made this capital shortage even more acute.

To manage and mobilize resources, socialist governments in developing countries, including China and Cuba, nationalized their economies. By the eighties, this model had lost much of its appeal, having led to the development of a privileged bureaucratic elite and condemning each country to isolation from potential markets, sources of capital, and modern technology.

Revolutions following the Vietnam War looked for models that might generate less social dislocation and more rapid economic growth. Nicaragua and Zimbabwe were prime examples of experiments on a more moderate road toward socialism.[6,7] The strategy paid off for both countries, albeit in limited ways. Providing loans and credits to the private sector in Nicaragua stimulated the economy in the early eighties and may have reduced or delayed hostile acts, including a possible direct U.S. military intervention. It permitted the combined growth of socialist government health initiatives, populist health promotion policies, and a thriving private sector in health. One drawback was that this moderate, mixed public–private road toward socialism in health led to a more capital-intensive, doctor-based health system than might otherwise have occurred. Thus, when the UNO coalition won, conditions were ripe for a return to the exploitation and neglect that had accompanied capitalism before.

THE HEALTH AGENDA

Health had been a high priority in the Sandinista political agenda at least since the elaboration of the "Historic Program of the FSLN" in 1969.[8–16] That agenda proposed to empower people to identify their health needs, organize them to realize their health goals, and involve them in the institutions and programs that developed. The agenda preceded the primary health strategy, which was elaborated at Alma Ata a decade later. It has sometimes evolved in unexpected ways. Sandinista government plans were often modified under pressure from doctors, community groups, or other ministries. Ironically, it is only under the UNO government that community groups are independently defining and meeting their health needs. Although the Sandinistas developed the conditions for this independence, it was not until the UNO government's de facto privatization that it was forced to mature.

Health programs that increased access to hospital care and medicines in the first years of the revolution responded well to people's felt needs.[17,18] The health system was living testimony that the revolutionaries had made good on their promises. It also created expectations that the system was unable to meet. The "have-nots" rapidly became enthusiastic consumers of modern health services. While people could be mobilized for massive, government-led campaigns, they were often not sufficiently empowered to develop and direct day-to-day services. To many pro-FSLN activists, involvement in health became an expression of faith in the revolution and loyalty to the government. Attempts at further health reform seemed to question that faith.

Like socialist revolutions in other countries,[19] the Sandinistas went through two stages in developing the health service. The first was a rapid expansion in coverage of conventional care, responding to prerevolutionary goals and plans. The second was a reformulation of health plans in response to the revolutionary economic, political, and social environment. Some countries did this under conditions of extreme scarcity, such as the USSR during its New Economic Plan in the twenties. Others, like Cuba and its community medicine program starting in 1976, did it during relative affluence. Nicaragua reformulated its health system between 1983 and 1986 in response to scarcity and war, without nationalization or affluence. The major successes of this reorientation provide important lessons for other countries attempting to do more for health with less money. Successes include:

1. Decentralization of budgeting and priority-setting, leading to improved intersectoral coordination, resource generation, and responsiveness to the community.
2. The modification of developed-country technologies to developing-country conditions. A few examples of appropriate technologies described in this book include oral rehydration centers, the midwifery training program, the herbal medicine development, and the approach to cervical cancer screening and treatment.
3. Encouragement and coordination of volunteer efforts, including

Health Day campaigns, mothers' clubs, *barrio* doctors, *brigadistas,* and involvement of mass organizations in health promotion.

4. Careful utilization of both large-scale and small-scale international support for finance, personnel, training, and treatment.
5. Coordination of public and private health services.
6. A slow shift from free access to services for all to a focus on the groups and individuals most in need and most likely to benefit from services.

The election of Chamorro changed several of these components:

1. Small-scale international assistance declined.
2. Intersectoral coordination disappeared.
3. Attention to primary care declined as interest shifted to doctors and hospitals.
4. The private sector grew while the system of public care declined.
5. Community participation shifted toward defending the poor from rather than collaborating with the public health system.

INVESTING IN HEALTH

Ten years before the Sandinistas came to power, Costa Rica began to invest heavily in health services. Twenty years earlier, Cuba began a new health system with the advent of its socialist revolution.[20] In each country, expanded services and improved health were apparent within seven years (see Table 14–2). Costa Rica was able to build on sixty years of investments in education and infrastructure. Cuban resources were mobilized through nationalization and Soviet assistance. The improvements in Nicaragua have been no less dramatic despite worse underlying health conditions and far more limited resources.

Sandinista supporters often point to the rapid expansion of the health system in the early eighties as one of the revolution's outstanding achievements. The reorganization in the late eighties, however, may well be a more useful example for other developing countries.

Large investments in modern health services cannot be sustained in a developing country with a deteriorating economy. This became apparent in 1983, when popular pressure forced the government to reevaluate the health system it had built. To continue the doctor-run, hospital-based programs of the early eighties would have effectively excluded many people from the system. The number of medical visits and supervised births were already declining by 1984. A new approach was needed that would provide services more efficiently and generate additional resources for the health system.

Table 14–2   Cuba, Costa Rica, and Nicaragua on the eve of change and seven
years later

	Cuba		Costa Rica		Nicaragua	
	1959	1966	1969	1976	1979	1986
Doctors per 10,000 population	9.0	8.5	5.6	6.6	5.0	5.4
Infant mortality rate	62	40	69	28	90[a]	76
Life expectancy at birth	63	68	65	70	55	60
Diarrhea deaths per 100,000 population	70	20	130	19	200[a]	100[a]
Beds per 10,000 population	42	47	40	35	18	15
Percent of births attended	63	78	70	82	37	40
Medical visits per capita	2.0	2.8	2.0	2.9	0.8	2.3

Sources:

Danielson, R. Cuban Medicine. New Brunswick, Transaction Books, 1979.

Mohs, E. Infectious diseases and health in Costa Rica: The development of a new paradigm. Ped Infect Dis 3:212–15, 1982.

Saenz, L. Salud sin riqueza: El caso de Costa Rica. San Jose, Ministerio de Salud, 1985.

[a]Estimated.

Examples of the new approach emerged clearly by 1988. They include the Campaign to Defend the Lives of Children, the *barrio* doctor program, decentralization of health administration to the municipalities, and new roles for health volunteers and traditional birth attendants. These were remarkably moderate responses to a political situation that might have provoked more radical actions, including the nationalization of all health resources.

Around the world, "the gap between health 'haves' and 'have-nots' has not narrowed in spite of the revolution [in primary care] . . . which started in Alma Ata ten years ago," according to World Health Organization Director Hiroshi Nakajima.[21] In Nicaragua this gap has narrowed. To achieve this, many components of the health system have been limited, cut back, or reorganized. What is left in towns, neighborhoods, and villages throughout the country is a health service that is more modest and more sustainable.

Investments in medicines, doctors, and hospitals are less efficient in improving the quality of life than spending on food, latrines, and basic education. Expansion of health services, however, visibly responds to the desires of the people and the interests of the government. Myrna Cunningham, physician and governor of northern Zelaya, observed:[22] "Many things the revolution would like to do are slow. You can't build a road or make good nutrition overnight. But health is something you can do in every village, and right away. It is a way for the revolution to get to everybody, anywhere in Nicaragua."

Investments in health care also make sense as part of the government's long-range strategy. Improved health might result even without government involvement if the economy experienced sustained, balanced growth. But the government was not able to mobilize adequate resources or control the conditions of the economy. It has, however, mobilized more modest resources and coordinated nonpublic resources to provide health care. Such care provided a safety net to protect people from some of the threats to health that result from a decline in living conditions. The very existence of this safety net is threatened by the policies of the UNO government.

THE NICARAGUAN MODEL

International participation in the Nicaraguan health system is widespread. It includes unpaid European volunteers who staff church and government clinics, solidarity committees that collect equipment and medicines to supply to health facilities, and bilateral and multilateral programs to build and run hospitals, train and equip traditional birth attendants, and supply nutritional supplements.

Small-scale donations from religious and political groups in the United States, for example, provided a quarter of the operating budget of the national children's hospital during the late eighties. From 1981 to 1985, Cuban physicians provided 24 percent of all public medical consultations in the country.[23] The Swiss, East German, Soviet, Dutch, and Norwegian governments have each built or are currently running a hospital. "But even more than the money," says former Health Minister Dora María Tellez, "we depend on international solidarity for human values and the experience that people bring. This is their revolution, too." At least five foreign health workers were among the more than thirty *internacionalistas* killed in the Contra war.

The efficiency of investments in health has improved. Primary care began with plans for comprehensive care, formalized in the eighteen programs of PIASS. Step by step, these lofty goals have been revised. Programs for universal coverage have been restricted to focus on groups at special risk, particularly pregnant women and children under five years of age. Priorities have been trimmed to focus primarily on the major causes of preventable death, including diarrhea, respiratory disease, violence, and accidents. Education has been given precedence over more costly strategies of improved sanitation, water supply, and nutrition.

The limitations that have evolved in the primary care system hardly represent the "selective" strategy some experts advocate for primary care in poor countries.[24-26] The "selective" model usually involves a package of services provided in a uniform manner (vertically) by national-level administrators. By contrast, the Nicaraguan approach has primarily evolved from local needs and interests (horizontally). It is administered regionally or subregionally via "territorial health systems" and municipal government offices, and depends on decisions and resources that are generated in part from local offices of government ministries and community organizations. This approach resembles the "comprehensive" primary health care approach intended to provide a full array of services. The Nicaraguan system thus appears to be a unique hybrid: A selective primary health program in its technologic limitations and a comprehensive primary health program in its social and political dynamics. The Nicaraguan experience demonstrates, as many around the world in the eighties learned, that implementation of a primary care system is far more complex and difficult than is reflected in the philosophical documents produced at Alma Ata.[27]

The system is far from ideal. Despite claims of a unified national health system, Nicaragua by 1989 had what was effectively a two-tiered system. In rural areas, services are provided mainly at public facilities staffed by professionals doing social service, local auxiliary staff, or volunteers with a medical bag. Urban options include public and private doctors, health centers, pharmacies, and hospitals. The de facto privatization of some of these services in 1990 and 1991 led toward a creeping third tier of the health system. Some observers believe that MINSA would have been able to do more for health if it had not taken on the entire health system. This option would have left intact a formal two-tiered system, with the government reimbursing municipal or private hospitals and clinics for care provided to public patients. Under this scenario, the Social Security system would have remained independent and private health insurance schemes would probably have multiplied. While surely more manageable, such a system would not have permitted the development of important innovations in the primary care system, international assistance, or community participation. In both the urban and rural areas, coordination between primary and secondary care has proven difficult. For problems including diarrhea, childbirth, and cervical cancer, a good mix of simple curative and specialized backup services has evolved. Other problems, including nutrition, abortion, and respiratory diseases, are still dealt with in a more haphazard and less effective manner.

Primary health care has proved to be no panacea. It may be cheaper than sophisticated medical care, but it is not cheap. It depends on a strong administrative infrastructure, which is itself costly to develop and maintain, brings results that are often not as dramatic as leaders expect, and at best responds only to part of the seemingly bottomless pit of potential demand for care.

The unique power of doctors to make or break this system has become apparent. Nicaragua is still producing doctors with a curative, clinical orientation.[28] The health of groups still seems less important than the treatment of individual cases. MINSA attempted to placate organized medicine by pushing only limited reforms in medical schools and hospitals. An unintended result of this was to limit the potential of preventive medicine and community health efforts, since doctors in positions of leadership never overcame their curative focus.

Defining Rights

In 1979, the FSLN declared that health care was a right of the people and a responsibility of the government. The war and economic decline forced a change in philosophy. According to Health Minister Tellez, in 1988 it was "still the responsibility of the government to provide health care, but only to the degree that the people are willing to take part. Health is a shared responsibility of the government and people. Our responsibility is to respond to people's concerns and focus their resources."

In 1990, conservatives tried to make health what Tellez then called "the right of those with money." By contrast, Minister Salmeron viewed the situation in more popular, more charitable terms: "Eighty percent of Nicaraguans are very poor . . . this ministry exists to serve that 80 percent."

For Whom Is Nicaragua Relevant?

Nicaragua began the eighties as a middle-income developing country with an infant mortality rate characteristic of poorer developing countries. The revolution was associated with both an improvement in the infant mortality rate and a serious deterioration of income levels[29-31] (see Table 14-3).

It was one of thirty-one poor countries, with a combined population of 1 billion people, that suffered sustained economic declines during the eighties.[32,33] Although Central America is the poorest region of Latin America, it is by no means the only one where misery is common (see Table 14–4). Most of these countries experienced a similar deterioration in health status. In Latin America alone, it is estimated that 130 million people lack access to basic modern health services. Primary health care in such areas "demands new forms of dialogue between communities, health professionals, and social and political groups . . ."[34] This book highlights a decade of such dialogue.

Many countries have enjoyed improved systems for primary health care, but few of these are among the thirty-one countries suffering declines. The major examples of primary care development occurred in countries that were either very poor and therefore have little legacy of doctors and hos-

Table 14–3 Demographic indicators for groups of countries, around 1985

Countries	Annual per capita income ($U.S.)	Annual population growth rate (%)	Life expectancy at birth (yr)	Infant mortality per 1000
Low income (39)*	250	2.3	52	121
Lower middle income (40)	714	2.5	55	94
Nicaragua	860	3.4	63	64
Upper middle income (39)	2058	2.4	60	69
High income (52)	9364	0.7	74	17

*Excluding China

pitals, or had long enjoyed enlightened policies to promote human well-being with roads, schools, and social welfare promotion.[24]

Such examples are of only limited value. Like Nicaragua, most developing countries have little social infrastructure upon which to build, while many of their people have already been exposed to doctors, hospitals, and modern pharmaceuticals. And like Nicaragua, the leaders of most countries feel the need to show quick results from their social investments. In this situation, it may be much harder to make primary health care work. China tried unsuccessfully to reorient its health system through suppression of conservative medical forces. Cuba tried not to overcome but to reform professional medicine; it was more successful in orienting its practitioners to provide good quality care under very difficult conditions despite low public salaries. Nicaragua, by contrast, seems more successful in gradually

Table 14–4 Unmet basic needs in some Latin-American capital cities, 1980–1989

City	Year	Percent of households with			
		Inadequate housing	Insufficient services	Cramped housing	Low education
Managua	1985	—	7.8	23	5.8
Managua	1989	11.8	6.3	21.6	5.3
Buenos Aires	1980	3.8	0.3	1.5	0.7
Bogotá	1985	3.3	1.3	12.8	2.5
Montevideo	1985	3.7	5.1	7.2	1.2
Quito	1982	3.0	12.6	14.2	—
Tegucigalpa	1988	12.3	33.4	38.2	5.3

Source: World Bank, Regional Project on Poverty (RLA/86/004).

shifting popular demand away from excessive medication and sophisticated treatments, in favor of more modest health facilities and more preventive health programs.

Parallel to What?

To the first Sandinista health leaders, the Cuban medical model stood out very prominently. This was a state socialist model of central management for equitable distribution of scarce health resources. Under state direction, a motivated and disciplined population could reduce individual consumption to facilitate greater collective well-being.

An alternative model is that of a populist capitalist government, which promotes general well-being only indirectly, through the promotion of private initiative. Individuality rather than collective benefits are stressed. The state's main job is not to manage the economy but to mediate conflicts among various private forces.

The process thus far has contributed considerably to the enfranchisement and political empowerment of citizens who before neither consumer nor directed health benefits. At the local level, it has thus been part of the development of a political consensus that has stabilized and matured the political institutions of the country. Such processes are hard to turn back; the decentralized approach will likely continue even when the crisis ends and despite the presence of those who would abolish the public health system altogether.

New leaders have wisely chosen to continue many aspects of the Sandinista health program. It appears that much of the Sandinista health program is administratively and politically sustainable, at lower levels of activity, even under a radically different government. A planning document from USAID eloquently described it in 1990:

> The health system which has developed over the last ten years is far superior to the health system which existed under the Somoza government. . . . It has achieved one of the highest levels of community participation in the region. It has achieved a level of administrative decentralization also unparalleled in the Central American subregion. It has extended coverage and is the only Central American country to have eliminated polio from its territory. It has prioritized its resources in order to achieve maximum impact on the primary causes of infant, child, and maternal ill health, often at the expense of its secondary and tertiary hospitals—always a politically difficult task to accomplish. Despite the partial marginalization of the hospitals, they have achieved a notable decline in neonatal mortality rates in some of the hospital neonatal units. MINSA's epidemiologic surveillance system is actually used for program decisions at the regional, area, and health center level. The fact that it has accomplished all of this while at the same time fighting a civil war is even more remarkable.[35]

During the eighties, the system grew to resemble Cuba's less. It was less dependent on doctors, more focused on primary health, interested in breaking the "culture of medicines," favored folk practices and folk practitioners, depended increasingly on the private sector and international assistance, and provided for expanded priority-setting at the local level. Such decentralized health programs resemble Yugoslavia's, Finland's, and other Scandinavian countries' more than Cuba's or China's.

This same decentralization, under a different government, facilitated the partial dismembering of the public system of health care. In much of the developing world, economic decline in the 1980s led to policies that increased financial and disease burdens on the poor through inappropriate or excessive privatization of social services. Nicaragua stood as a shining example of the role of government in defending the poor. Even under the Chamorro administration, many health policies of a government-for-the-poor continue. These are reinforced by groups that coalesced during the Sandinista administration: health worker unions, public health professional organizations, the University, and solidarity committees in developed countries.

Despite these supports, a rapid shift toward excessive privatization occurred during the first 18 months of the Chamorro government. This shift demonstrates the system's dependence on foreign funds and materials. More funds would permit the reduction of growing inequalities that have resulted from increasing dependence on the private sector and international assistance. A healthy competition between public and private sectors could ensue, benefiting the entire population. These conditions will only occur if the Left and its allies remain prominent in the UNO-led health system. Otherwise, Nicaragua could slowly devolve to the status of so many other developing countries, where economic growth leads to few benefits for the general population. Even with optimal policies, the solution will not come quickly. Improvement will require continued support from the international community for years to come.

Appendices

Appendix A General health data, 1974–1990

	1974	1975	1976	1977	1978	1979	1980	1981	1982	1983	1984	1985	1986	1987	1988	1989	1990
1. Population (000s)†																	
Total	2,200	2,282	2,367	2,456	2,545	2,638	2,750	2,838	2,942	3,052	3,166	3,281	3,445	3,612	3,779	3,907	4,087
Rural	1,100	1,141	1,160	1,180	1,222	1,240	1,286	1,305	1,324	1,343	1,361	1,378	1,396	1,414	1,431	1,463	1,490
Towns	374	365	379	393	407	422	424	426	441	458	475	492	526	558	575	600	624
Cities	726	776	828	883	916	976	1,040	1,107	1,177	1,251	1,330	1,411	1,523	1,640	1,771	1,844	1,973
2. Population under five years old (000s)†																	
	374	388	402	418	433	448	481	511	544	565	586	591	620	632	661	703	736
3. Coverage of vital events (%)†																	
Births	—	—	—	—	—	—	80	82	80	77	73	68	88	79	71	67	—
Deaths	—	—	—	—	—	—	42	32	30	41	38	32	47	48	39	35	—
4. Real salary relative to 1980																	
	—	—	—	—	—	1.04	1.00	0.91	0.81	0.70	0.68	0.52	0.19	0.12	0.07	0.05	0.05
5. Rate of inflation (%)																	
	—	—	—	—	—	48	35	24	25	31	35	219	682	1,250	3,600	1,500	13,490
6. Per capita national product in 1988 dollars																	
Nicaragua	—	—	—	—	1,581	1,130	1,147	1,171	1,124	1,137	1,082	1,003	960	921	819	777	712
Rest of Central America	—	—	—	—	1,648	1,664	1,654	1,601	1,517	1,474	1,468	1,451	1,444	1,456	1,408	1,406	1,399

7. Source of MINSA funds (%)																	
Social Security	—	—	—	—	65	48	30	26	29	28	26	20	19	—	—	—	—
National lottery*	—	—	—	—	3	3	4	4	4	4	4	4	4	—	—	—	—
Central government	—	—	—	—	32	49	67	51	51	56	65	77	78	—	—	—	—
8. Health spending as percent of gross domestic production	—	—	—	—	1.8	2.5	3.2	4.7	4.9	4.7	4.8	6.0	7.0	7.8	7.1	—	—
9. Proportion of governmental budget to (%)																	
Health	—	—	—	—	8	10	11	13	11	9	7	9	11	9	8	—	—
Other social	—	—	—	—	—	15	16	14	13	13	14	15	15	—	—	—	—
Defense	—	—	—	—	—	20	22	19	20	23	35	38	46	—	—	—	—
Production	—	—	—	—	—	52	49	56	58	57	42	36	30	—	—	—	—
10. MINSA total budget in millions of 1980 dollars	—	—	—	—	—	—	97	123	143	117	116	130	150	162	147	91	83
11. MINSA foreign expenditures in millions of dollars																	
Dollar spent	—	—	—	—	—	—	46	64	48	58	29	55	41	23	20	—	—
MINSA debt	—	—	—	—	—	—	—	0	0	0	11	15	20	18	18	19	17
Donations received	—	—	—	—	—	—	12	13	6	21	12	9	6	8	—	—	—
12. Doctors	928	911	1,131	1,319	1,492	1,345	1,212	1,151	1,951	2,081	2,172	2,142	2,272	2,200	2,205	2,462	2,417

cont.

Appendix A General health data, 1974–1990—Continued

	1974	1975	1976	1977	1978	1979	1980	1981	1982	1983	1984	1985	1986	1987	1988	1989	1990
13. Nurses	379	395	442	566	379	640	808	900	795	1,182	1,271	1,152	1,259	1,255	1,345	1,580	1,589
14. Dentists	72	86	96	139	153	179	190	183	191	229	222	260	305	263	278	289	261
15. Auxiliary nurses	1,870	2,120	2,261	2,940	1,873	3,176	3,879	3,884	3,995	4,226	4,378	4,116	4,421	5,296	3,899	5,245	5,398
16. Other technical staff	—	—	—	—	—	—	—	—	—	—	9,610	9,438	9,498	5,160	5,933	4,130	4,784
17. Administrative staff	—	—	—	—	—	—	—	—	—	—	3,879	5,233	5,624	7,570	4,843	8,485	8,233
18. New graduate doctors	50*	50*	50*	50*	60	72	80	172	121	117	213	341	274	261	271	257	263
19. New graduate nurses	79	56	76	73	106	136	150	197	110	162	192	177	125	279	205	160	103
20. New graduate auxiliary nurses	103	128	131	54	167	230	603	738	574	338	234	321	452	586	487	436	613
21. Total MINSA labor force (00s)	—	—	—	69	—	—	155	154	179	208	216	222	231	213	183	222	231

Indicator																		
22. Left MINSA labor force (00s)	—	—	—	—	—	—	—	—	—	—	23	56	60	74	70	82	78	—
23. Health workers mobilized to the army	—	—	—	—	—	—	—	—	—	—	—	—	510	710	1,570	1,960	1,530	—
24. Regional variation in health personnel per 10,000 population	—	—	—	—	—	—	—	—	—	—	—	—	—	—	—	—	—	—
Region with highest rate of doctors	—	—	—	—	—	—	—	9.0	7.9	8.2	9.3	10.6	9.6	8.6	9.1	8.0	5.7	10.8
Region with lowest rate of doctors	—	—	—	—	—	—	—	1.4	1.9	3.0	4.1	4.0	3.6	2.6	2.0	3.5	2.1	2.1
Region with highest rate of nurses	—	—	—	—	—	—	—	3.4	5.2	4.6	3.5	6.6	5.7	3.7	4.3	4.5	6.1	7.4
Region with lowest rate of nurses	—	—	—	—	—	—	—	0.1	1.2	1.8	1.9	2.5	2.6	1.8	2.3	2.2	1.5	2.2
Region with highest rate of auxiliary nurses	—	—	—	—	—	—	—	12.4	19.3	17.2	17.0	19.3	16.6	16.1	13.7	13.9	20.0	18.0
Region with lowest rate of auxiliary nurses	—	—	—	—	—	—	—	1.4	7.8	8.6	7.6	6.0	7.0	8.9	7.8	7.3	5.7	5.6
25. Prescriptions filled (0000s)	—	575	560	726	778	680	788	896	1,039	1,161	1,303	1,458	1,545	1,439	1,338	1,176	900	845
Of which, in health areas	—	—	—	—	—	—	—	329	472	631	627	881	941	862	828	681	489	452
26. Lab exams (00s)	—	—	1,420	1,539	1,929	2,452	2,351	3,046	3,133	3,625	3,822	3,741	3,617	3,846	3,869	4,046	4,159	4,173
Of which, health areas	—	—	—	—	—	—	—	872	1,216	1,547	1,646	1,346	1,424	1,627	1,627	1,625	1,575	1,578

cont.

Appendix A General health data, 1974–1990—Continued

	1974	1975	1976	1977	1978	1979	1980	1981	1982	1983	1984	1985	1986	1987	1988	1989	1990
27. X-rays (00s)	1,370	1,680	2,100	2,590	2,350	2,270	3,090	3,370	4,050	3,940	3,640	3,290	3,657	3,634	3,499	2,914	2,794
Of which, health areas (00s)	—	—	—	—	—	—	466	600	123	769	99	70	90	105	99	63	67
28. Beds in public hospitals	3,991	4,115	4,272	4,313	4,409	4,000	4,677	4,729	4,765	4,897	5,045	5,083	4,925	4,904	4,762	4,731	4,720
29. Inpatients (000s)	107	108	121	125	136	155	178	191	197	207	200	202	215	223	233	235	236
Of which, in health centers (000s)	—	—	—	—	—	—	8	10	13	14	17	19	21	27	28	29	30
30. Surgical procedures (000s)	24	28	35	36	25	—	54	54	56	54	56	56	61	66	67	60	58
Of which, emergencies	—	—	—	—	—	—	—	—	—	24	30	31	18	13	28	22	34
Of which, in health areas (00s)	—	—	—	—	—	—	3	1	2	4	4	4	3	2	5	4	8
31. Dental visits (00s)	1,240	1,530	1,770	2,040	1,790	1,100	2,590	3,320	4,170	4,400	4,290	4,600	5,230	5,599	4,796	4,567	3,860

32. Births in health institutions (00s)	320	350	360	419	400	—	516	556	597	602	582	579	614	591	540	692	688
Of which, in health areas (00s)	—	—	—	—	—	—	40	24	33	47	38	42	77	78	116	146	147
Of which, high risk (00s)	—	—	—	—	—	—	—	90	190	220	210	190	220	190	240	350	—
33. Nursing visits (000s)	—	—	—	—	—	—	—	—	—	185	490	680	793	836	849	534	617
34. Medical visits (000s)	1,837	1,939	1,953	2,433	1,769	2,117	4,982	5,411	6,034	6,334	6,045	5,654	6,150	6,460	6,359	6,244	6,061
35. Medical visits at (000s) Clinics and health posts	—	—	—	—	—	—	3,025	3,122	3,825	4,273	3,799	3,609	4,479	4,913	4,525	4,479	4,338
Of which, emergency	—	—	—	—	—	—	—	—	—	—	41	60	65	76	90	88	114
Hospitals	—	—	—	—	—	—	1,925	2,289	2,209	2,061	2,246	2,045	1,671	1,547	1,834	1,768	1,724
Of which, emergency	—	—	—	—	—	—	—	—	—	—	903	963	957	907	919	882	896

cont.

Appendix A General health data, 1974–1990—Continued

	1974	1975	1976	1977	1978	1979	1980	1981	1982	1983	1984	1985	1986	1987	1988	1989	1990
36. Per capita medical visits																	
Region 1	—	—	—	0.2	—	—	1.4	1.7	2.1	2.4	2.1	1.9	1.9	1.7	1.6	1.4	1.1
Region 2	—	—	—	0.9	—	—	1.5	1.4	1.6	1.9	1.7	1.7	1.8	1.8	1.8	1.7	1.9
Region 3	—	—	—	2.1	—	—	2.8	2.9	2.6	3.0	2.3	2.2	2.0	2.1	2.1	2.0	1.9
Region 4	—	—	—	0.5	—	—	1.7	1.8	1.9	2.0	1.8	1.3	1.6	1.7	1.5	1.6	1.5
Region 5	—	—	—	0.2	—	—	1.4	1.1	1.4	1.2	1.3	1.2	1.4	1.8	1.7	1.5	1.3
Region 6	—	—	—	0.3	—	—	0.7	1.3	1.8	1.6	1.8	1.8	1.9	1.8	1.6	1.3	1.2
Autonomous zone	—	—	—	0.9	—	—	2.2	2.4	2.9	2.0	2.2	2.0	2.2	1.8	1.6	1.6	1.6
37. Per capita medical visits by age, national																	
Under-1-year-olds	—	—	—	—	—	—	—	—	—	3.8	3.2	2.4	4.4	4.6	4.4	5.7	5.2
1–4-year-olds	—	—	—	—	—	—	—	—	—	1.6	1.5	1.0	1.8	1.8	1.9	2.1	2.2
5–14-year-olds	—	—	—	—	—	—	—	—	—	0.9	0.8	0.8	0.9	0.9	0.8	0.9	0.9
Over age 15	—	—	—	—	—	—	—	—	—	1.5	1.4	1.3	2.0	2.1	1.9	1.7	1.5
38. Per capita medical visits by age, Managua																	
Under-1-year-olds	—	—	—	—	—	—	—	—	—	7.0	5.2	4.0	3.7	3.8	4.7	6.9	—
1–4-year-olds	—	—	—	—	—	—	—	—	—	2.9	2.8	1.8	1.7	1.5	2.3	2.6	—
5–14-year-olds	—	—	—	—	—	—	—	—	—	1.1	0.9	0.8	0.6	0.7	0.8	1.0	—
Over age 15	—	—	—	—	—	—	—	—	—	3.7	3.5	2.7	2.6	2.8	2.4	2.1	—

39. Visits for nutritional monitoring (000s)	105	456	294	441	493	430	404	439	288	128	—	—	—	—	—	—
40. Visits for growth and development (000s)	816	1,163	799	976	1,006	879	858	841	630	328	—	—	—	—	—	—
41. Well-child visits (000s)	670	770	728	467	495	429	403	438	287	128	—	—	—	—	—	—
42. Visits for prenatal care (000s)	336	355	342	365	360	316	318	303	245	138	—	—	—	—	—	—
43. Visits for birth control (000s)																
Total	325	290	278	292	264	201	137	142	81	24	—	—	—	—	—	—
Pills	241	225	220	234	222	161	104	106	60	15	—	—	—	—	—	—
IUDs	45	39	25	27	24	21	17	15	8	2	—	—	—	—	—	—
Other	39	36	33	25	19	20	16	22	13	6	—	—	—	—	—	—
44. Visits for puerperal care (000s)	49	52	51	60	60	47	43	43	25	7	—	—	—	—	—	—
45. Visits for Pap smears (000s)	64	63	56	59	54	41	26	22	22	7	—	—	—	—	—	—
46. Abortions in health institutes (00s)	98	108	108	92	76	75	75	75	84	75	72	—	—	—	—	—

cont.

251

Appendix A General health data, 1974–1990—Continued

	1974	1975	1976	1977	1978	1979	1980	1981	1982	1983	1984	1985	1986	1987	1988	1989	1990
47. Gastroenteritis treatments among																	
Hospital inpatients (000s)	—	—	—	—	—	—	14	15	15	17	15	15	15	15	15	—	—
Hospital outpatients (000s)	—	—	—	—	—	—	42	52	67	76	79	99	99	81	87	—	—
Health centers (000s)	—	—	—	—	—	—	157	191	237	265	266	257	266	243	289	—	—
Oral rehydration centers (000s)	—	—	—	—	—	—	72	96	141	172	173	202	248	264	271	310	267
48. Gastroenteritis treatments in oral rehydration centers																	
Referred for IV treatment (000s)	—	—	—	—	—	—	2	2	3	3	2	3	3	3	4	7	5
Oral treatment, referred to home (000s)	—	—	—	—	—	—	29	42	60	90	99	103	101	101	83	60	52
Oral treatment, at URO (000s)	—	—	—	—	—	—	40	52	77	78	71	96	144	159	184	243	210
49. Health volunteers trained (000s)	—	—	—	—	—	—	—	—	20	21	20	14	12	12	12	12	10

50. Birth attendants trained (00s)	—	—	—	—	—	—	—	—	—	—	—	—	13	13	13	13	22
51. Health centers without beds	92	116	127	152	163	146	88	89	85	87	86	83	76	82	81	78	82
52. Health centers with beds	1	1	1	1	1	1	11	15	13	17	18	22	24	23	25	24	26
53. Health posts	38	0	0	19	25	25	267	358	354	348	323	281	249	348	484	541	537
54. War-affected health posts	—	—	—	—	—	—	0	0	8	36	59	82	102	119	—	—	—
55. Hospitals	33	34	37	37	35	34	31	31	31	31	31	31	31	31	31	31	30
56. Hospitals inaugurated	—	—	—	—	—	0	0	1	0	3	0	1	1	0	1	0	1
57. Amputations performed, by reason																	
Mines and explosives	—	—	—	—	—	13	3	5	6	10	23	28	20	132	50	—	—
Other	—	—	—	—	—	7	4	11	6	5	10	17	109	79	15	—	—
58. Number of people displaced by Contra war (000s)	—	—	—	—	—	—	—	—	—	91	143	120	97	81	24	5	—

cont.

Appendix A General health data, 1974–1990—Continued

	1974	1975	1976	1977	1978	1979	1980	1981	1982	1983	1984	1985	1986	1987	1988	1989	1990
59. Number of casualties among health workers																	
Wounded	—	—	—	—	—	—	0	0	0	5	2	5	4	9	0	—	—
Kidnapped	—	—	—	—	—	—	0	3	0	4	10	11	1	2	0	—	—
Killed	—	—	—	—	—	—	1	1	3	13	11	11	2	3	0	—	—
60. Number of casualties among general population (000s)																	
Wounded	—	—	—	—	—	—	1	24	164	943	1,461	1,863	2,116	3,974	3,319	—	—
Kidnapped	—	—	—	—	—	—	1	3	160	586	1,661	1,455	2,389	971	249	—	—
Killed	—	—	—	—	—	—	2	46	205	870	1,408	1,452	969	1,808	1,413	—	—
61. Reported cases of whooping cough	2,219	1,390	853	791	623	267	2,469	1,935	395	97	60	150	223	293	145	—	—
62. Reported cases of measles	853	1,765	1,361	901	161	1,270	3,784	224	226	112	153	956	2,021	794	315	157	16,302
63. Reported cases of tetanus	72	59	13	18	13	—	89	132	115	177	97	76	73	44	51	—	31
64. Reported tetanus deaths	207	227	229	237	109	—	153	127	109	120	50	42	49	37	52	—	—

65. Reported cases of malaria and dengue (00s)

Malaria	122	247	262	116	106	184	255	174	156	129	157	151	202	169	307	460	227
In nonwar zone	—	—	—	—	—	—	—	—	91	26	35	32	40	31	—	—	—
In war zone	—	—	—	—	—	—	—	—	65	103	122	119	130	138	—	—	—
Dengue	—	—	—	—	—	—	—	—	—	—	—	175	5	1	2	7	—

66. Reported cases of polio

	43	40	1	36	1	101	21	45	0	0	0	0	0	0	0	0	0

67. Measles vaccine doses administered by

Volunteers (000s)	—	—	—	—	—	—	—	132	125	153	175	130	108	78	178	93	75
Health system (000s)	—	—	—	92	—	—	102	96	80	81	98	157	142	114	138	158	248

68. Polio vaccine doses administered by

Volunteers (000s)	233	—	—	—	—	—	—	642	1,123	1,343	1,643	1,649	1,708	1,256	1,408	915	812
Health system (000s)	504	757	504	643	384	—	538	521	367	473	429	540	552	499	512	697	761

69. Diphtheria, tetanus, pertussis doses administered by

Volunteers (000s)	—	—	—	—	—	—	180	0	505	0	0	0	0	236	219	266	271
Health system (000s)	—	—	—	—	—	—	385	409	375	342	529	642	791	676	539	591	604

cont.

Appendix A General health data, 1974–1990—Continued

	1974	1975	1976	1977	1978	1979	1980	1981	1982	1983	1984	1985	1986	1987	1988	1989	1990
70. Coverage among children under one year of age with vaccines against (%)																	
Diphtheria, pertussis, tetanus (DPT)	—	—	—	—	18	—	15	23	26	24	33	42	45	51	47	68	70
Tuberculosis	—	—	—	—	24	—	33	65	82	88	98	99	99	94	91	94	84
Polio	—	—	—	—	17	—	21	24	70	82	77	84	94	98	91	87	90
Measles	—	—	—	—	—	—	15	20	40	42	47	51	49	43	57	63	83
71. Numbers of children served by social welfare centers (0s)																	
Urban food centers	—	—	—	—	—	—	—	178	179	121	170	200	230	440	286	—	—
Rural food centers	—	—	—	—	—	—	—	150	395	487	1,000	1,400	1,650	1,913	2,172	—	—
Urban child care	—	—	—	—	—	—	62	163	206	294	300	330	354	412	426	—	—
Rural child care	—	—	—	—	—	—	—	67	187	267	190	290	390	446	348	—	—
72. Percent of population illiterate over 12 years old*																	
	40	—	—	—	39	40	13	—	—	—	—	—	—	—	—	—	—
Urban	18	—	—	—	17	—	—	—	—	—	—	25	—	26	—	—	—
Rural	66	—	—	—	63	—	—	—	—	—	—	40	—	—	—	—	—
Women	43	—	—	—	38	—	—	—	—	—	—	26	—	—	—	—	—

73. Estimated infant mortality rate (per 1000 live births)†

Nation	99	97	94	92	90	89	85	81	77	73	72	70	67	66	65	65	62
Rural	105	103	100	97	95	92	89	86	83	80	78	76	74	74	72	72	70
Urban	82	81	79	78	77	76	75	73	71	68	68	66	63	62	60	60	58

74. Value of exports in millions of current dollars

Coffee	—	—	—	—	—	158	166	137	124	153	122	118	110	133	—	—	—
Cotton	—	—	—	—	—	136	30	123	87	110	134	91	44	46	53	—	—
Beef	—	—	—	—	—	94	59	23	34	31	18	11	5	15	19	—	—
Sugar	—	—	—	—	—	20	20	51	36	34	21	7	18	20	—	—	—
Bananas	—	—	—	—	—	6	8	21	10	15	12	16	15	14	15	—	—
Manufactured goods	—	—	—	—	—	115	91	82	58	57	51	31	31	35	31	—	—
Total exports	—	—	—	—	—	572	451	508	405	431	385	299	252	295	235	—	—

75. Per capita food availability

Eggs (dozens)	—	—	—	10	—	—	—	11	14	13	13	14	10	10	8	5	—
Milk (liters)	—	—	—	90	—	—	—	61	74	85	88	85	81	67	54	48	—
Oil (liters)	—	—	—	9	—	—	—	12	10	15	11	9	11	10	9	9	—
Meat (pounds)	—	—	—	39	—	—	—	39	41	42	42	42	35	34	32	22	—
Beans (pounds)	—	—	—	35	—	—	—	31	28	38	40	33	28	26	24	30	—
Rice (pounds)	—	—	—	37	—	—	—	81	64	70	73	76	71	63	45	54	—
Sugar (pounds)	—	—	—	97	—	—	—	90	102	104	100	119	102	90	67	62	—
Maize (pounds)	—	—	—	158	—	—	—	123	124	149	129	135	123	123	112	117	—

cont.

Appendix A General health data, 1974–1990—Continued

	1974	1975	1976	1977	1978	1979	1980	1981	1982	1983	1984	1985	1986	1987	1988	1989	1990
76. Percent of population with access to piped water																	
Urban	72	—	—	—	—	63	—	—	—	—	—	76	—	76	—	—	—
Rural	6	—	—	—	—	6	—	—	—	—	—	11	—	15	—	—	—
77. Hundreds of metric tons of food imported																	
Maize	1	10	46	11	38	3	114	73	54	300	76	119	109	54	16	24	—
Beans	7	3	0.2	0.2	2	2	27	58	5	6	24	28	11	16	42	14	—
Rice	—	—	—	—	—	—	80	49	1	10	38	71	67	75	83	62	—
78. Hundreds of metric tons of food produced																	
Maize	415	414	417	437	394	611	317	400	420	360	452	458	424	470	616	675	621
Beans	74	101	96	117	89	187	64	62	90	103	122	126	101	129	74	123	135
Rice	112	146	122	82	105	118	136	138	195	213	223	194	177	173	150	140	168
Coffee	—	—	—	—	—	126	123	128	133	157	107	112	77	94	84	—	—
Sugar	—	—	—	—	—	298	236	267	312	299	313	258	279	262	223	—	—

79. Per capita health spending relative to national per capita average

	1972	1986	1988
Region 1	37	64	82
Region 2	312	84	97
Region 3	530	133	130
Region 4	116	69	78
Region 5	63	64	65
Region 6	46	49	72
Autonomous zone	93	128	180

80. Infant deaths per 1000 births 1985/86 by cause

	Vaccine-preventable infections	Respiratory	Gastroenteritis	Perinatal	Other
Nicaragua	0.5	8.4	22.8	25.6	9.9
Honduras	8.2	14.3	30.8	15.7	12.0

81. Deaths per 10,000 children aged 1 to 4 years old, Nicaragua

	Vaccine-preventable infections	Respiratory	Gastroenteritis	Violence	Other infections	Other
1975/76	6	18	48	6	14	16
1985/86	10	15	22	10	8	21

82. Infant deaths per 1000 live births by mother's education

	No School	Illiterate	Literate	Primary	Secondary
1966/67	136			108	57
1973/74	112			91	47
1982/83		91	73	71	46

cont.

Appendix A   General health data, 1974–1990—Continued

1974	1975	1976	1977	1978	1979	1980	1981	1982	1983	1984	1985	1986	1987	1988	1989	1990

83. Reported and estimated rate of death per 1000 population, by age, 1986

Age	Deaths registered in hospitals	Total deaths registered	Total estimated number of deaths
Under 1 year	16	31	55
1–4 years	1	1.5	9
5–14 years	0.2	0.5	2
15–49 years	0.5	2.1	3
5 years or more	4	16	27

84. Percent of all health personnel working in primary care

	1971	1981	1986	1990
Nurses	11	30	28	27
Doctors	12	36	30	34
Auxiliary nurses	9	30	47	47

Key: *Data estimated; — Data unavailable; †Differs from official sources.

Appendix B Comparative data on health and social conditions in Central America (1984 or 1985 unless otherwise stated)

	Nicaragua	Honduras	Costa Rica	El Salvador	Guatemala
85. Population in millions	3.2	4.3	2.6	5.5	7.9
86. Percent rural	43	60	52	47	62
87. GNP per capita in current dollars	880	670	1670	680	1110
88. Last year in which real per capita income was as low as 1985	1962	1971	1975	1965	1974
89. Percent value of currency compares with 1979 value	3	53	16	37	38
90. Literacy rate 1980/1985	88/85	67/59	90/94	57/72	57/55
91. Infant mortality rate/1,000	72	82	20	71	68
92. Life expectancy at birth	60	60	73	65	59
93. Population per doctor	1800	3120	1460	3220	8610
94. Rate of population growth	3.4	3.4	2.7	3.0	2.9

cont.

261

Appendix B Comparative data on health and social conditions in Central America—Continued

	Nicaragua	Honduras	Costa Rica	El Salvador	Guatemala
95. Percent of population indigenous	2	3	1	2	60
96. Population per square kilometer	24	39	51	265	73
97. Public spending as percent of GNP	58	25	18	21	11
98. Percent population poor and very poor in 1980	62	68	25	68	71
99. Percent population very poor in 1980	35	57	14	50	40
100. Percent of national income going to poorest 40% of population around 1975	9	7	12	16	13
101. Percent of national income going to richest 20% of population around 1975	65	68	55	47	60

102. Percent of urban population with adequate water access in 1979	81	92	100	67	89
103. Percent of urban population with toilets in 1979	31	43	43	47	34
104. Percent of children fully immunized against polio at age 1	70	58	75	54	21
105. Percent of births medically assisted	38	34	96	34	16
106. Population age structure:					
0–9	34	34	26	32	33
10–19	24	24	21	25	23
20–64	40	39	49	39	41
65 +	3	3	4	3	3

263

Appendix C Principal causes of death among hospitalized patients, 1980–1987

Diagnosis/ICD Code	1980	1981	1982	1983	1984	1985	1986	1987
Intestinal infections (015, 016)	510(1)	291(3)	216(7)	331(4)	286(6)	325(5)	545(1)	716(1)
Pneumonia (321)	498(2)	281(4)	220(6)	342(3)	292(5)	304(6)	429(4)	406(4)
Septicemia (038)	434(3)	321(1)	333(2)	385(2)	330(4)	364(4)	253(7)	163(7)
Late fetal growth and malnutrition (452)	292(4)	300(2)	399(1)	306(6)	262(7)	275(7)	277(6)	263(5)
Perinatal causes (459)	266(5)	257(5)	227(5)	318(5)	375(2)	451(2)	447(2)	479(3)
Hypoxia and other neonatal causes (454)	214(6)	257(6)	283(3)	401(1)	440(1)	373(3)	435(3)	521(2)
Poorly defined causes (468, 469)	162(7)	189(7)	234(4)	303(7)	413(3)	512(1)	414(5)	176(6)

Number in parentheses indicates rank as cause of death in hospitals.

Appendix D Demographic variables, 1950–1990

	1950–55	1955–60	1960–65	1965–70	1970–75	1975–80	1980–85	1985–90
Total fertility rate (Average number of total children per woman)	7.3	7.3	7.3	7.1	6.7	6.3	5.9	5.6
Crude birth rate (births per 1000 inhabitants)	54	52	50	48	47	46	44	41
Crude death rate (deaths per 1000 inhabitants)	23	20	17	15	13	12	10	8
Population growth rate (percent annual increase in the population)	3.1	3.2	3.2	3.2	3.2	3.4	3.5	3.4
Life expectancy at birth (in years)	42	45	49	52	55	56	60	63

Appendix E Hospital admissions and mortality rates for diarrheal diseases (ICD No. 015 and 016), 1980–1987

Age at admission	1980	1981	1982	1983	1984	1985	1986	1987
1–27 days	964(6.7)	757(6.5)	944(3.3)	961(4.3)	859(4.1)	689(3.5)	758(5.8)	14,493(3.8)
28 days to 11 months	9,013(3.6)	9,271(1.9)	9,514(1.6)	11,347(1.9)	10,065(2.1)	8,702(2.7)	7,969(3.7)	3,176(3.5)
1–4 years	2,904(3.6)	3,079(1.9)	3,362(1.8)	3,284(1.5)	2,926(1.1)	2,441(2.0)	2,103(2.4)	363(3.9)
5–14 years	453(3.8)	433(1.6)	380(0.8)	380(1.3)	304(1.3)	304(1.0)	266(2.1)	795(1.5)
15–49 years	762(0.4)	737(0.4)	680(0.1)	710(1.5)	613(0.5)	641(0.5)	528(0.9)	737(3.0)
50+ years	323(1.9)	362(1.9)	355(2.3)	415(3.4)	488(2.5)	468(1.7)	467(3.2)	
Total	14,419(3.7)	14,639(2.1)	15,235(1.5)	17,097(2.0)	15,255(2.0)	13,245(2.5)	12,091(3.5)	19,564(3.7)

Appendix F Recorded deaths by cause, 1983–1988

Diagnosis/ICD code	1983	1984	1985	1986	1987	1988	1989
Intestinal infections (04)	1,522	1,406	1,386	1,670	1,747	1,942	1,946
Pulmonary diseases and other heart diseases (54)	976	880	1,008	862	1,687	1,622	1,842
Cerebravascular diseases (55)	751	743	825	848			
Pneumonia (58)	819	634	706	758	843	755	1,242
Malignant tumors (26–34)	930	893	813	825	898	894	954
Late fetal development, malnutrition, and prematurity (80)	466	609	696	708	163	120	99
Wounds resulting from war (98)	453	501	644	603	1,149	404	120
Total deaths registered			14,606	14,227	13,985	13,315	12,389

Scottish Medical Aid Campaign
c/o Guilliene Breir

Nicaragua Health Fund
c/o Sarah Jackson, 83 Margaret Street,
London, UK W1N 7HB

National Central America Health Rights
Network
853 Broadway, Room 416, New York,
NY 10003 (212) 420–9635

Project Hope
Millwood, VI 22646

International Medical Corps
5933 West Century Boulevard,
Suite 310, Los Angeles, CA 90045

Association Medicale pour l'Amerique
Latine et les Caribes
c/o Raymond Herrera, CP 458, Station
H, Montreal, Quebec, Canada H3G 2L1

Gesundheitsbrigade Schweiz-Nicaragua
c/o Zentralamerikasekretariat,
Baslerstrasse 106, CH-8048 Zurich,
Switzerland

Comitato Solidarieta Medica con il
Nicaragua
Casella Postale 2536, CH-6500
Bellinzona, Switzerland

COBRISA (Brigada de Salud Aleman)
c/o Gesundheitsladen Berlin, D-1 Berlin
61, Federal Republic of Germany

Nicaragua Health Aid
G.P.O. 5421CC, Melbourne, Victoria,
3001, Australia

CARE
60 First Avenue, New York, NY 10016

Adventist Development and Relief
Agency
6840 Eastern Avenue, NW, Washington,
DC 20012

Partners of the Americas
1424 K Street, NW, Suite 700,
Washington, DC 20005

World Rehabilitation Fund
400 East 34th Street, New York, NY
10016

Notes

PREFACE

1. Nicaragua Health Study Collaborative at Harvard, CIES, UNAN. Health effects of the war in two rural communities in Nicaragua. Am J Public Health 79(4):424–29, 1989.

2. Myers, A. Diarrhea and the revolution. Links 2(4):3, 1985.

3. See for example: Braveman, PA and Roemer, MI. Health personnel training in the Nicaraguan health system. Int J Health Services 15(4):699–705, 1985. The highest published figure I have seen was 280 deaths per 1,000 live births; the lowest was 45.

4. Leiken, R. Nicaragua's untold stories. *The New Republic* (October 4), 1984.

5. Anonymous. The Leon Document, UNO Health Committee Recommendations. *Mimeo* (14 March 1990).

6. UNICEF/WHO Joint Committee on Health. National decision-making for primary health care. Geneva, World Health Organization, 1981.

7. WHO. Alma-Ata 1978: Primary health care. Health for All (series). Geneva, WHO, 1978.

CHAPTER 1

1. Espinosa, H, Murguia, W, and Perez, E. La situacion de la salud en la economia Nicaraguense post-terremoto. Managua, Master's thesis, UNAN, 1975.

2. Vijil, C. The earthquake in Managua. Lancet 1:146, 1973.

3. ECLA. Nicaragua: Economic Repercussions of Recent Political Events. Santiago de Chile, United Nations, 1979.

4. Rosset, P and Vandermeer, J, eds. Nicaragua: Unfinished Revolution. New York, Grove Press, 1986.

5. Vilas, CM. Perfiles de la revolucion Sandinista. Buenos Aires, Editorial Legasa, 1984.

6. Equipo Interdisciplinario Latinoamericano. Teoria y Practica Revolucionaria en Nicaragua. Managua, Ediciones Contemporaneas, 1983.

7. Described well in Ruchwarger, G. People in Power: Forging a Grassroots Democracy in Nicaragua. South Hadley, Bergin & Garvey, 1987.

8. Chavez, R. Urban planning in Nicaragua, the first five years. Latin American Perspectives 14(2):226–36, 1987.

9. Wilson, PA. Regionalization and decentralization in Nicaragua. Latin American Perspectives 14(2):237–54, 1987.

10. IADB. Economic and social progress in Latin America. Washington, DC, IADB, 1977.

11. Garfield, RM and Rodriguez, PF. Health and health services in Central America. JAMA 254:936–43, 1985.

12. The rector was Carlos Tummerman, who went on to become Sandinista minister of education and, later, ambassador to the United States.

13. MINSA/FETSALUD. Los trabajadores de la salud, su lucha historica y su participación en las jornadas populares de salud. Primer Congreso Nacional JPS. Managua, MINSA, 1984.

14. Bolanos, AD. El interrogatorio. Masaya, Libreria Loaisiga, 1979.

15. Fox, RW and Huguet, JW. Population and Urban Trends in Central America and Panama. Washington, DC, Inter-American Development Bank, 1977.

16. Escudero, JC. Starting from year one: The politics of health in Nicaragua. Int J Health Services 10(4):647–56, 1980.

17. Nunez, O. Las politicas de salud del estado en Nicaragua: sobre-explotacion, deterioro fisico-mental de la fuerza de trabajo y reserva infantil de mano de obra. Congreso Centroamericano de Sociologia 1978. Tegucigalpa, Honduras, 1978.

18. See for example: Braveman, PA and Roemer, MI. Health personnel training in the Nicaraguan health system. Int J Health Services 15(4):699–705, 1985.

19. Anonymous. The health situation in revolutionary Nicaragua. *Envio,* 1983.

20. JGN. La salud en Nicaragua antes y despues de la revolucion. Managua, MINSA, 1980.

21. Halperin, D and Garfield, R. Developments in health care in Nicaragua. N Engl J Med 307:388–92, 1982.

22. Tefel, RA, Mendoza, H, and Flores, J. Social welfare. In Walker, T, ed. Nicaragua: The First Five Years. New York, Praeger, 1985.

23. Garfield, unpublished. Based on data drawn from INSS. Anuario Estadistico, 1974–1980.

24. USAID. Health sector assessment for Nicaragua. Managua, USAID Mission, 1976.

25. USHEW. Syncrisis: The dynamics of health. Publication No. (OS)74-50007, Washington, DC, USGPO, 1978.

26. Saenz, L. Integracion y coordinacion de los servicios de salud de Centroamerica. San Salvador, ODECA, 1971.

27. Paredes, JA. Los recursos de la salud publica en Centro America. San Salvador, ODECA, 1968.

28. Kuhl, CA. Report on the health situation in Nicaragua to the 33rd World Health Assembly. Managua, MINSA, 1980.

29. Kuhl, CA. Informe de la situation de salud de Nicaragua. Managua, MINSA, 1980.

30. Cabezas, O. Fire from the Mountain. New York, Crown Publishers, 1985.

31. Bollag, U. Utilization of local first aiders in the provision of health care for prisoners by the international committee of the Red Cross in Nicaragua. J Community Health (10)1:17–21, 1985.

32. Zembrana, DR and Huertas, P. Aportes para la comprension del comportamiento del sistema de salud en el marco de las guerras populares de liberacion. Revista Centroamericana de Ciencias de la Salud 17:135–42, 1980.

33. MINSA. Logros y Limitaciones en Salud. Managua, MINSA, 1980.

34. Cruz, JMC. La salud en la revolucion. *El Nuevo Diario* (27 November 1980), p. 4.

35. Echavarria, F. Oficial Cubano de la salud publica habla de los problemas de salud. *Bohemia* (8 February 1980), pp. 60–63.

36. MINSA. Reglamento general del servicio social rural. Managua, MINSA, 1980.

CHAPTER 2

1. Published in JGN. The philosophies and policies of the government of Nicaragua. In Rosset, P and Vandermeer, J, eds. The Nicaragua Reader. New York, Grove Press, 1983.

2. Kuhl, CA. Mensaje del companero ministro de salud. Boletin Informatica No. 1 (7 September 1979), p. 3.

3. Anonymous. Competitor or partner? Private practice in Nicaragua. Nicaragua Health Fund Newsletter 8:8–9, 1989.

4. Antillon, JJ. Changes in health care strategies in Costa Rica. PAHO Bull 21(2):136–47, 1987.

5. Casas, A and Vargas, H. The health system in Costa Rica: Toward a national health service. J Public Health Policy 1:177–86, 1980.

6. Jaramillo, J, Pineda, C, and Contreras, G. Primary health care in marginal urban areas: The Costa Rican model. PAHO Bull 2:107–14, 1984.

7. Rosero-Bixby, L. Las politicas socio-economicas y su efecto en el descenso de la mortalidad Costarricense. In Association Demografico Costarricense. Mortalidad y Fecundidad en Costa Rica. ADC, San Jose, 1984.

8. Rosero-Bixby, L. Infant mortality decline in Costa Rica. In Halstead, SB, Walsh, JA, and Warren, KS, eds. Good Health at Low Cost. New York, Rockefeller Foundation, 1985.

9. Mohs, E. Infectious diseases and health in Costa Rica: The development of a new paradigm. Pediatr Infect Dis 3:212–15, 1982.

10. Haines, MR and Avery, RC. Differential infant mortality in Costa Rica: 1968–1973. Population Studies 36(1):31–44, 1982.

11. Gomes, M. Servicos de saude para todos: O caso da Costa Rica. Boletin de la Oficina Sanitaria Panamericana 101(1):58–73, 1986.

12. Saenz, L. Salud sin riqueza: El caso de Costa Rica. San Jose, Ministerio de Salud, 1985.

13. Stein, Z and Susser, M. The Cuban health system: A trial of a comprehensive service in a poor country. Int J Health Services 2(4):551–66, 1972.

14. Danielson, R. Cuban Medicine. New Brunswick, Transaction Books, 1979.

15. Conover, S, Donovan, S, and Susser, E. Reflections of health care in Cuba. Lancet 2:958–60, 1980.

16. Navarro, V. Health services in Cuba: An initial appraisal. N Engl J Med 287:954–59, 1972.

17. Ubell, RN. High-tech medicine in the Caribbean: 25 years of Cuban health care. N Engl J Med 309(23):1468–72, 1983.

18. Muller, F and Vila, E. Participacion popular en la atencion sanitaria primaria en un area rural de Cuba, 1978. Revista Cubana de Administracion de Salud 5(3):181–209, 1979.

19. Werner, D. Health care in Cuba: A model service or a means of social control—or both? In Morley, D, Rohde, J, and Williams, G, eds. Practicing Health for All. Oxford University Press, 1983.

20. LeoGrande, WM. The revolution in Nicaragua: Another Cuba? Foreign Affairs 58:1, 1979.

21. Grant, J. State of the World's Children Report 1981/82. New York, Oxford University Press, 1982.

22. PAHO. Child Survival: Priority Health Needs in Central America and Panama. Washington, DC, PAHO, 1984.

23. Acuna, HR. Toward 2000: The quest for universal health in the Americas. Washington, DC, PAHO, 1983.

24. Acuna, HR. Steps toward "health for all by the year 2000": A review of PAHO's plan of action. Bull PAHO 16(1):1–6, 1982.

25. Montis, M, Molina, G, Tercero, I, Jarquin, C, Jaramillo, H, Bisso, JM, Garcia, N, and Capote, R. Estrategias de atencion primaria de la salud en la republica de Nicaragua. Managua, MIPLAN/MINSA, 1981.

26. Bohoslavsky, A. La transformacion de la medicina en Nicaragua. *Barricada* (25 September 1982), p. 3.

27. Anonymous. Salud: Metas y objectivos para 1980. *Barricada* (24 December 1979), p. 1.

28. Bossert, TJ. Health care in revolutionary Nicaragua. In Walker, TW, ed. Nicaragua in Revolution. New York, Praeger, 1982.

29. Jones, M. Nicaragua invests in health. World Health 12:15–27, 1981.

30. Chamorro, A. Programa de extension de servicies de salud. Managua, MINSA, 1980.

31. MINSA. Cartilla de salud para el alfabetizador. Managua, MINSA, 1979.

32. Anonymous. MINSA apoya la cruzada de alfabetizacion con 25 milliones de cordobas. MINSA Boletin Informativa No. 8 (29 January 1980), p. 1.

33. Velasquez, E, Hassan, A, Belmar, R, Drucker, E, and Michaels, D. Occupational mercury poisoning in Nicaragua. Morbidity and Mortality Weekly 29(33):393–95, 1980.

34. Amador, R, Lopez, J, and Garcia, R. Research and development at the department of preventive medicine at the medical school of UNAN, Leon, Nicaragua. Scand J Soc Med 16:235–36, 1988.

35. Aragon, A, Pena, R, Svanstrom, L, and Thorn, A. Development of a community intervention programmer on miners' health and working environment in Nicaragua. Scand J Soc Med 16:237–40, 1988.

36. This and other quotes from Antonio Dajer are drawn from an unpublished manuscript from which he generously permitted us to draw.

37. MINSA. El sistema nacional unico de salud: Tres años de revolucion 1979–1982. Managua, MINSA, 1983.

38. Cuan, M and Lopez, MA. Evolucion y analysis de los servicios hospitalarios en Nicaragua. Master's thesis. Managua, CIES, 1984.

39. Anonymous. Salud va llegando poco a poco a todos los rincones. *El Nuevo Diario* (5 December 1982), p. 4.

40. Eitel, J. Health care revisited. Nicaraguan Perspectives 12:30–36, 1986.

41. Convenio INSS-MIDA-INRA: Centros de salud para unidades productivas. *El Nuevo Diario* (10 October 1980), p. 9.

42. Anonymous. Cada diez minutos una consulta medica. *Barricada* (3 March 1982), p. 1.

43. Miller, V. Between Struggle and Hope: The Nicaraguan Literacy Crusade. Boulder, Westview Press, 1985.

44. MINSA. Cartilla de malaria para los brigadistas de la campana de alfabetizacion. Managua, MINSA, 1979.

45. Anonymous. Escuela se convierte al instituto de salud. *Barricada* (4 July 1980), p. 1.

46. Garfield, RM and Taboada, E. Health service reforms in revolutionary Nicaragua. Am J Public Health 74:1138–44, 1984.

47. Lopez, C. Programa de extension de cobertura, regionalizacion, de los servicios de salud, segun region y area de salud. Managua, MINSA, 1980.

48. MIPLAN. Analisis del informe trimestral Enero–Marzo 1981. Managua, MINSA, 1981.

49. Anonymous. Sorpresa: Renuncia Amador. *La Prensa* (8 May 1980), p. 1.

CHAPTER 3

1. Acuna, HR. Community participation in the development of primary health services. PAHO Bull 9(2):95–99, 1977.

2. ECLAC. Popular participation in development. Community Dev J 2:77–92, 1973.

3. Gallardo, LD. Algunas tendencias de la educacion y participacion comunitarias en salud en America Latina. Boletin Oficial de la Organizacion Sanitaria Panamericana 96(4):314–24, 1984.

4. Muller, F. Participacion popular en programas de atencion sanitaria primaria en America Latina. Medellin, Universidad de Antioquia, 1979.

5. Storms, DM. Training and use of auxiliary health workers: Lessons from developing countries. Washington, DC, APHA International Health Programs, 1979.

6. Stinson, W, Favin, M, and Bradford, B. Training community health workers. Washington, DC, World Federation of Public Health Associations, 1983.

7. Hakim, P. Lessons from grass-roots development experience in Latin America and the Carribbean. Assignment Children 59/60:137–44, 1982.

8. WHO. The Community Health Worker. Geneva, WHO, 1987.

9. Ministerio de Salud. Politicas, estrategias y organizacion de la division de educacion para la salud. Managua, Ministerio de Salud, 1975.

10. USHEW. Syncrisis: The Dynamics of Health. Publication No. (OS)74-50007, Washington, DC USGPO, 1978.

11. DECOPS. Aportes para el analisis historico de la educacion y la participacion popular en salud. Managua, MINSA, 1980.

12. de Keyzer, B and Ulate, J. Educacion, participacion en salud e ideologia: Nicaragua pasado y presente. Revista Centroamericana de Ciencias de la Salud 17:143–58, 1981.

13. Le Boterf, G. The challenge of mass education in Nicaragua. Assignment Children 65/68:247–66, 1984.

14. DECOPS. Educacion y participacion comunitaria en la salud: Lineamientos generales. Managua, DECOPS, 1980.

15. DECOPS. Las jornadas populares: Un proyecto de participacion popular en Nicaragua. Revisita Centramericano de Ciencias de la Salud 17:173–84, 1980.

16. DECOPS. Manual operativo del capacitador, multiplicador, y brigadista popular de salud. Managua, DECOPS, 1981.

17. Donahue, JM. The Nicaraguan Revolution in Health. South Hadley: Bergin & Garvey, 1986.

18. Frieden, T and Garfield, R. Popular participation in health in Nicaragua. Health Policy and Planning 2(2):162–70, 1987.

19. MINSA. Objectivos, estructura, y funciones de la comision popular de salud. Managua, MINSA, 1980.

20. Anonymous. Primer consejo popular de salud del area #1 del centro de salud La Primavera. MINSA Boletin Informativa No. 11 (25 April 1980), p. 1.

21. Comision de Salud de León. Programa de capacitacion popular en salud. León, Comision de Salud de León, 1979.

22. MINSA/Consejo Popular de Salud de Region 4. El papel de los consejos populares de salud en las jornadas populares de salud. Primer Congreso Nacional JPS. Managua, MINSA, 1984.

23. DECOPS. La educacion popular y las organizaciones de masas en la gestion de salud en Nicaragua. Revista Centroamericano de Ciencias de la Salud 17:159–72, 1980.

24. Donahue, JM. The politics of health care in Nicaragua before and after the revolution of 1979. Human Organization 42:262–74, 1983.

25. Woznica, C. Community participation in health as an empowering process: A case study from Nicaragua. Ph.D. dissertation, University of Illinois, Chicago, 1987, p. 192.

26. Garfield, RM and Frieden, T. Social and demographic characteristics of Nicaraguan health volunteers. Int Q Community Health Education 7(2):123–34, 1986–87.

27. MINSA. La mujer Nicaraguense y su experiencia de participacion en salud. Managua, MINSA, 1984.

28. For example, in a Peruvian survey, half of all volunteers had stopped working after five years. See Christensen, PB and Karlqvist, S. Community health workers in a Peruvian slum area: An evaluation of their impact on health behavior. PAHO Bull 24(2):183–96, 1990.

29. Scholl, EA. An assessment of community health workers in Nicaragua. Social Science and Medicine 20:207–14, 1985.

30. Ruchwarger, G. People in Power: Forging a Grassroots Democracy in Nicaragua. South Hadley: Bergin & Garvey, 1987.

31. Cavallini, I. Una critica sana. *Barricada Internacional* (8 September 1988), p. 14.

32. MINSA/Comision Popular de Salud Zona Especial II. Abriendo la trocha: Brigadistas defienden salud y la revolucion en Zelaya Sur. Primer Congreso Nacional JPS. Managua, MINSA, 1984.

33. Rifkin, SB, Muller, F, and Wolfgang, B. Primary health care: On measuring participation. Soc Sci Med 26(9):931–40, 1988.

34. Ugalde, A. Ideological dimensions of community participation in Latin America health programs. Soc Sci Med 21(1):41–53, 1985.

35. de Kadt, E. Community participation for health: The case of Latin America. World Development 10:573–84, 1982.

36. Woznica, C. Community participation in health as an empowering process: A case study from Nicaragua. Ph.D. dissertation, University of Illinois, Chicago, 1987, p. 258.

37. Ibid., p. 243.

38. Ibid., p. 244.

39. Ibid., p. 281.

40. Shanks, K. Poetry, puppets, and the people's health. Nicaragua Health Fund Newsletter 7:7–9, 1988.

41. CIES. La participacion popular como componente y estrategia de atencion primaria. Managua, MINSA, 1983.

42. Walt, G, Perera, M, and Heggenhougen K. Are large-scale volunteer community health worker programs feasible? The case of Sri Lanka. Soc Sci Med 29(5):599–608, 1989.

43. Heiby, JR. Low-cost health delivery systems: Lessons from Nicaragua. Am J Public Health 71(5):514–19, 1981.

CHAPTER 4

1. Woznica, C. Community participation in health as an empowering process: A case study from Nicaragua. Ph.D. dissertation, University of Illinois, Chicago, 1987. p. 218–19.

2. PAHO. Health conditions in the Americas. Scientific publ. No. 364, Washington, DC, PAHO, 1978.

3. de Castro, JF. Mass vaccination against poliomyelitis in Mexico. Rev Infect Dis 6(Supp.2):397–99, 1984.

4. Risi, JB. The control of poliomyelitis in Brazil. Rev Infect Dis 6(Supp.2):404–12, 1984.

5. APHA. Nicaragua: 40,000 health volunteers vaccinate a nation. Salubritas 5(3):1–2, 1981.

6. MINSA. Plan nacional de medicina preventiva. Managua, MINSA, 1980.

7. Estimates from MINSA, as reported to PAHO and published in PAHO: Health conditions in the Americas 1977–1980. Scientific Publ. No. 427. Washington, DC, PAHO, 1982.

8. Fonseca, R. La polio no ha muerto, aun palpita. *Barricada* (28 January 1989), p. 2.

9. Anonymous. Reportan cuatro casos "sospechosos" de polio. *Barricada* (26 January 1989), p. 1.

10. Williams, G. Immunization in Nicaragua. Lancet 2:780, 1985.

11. Anonymous. "The León Document" of UNO Health Committee Recommendations. *Mimeo* (14 March 1990).

12. Wernsdorfer, WH. The importance of malaria in the world. In Kreier, JP, ed. Malaria, vol. 1. Epidemiology, Chemotherapy, Morphology, and Metabolism. New York, Academic Press, 1980.

13. Harrison, G. Mosquitoes, Malaria, and Man. New York, Dutton, 1978.

14. Anonymous. Sera como la alfabetizacion: Cruzada anti-malarica. *El Nuevo Diario* (19 September 1981), p. 1.

15. Garfield, RM and Vermund SH. Health education and community participation in mass drug administration for malaria in Nicaragua. Soc Sci Med 22(8):869–77, 1986.

16. Anonymous. Medicos ofrecen ayuda en plan anti-malarico. *La Prensa* (23 October 1981), p. 6.

17. Garfield, RM and Vermund, SH. Changes in malaria incidence after a mass drug administration in Nicaragua. Lancet 2:500–3, 1983.

18. Garfield, RM and Vermund, SH. Malaria in Nicaragua: An update. Lancet 1:1125, 1984.

19. Bruce-Chwatt, LJ. Mass drug administration for control of malaria. Lancet 2:688, 1983.

20. Foll, C. Mass drug administration for control of malaria. Lancet 2:1022, 1983.

21. PAHO. Status of malaria control programs in the Americas: 36th annual report. Washington, DC, PAHO, 1988.

22. Garfield, RM, Prado, E, Gates, JR, and Vermund, SH. Malaria in Nicaragua: Community-based control efforts and the impact of war. Int J Epidemiol 18(2):1989.

23. Sweezey, SL, Murray, DL, and Daxl, RG. Nicaragua's revolution in pesticide policy. Environment 28(1):6–36, 1986.

24. Arguello, L, Castillo, O, Chavarria, J, Cuadra, I, and Heldel, E. Short course chemotherapy of TB: The Nicaraguan experience. Bulletin of the International Union against TB and Respiratory Diseases 64(3):46–49, 1989.

25. See also Loevinsohn, BP and Loevinsohn, ME. Well child clinics and mass vaccination campaigns: An evaluation of strategies for improving the coverage of primary health care in a developing country. Am J Public Health 77(11):1407–11, 1987.

CHAPTER 5

1. JGN. Contrarevolucion: Dessarrollo y conscuencias, datos basicos, 1980–1985. JGN, Managua, 1985.

2. INSSBI. 48 meses de aggression extranjera. Managua, INSSBI, 1984.

3. Perez, B. Efectos epidemiologicos de la guerra de aggression. Presentation at the 3rd annual U.S.–Nicaragua Health Colloquium, Managua, November 1985.

4. CAHI. Nicaragua 1984: Human and material costs of the war. In Rosset, P and Vandermeer, J, eds. Nicaragua: Unfinished Revolution. New York, Grove Press, 1986.

5. Kornbluh, P. Nicaragua, the price of intervention: Reagan's war against the Sandinistas. Washington, DC, Institute for Policy Studies, 1987.

6. Garfield, RM. Health and the war against Nicaragua, 1981–1984. J Public Health Policy 6(1):116–31, 1985.

7. Garfield, RM, Frieden, T, and Vermund, SH. Health related outcomes of war in Nicaragua. Am J Public Health 77(5):615–18, 1987.

8. Siegel, D, Baron, R, and Epstein, P. The epidemiology of aggression. Lancet 1:1492–93, 1985.

9. Garfield, R. Health consequences of war in Nicaragua. Lancet 2:392, 1985.

10. INEC. Efectos socio-economicos de la guerra de aggression. Managua: INEC, 1988.

11. Personal communication, Tim Takaro and MINSA workers in region 6.

12. INSSBI. Repercusion del terrorismo de estado de la administracion Reagan en la vida del pueblo Nicaraguense. Managua, Comite Nacional de Emergencia, 1984.

13. Kinzer S. Casualties in Nicaragua: Schools and health care. New York Times (23 March 1987), p. 10.

14. MINSA. Repercusion de la agresion en la situacion de salud del pais. El Nuevo Diario (9 August 1983), p. 13.

15. Almasi, MS. Desarrollo del sector farmaceutico de Nicaragua. Geneva, United National Industrial Development Organization, 1985.

16. Leahy, S. Captured by the Contra. Nicaragua Health Fund Newsletter 2:3–5, 1987.

17. JGN. The philosophies and policies of the government of Nicaragua. In Rosset, P and Vandermeer, J, eds. The Nicaragua Reader. New York, Grove Press, 1983.

18. Garfield, RM. War-related changes in health and health services in Nicaragua. Soc Sci Med 28(7):669–76, 1989.

19. Sivard, RL. World military and social expenditures 1985. Washington, DC, Worldwatch Institute, 1985.

20. See for example Donahue, JM. The Nicaraguan Revolution in Health. South Hadley: Bergin & Garvey, 1986.

21. Siegel, D, Baron, R, and Eitel, J, eds. Health Consequences of War in Nicaragua. Committee for Health Rights in Central America: San Francisco, 1985.

22. MINSA. Plan de salud 1987. Managua, MINSA, 1986.

23. Kinzer, S. Land mines in Nicaragua cause rising casualties. New York Times (19 July 1986), p. 5.

24. Anonymous. Manejo integral del herido de guerra de la lucha irregular en el

teatro de operaciones militares de Nicaragua, 1984–1986. Primera Conferencia Cientifica de los Servicios Medicos E.P.S. Mimeo, 1986.

25. Gogstad, A. Rehabilitation in war-ravaged developing countries. Rehabilitation Literature 38:5–8, 1978.

26. Braveman, P and Siegel, D. Nicaragua: A health system developing under conditions of war. Int J Health Service 17:169–78, 1987.

27. MINSA/Comision Popular de Salud Zona Especial II. Abriendo la trocha: Brigadistas defienden salud y la revolucion en Zelaya Sur. Primer Congreso Nacional JPS. Managua, MINSA, 1984.

28. Meyer, H. Physician's war in Nicaragua. *American Medical News* (13 November 1987), p. 3.

29. CAHI. The other side of the border: Nicaragua's internal refugees. CAHI Update 14:1–4, 1985.

30. Garfield, RM, Prado, E, Gates, JR, and Vermund, SH. Malaria in Nicaragua: Community-based control efforts and the impact of war. Int J Epidemiology 18(2), 1989.

31. Dudley, HAF, Knight, RJ, McNeur, JC, and Rosengarten, DS. Civilian battles casualties in Vietnam. Br J Sur 55:332, 1968.

32. Hartigan, RS. The Forgotten Victim: A history of the Civilian. Chicago: Precedent Publishing, 1982.

33. Humphries, SV. The mental effects of guerrilla warfare. Central African J Med 24:37–39, 1978.

34. Summerfield, D. Nicaragua: War and mental health. Lancet 2:914, 1987.

35. Summerfield, D. The psychological war. Nicaragua Health Fund Newsletter 2:3–5, 1987.

36. Whitford, JD. Consecuencias psicologicas derivadas de la situacion de guerra. Psicologia en Nicaragua 1(1):10–15, 1987.

37. CARE. Children's survival assistance program. Needs assessment team field report: Nicaragua. New York, CARE, 1988.

38. Nelson, H. War takes toll on children in Nicaragua. *American Medical News* (17 February 1989), p. 3.

39. Anonymous. Barcos yanquis bloquean medicinas para el pueblo. *El Neuvo Diario* (7 October 1983), p. 1.

40. Schwartzberg, P. The U.S. embargo demystified. Links 2(4):8, 1985.

41. ECLAC. Notas para el estudio de America Latina y El Caribe, 1987: Nicaragua. Mexico City, ECLAC, 1987.

42. Cahill, KM. A bridge to peace. New York: Haymarket Doyma, 1988, p. 15.

43. Taylor, JA. Military medicine's expanding role in low-intensity conflict. Military Rev 1:26–34, 1985.

44. ECLA. Nicaragua: Economic Repercussions of Recent Political Events. Santiago de Chile, United Nations, 1979.

45. Cliff, J and Noormahomed, AR. Health as a target: South Africa's destabilization of Mozambique. Soc Sci Med 27(7):717–22, 1988.

46. Walt, G and Melamed, A, eds. Mozambique: Towards a People's Health Service. London, Zed Press, 1984.

47. Waghelstein, JW. Post-Vietnam counterinsurgency doctrine. Military Rev 1:42, 1985.

48. Keegan, J. The Face of Battle. Penguin, New York, 1976.

49. Anonymous. Plan de atencion medica antes un eventual invasion. *Barricada* (22 November 1984), p. 12.

50. Jackson, S. How to bring health care to war zone communities. Nicaragua Health Fund Newsletter 8:4–7, 1988.

51. Anonymous. The challenge of health care in the Nicaraguan countryside. CEPAD Report 1:1–4, 1989.

52. Schneider, ML. Health as a bridge for peace. World Health 10:5–6, 1987.

53. CIAV. Programa de asistencia urgente a los desmobilizados y familias de la resistencia Nicaraguense. CIAV Boletin Informativo 1990 No. 6, pp. 1–3.

54. Halbert, RJ, Simon, RR, and Hood, H. Providing health care in war-torn rural Afghanistan. Lancet 2:1214–15, 1988.

CHAPTER 6

1. Ortega, D. Daniel y los medicos de Nicaragua: Problemas, medidas y compromiso. Managua, Direccion de Informacion y Prensa de la Presidencia de la Republica, 1985.

2. Tamayo, JO. Public health system is ailing Nicaragua. *Miami Herald* (30 November 1985), p. 1.

3. UNICEF. Datos basicos e indicadores economicos, humanos, politicos, y sociales sobre Nicaragua. Managua, UNICEF, 1988.

4. Gariazzo, A, Acosta, M, and Bermudez, A. Analisis de la situacion economico-social de Nicaragua. Managua, UNICEF, 1984.

5. Braveman, P. Primary health care takes root in Nicaragua. World Health Forum 6:369–72, 1985.

6. Bossert, T. Nicaraguan health policy: The dilemma of success. Med Anthropol Q 15(3):73–74, 1984.

7. Bosche, MA. Development of primary health care in Nicaragua: Achievements and difficulties. Managua, MINSA, 1983.

8. MIPLAN/MINSA. Estrategias de atencion primaria de la salud en la Republica de Nicaragua. Managua, MIPLAN y MINSA, 1981.

9. MINSA. Guia de programacion de actividades para el desarrollo de la estrategia de atencion primaria a nivel de region y area de salud. Managua, MINSA, 1983.

10. MINSA. Plan integral de actividades del area de salud—libro rojo y negro. Managua, MINSA, 1982.

11. MINSA. Plan de salud 1987. Managua, MINSA, 1986.

12. Kinzer, S. Casualties in Nicaragua: Schools and health care. *New York Times* (23 March 1987), p. A10.

13. Slater, RG. Reflections on curative health care in Nicaragua. Am J Public Health 79(5):646–51, 1989.

14. Anonymous. Lea Guido: Hay sectores inmaduros e incomprensivos. *El Nuevo Diario* (7 August 1981), p. 6.

15. Anonymous. Comentan nombramiento en salud. *La Prensa* (2 July 1985), p. 1.

16. Wilson, PA. Regionalization and decentralization in Nicaragua. Latin American Perspectives 14(2):237–54, 1987.

17. OMS/OPS/UNICEF. Documentos basicos de coordinacion de la cooperacion interagencial en Nicaragua. Managua, OPS/UNICEF, 1985.

18. Wheelock, J. El sector agropequario en la transformacion revolucionaria. Revolucion y Desarrollo 1:14, 1984. For a more positive perspective, see Darrow, K and Pam, R. Appropriate Technology Sourcebook. Stanford, Volunteers in Asia, 1976.

19. Werner, D. Donde no hay doctor: Una guia para los campesinos que viven lejos de los centros medicos. Palo Alto, La Fundacion Hesperian, 1980.

20. Anonymous. A survival economy. *Envio* 4:52, 1985.

21. Borsari, A, Sessa, C, and Flores, B. Proyecto de un programa piloto de deteccion del cancer del cuello uterino en el area de salud No. 6 region III. Managua, MINSA, 1987.

22. Herdocia MM. La salud en Nicaragua. *La Prensa* (23 April 1990).

23. MINSA. Plan de salud 1988–1990. Managua, 1988.

24. Salmeron, E. Quien privatice salud, quiebra. *Barricada.*

25. Nicaragua is hardly unique in this area. About two-thirds of the world's population lives in areas where registration of births and deaths is poor, and even in the United States only 75 percent of maternal deaths are reported. For more on this, see Rubin, G, McCarthy, B, Shelton, J, Rochat, RW, and Terry, J. The risk of childbearing re-evaluated. Am J Publlic Health 71:712, 1981.

Yet even where vital statistics systems are poor at recording the total number of events, it is often possible to derive useful estimates from data trends by year. In the early sixties, for example, it is believed that about a quarter of all malaria cases were reported. By the eighties, this had increased to about half of all cases. Since reporting levels changed only gradually, the annual number of reported cases is probably a good indicator of changes in disease transmission. Also see Escudero, JC. Los sistemas de informacion en salud en America Latina. Revista Centroamericano de Ciencias de la Salud 14:109–22, 1979.

26. Palloni, A. Mortality in Latin America: Emerging patterns. Population Dev Rev 7(4):623–49, 1981.

27. Monto, AS and Johnson, KM. Respiratory infections in the American tropics. Am J Tropic Med Hyg 17(8):867–71, 1968.

28. Delgado, HL, Giron, EM, de Leon, H, and Hurtado, E. Epidemiology of acute respiratory infection in preschool children of rural Guatemala. PAHO Bull 22(4):383–93, 1988.

29. Oficina de Vigilancia Epidemiologica. Evaluacion de la vigilancia epidemiologica primer trimestre 1987. Boletin Epidemiologico Nicaraguense 2:1–3, 1987.

30. Cole, DC, McConnell, R, Murry, DL, and Anton, FP. Pesticide illness surveillance: The Nicaraguan experience. PAHO Bull 22(2):119–32, 1988.

31. MINSA. Analisis de la vigilancia epidemiologica del ano 1986. Boletin Epidemiologico Nicaraguense 1:1–3, 1987.

32. MINSA, Region 3. Algunas ideas sobre el medico del barrio. MINSA, Managua, 1989.

33. Danielson, R. Cuban Medicine. New Brunswick, Transaction Books, 1979.

34. See for example Donahue, JM. The Nicaraguan Revolution in Health. South Hadley, Bergin & Garvey, 1986.

35. Bossert, TJ. Health care in revolutionary Nicaragua. In Walker, TW, ed. Nicaragua in Revolution. New York, Praeger, 1982.

CHAPTER 7

1. Deighton, J, Horsley, R, Stewart, S, and Cain, C. Sweet Ramparts: Women in Revolutionary Nicaragua. London, War on Want, 1983.

2. MINSA. Normas de atencion prenatal. Managua, MINSA, 1984.

3. MINSA. Plan de salud 1988–1990. Managua, MINSA, 1987.

4. MINSA. Plan de salud 1986. Managua, MINSA, 1985.

5. Houtart, F and Lemercinier, G. Creencias y practicas que conciernen a la salud, en los grupos populares rurales y urbanos Nicaraguense. Louvain-la-Neuve, Universite Catholique de Louvain, 1984.

6. Norory, M. Abortion in Nicaragua. Nicaragua Health Fund Newsletter 4:7, 1987.

7. PAHO. Health of women in the Americas. Washington, DC, PAHO, 1985.

8. WHO. Maternal mortality rates. Geneva, WHO Bull 2, 1985.

9. Kwast, B. Maternal mortality: Levels, causes and promising interventions. J Biosoc Sci 10(suppl):51–67, 1989.

10. Anonymous. The health situation in revolutionary Nicaragua. *Envio,* 1983.

11. Guido, C, Garcia, M, and Navas, D. Analisis de 2746 abortos atendidos en el hospital general de Nicaragua. Int Surg 56(2):125–27, 1971.

12. Altamirano, L. Aborto inducido ilegalmente: Costos y consequencias. Presentation at Jornada Cientifica Nacional de Salud, Managua, November 1985.

13. ADN. Resultados de la encuesta sobre conocimiento, actitud, y practica hacia la educacion sexual y planificacion familiar. Managua, ADN, 1978.

14. Yopo, B. Nicaraguaneses menores en circunstancias especialmente deficiles. Managua, UNICEF, 1989.

15. UNICEF. Situacion de la ninez Nicaraguense. Managua, UNICEF, 1990.

16. MINSA. Campana defensa vida del nino. Boletin informativo 11:6–7, 1990.

17. Lebrun, JF. La imagen de los centros de salud en los medios populares de Nicaragua. Louvain-la-Neuve, Centro Tricontinental, 1984.

18. Heiby, JR. Low-cost health delivery systems: Lessons from Nicaragua. Am J Public Health 71(5):514–19, 1981.

19. Luisier, V. Te voy a ayudar nada mas . . . apuntes sobre las parteras empiricas en Nicaragua. MINSA, Nicaragua, 1985.

20. Pascoe, M and Stein, A. Midwifery work exchange project in Nicaragua. J Nurse-Midwifery 32(2):101–104, 1987.

21. Colectiva del libro de salud de las mujeres de Boston: Nuestros cuerpos, nuestras vidas: Un libro por y para las mujeres. Boston, The Boston Women's Health Book Collective, 1979.

22. Borge, T. Women's liberation in Nicaragua. Speech in León, Nicaragua, 29 September 1982. Translated and published in Intercontinental Press 1 November 1982, pp. 794–800.

23. Anonymous. Planning health care for women. Nicaragua Health Fund Newsletter 4:6–7, 1987.

24. Sandiford, P, Morales, P, Gorter, A, Coyle, E, and Smith, GD. Why do child mortality rates fall? An analysis of the Nicaraguan experience. Am J Public Health 81(1):30–37, 1991.

25. See for example Basch, PF. Textbook of International Health. Oxford University Press, New York, 1990, 158–161.

26. Caldwell, JC. Routes to decreased mortality in poor countries. Population Dev Rev 12(2):171–219, 1986.

CHAPTER 8

1. Miller, V. Between Struggle and Hope: The Nicaraguan Literacy Crusade. Boulder, Westview Press, 1985.

2. CIERA/PAN/CIDA. Informe del primer seminario sobre estrategia alimentaria. Managua, CIERA, 1983.

3. MINSA. El sistema nacional unico de salud: Tres años de revolucion 1979–1982. Managua, MINSA, 1983.

4. CELADE. La mortalidad en la niñez en Centroamerican, Panama y Belice: Nicaragua 1970–1986. San Jose, CELADE, 1988.

5. Silva, F. La salud del niño. Managua, Ministerio de Cultura, 1986.

6. Terra, JP. The major problems affecting children in Latin America. Assignment Children 47/48:79–91, 1979.

7. Puffer, RR and Serrano, CV. Patterns of mortality in childhood. Washington, DC, PAHO Sci Publ No. 262, 1973.

8. Grosse, RN. Interrelation between health and population: Observations derived from field experiences. Soc Sci Med 14c:99–120, 1980.

9. Baum, S and Arriaga, E. Levels, trends, differentials, and causes of early childhood mortality in Latin America. World Health Stat Q 34(3):147–67, 1981.

10. Behm, H. Mortalidad en los primeros años de vida en paises de America Latina. Costa Rica, CELADE, Serie A, No. 1024–1032 y 1036–1039, 1976–1978.

11. Behm, H. Mortalidad en America Central: Realidad actual y perspectivas. Revista Centroamericana de Ciencias de Salud 9:9–35, 1981.

12. MINSA. Programa control de enfermedades diarreicas. Managua, MINSA, 1980.

13. Scardino, PT. Bacterial diarrhea in eastern Nicaragua. Southern Med J 64(7): 823–29, 1971.

14. Zeldin, L. El impacto de la terapia de rehidratación oral en Nicaragua y perspectivas. Managua, MINSA/CIES, 1985.

15. Heiby, JR: Low-cost health delivery systems: Lessons from Nicaragua. Am J Public Health 71:514–19, 1981.

16. Braveman, P. Primary health care takes root in Nicaragua. World Health Forum 6:369–72, 1985.

17. Hirschhorn, N. Oral rehydration therapy: The programme and the promise. In Cash, R, Keusch, GT, and Lamstein, J, eds. Child Health and Survival. Helm, Wolfboro, 1987.

18. MINSA. Diarrhoeael diseases control programme. Weekly Epidemiol Rec 60:93–100, 1985.

19. Garfield, RM, Siu, C, Arguello, CA, Frieden, T, Vermund, SH, and Williams, G. Impact of diarrhea control programs in Nicaragua, 1980–1986. Unpublished.

20. Arostegui, J and Whitaker, E. Desarrollo del programa de monitoreo y evaluacion a traves de sitios centinela en Nicaragua 1984–1990. Managua, UNICEF, 1990.

21. Myers, A. Diarrhea and the revolution. Links 2(4):3, 1985.

22. Halperin, D and Garfield, R. Developments in health care in Nicaragua. N Engl J Med 307:388–92, 1982.

23. Anonymous. The health situation in revolutionary Nicaragua. *Envio,* 1983.

24. Williams, H. Organization and delivery of health care: A study of change in Nicaragua. In Morgan, JH, ed. Third World Medicine and Social Change. Lanham, University Press of America, 1983.

25. See also Rashad, H. Oral rehydration therapy and its effect on child mortality in Egypt.

26. Sequeira, M and Valdez, L. Estudio clinico epidemiologic de fallecidos menores de 5 años por enfermedad diarreica aguda en Region III, 1985. Boletin Epidemiologico Nicaraguense 1:10–11, 1987.

27. Torres, OD. Determinantes de la morbi-mortalidad por enfermedad diarreica de los menores de cinco años que acuden a los hospitales infantiles de Managua. Master's thesis, Managua, CIES, 1986.

28. MINSA. Manejo de la enfermedad diarreica aguda y la deshidratacion segun nivel de atencion. Managua, MINSA, 1985.

29. MINSA. Plan de salud 1988–1990. Managua, MINSA, 1987.

30. Watson, G. Desarrollo y perspectivas del programa atencion materno infantil. Boletin Nicaraguense de Higiene y Epidemiologia 1(2):33–43, 1984.

31. Anonymous. Interview with Dr. Fernando Silva. *Barricada Internacional* (8 September 1988), p. 4.

32. Ministerio de Salud. Sumario de estudios sobre el estratado nutricional de la poblacion. Managua, 1974.

33. From unpublished data generated as part of a study reported in Wolfe, BL and Behrman, I. Determinants of child mortality, health, and nutrition in a developing country. J Dev Economics 11:163–93, 1982.

34. Lindenberg, CS, Cabrera-Artola, R, and Jimenez, V. The effect of early postpartum mother-infant contact and breast-feeding promotion on the incidence and continuation of breast-feeding. Int J Nurs Stud 27(3):179–86, 1990.

35. MINSA. Primer taller nacional sobre lactancia materna. Managua, MINSA, 1980.

36. Area Materno-infantil. Programa de lactancia materna. Managua, MINSA, 1981.

37. O'Leary de Macias, G. A women's movement in Nicaragua, an advocate of breast-feeding. Assignment Children 55/56:117–30, 1981.

38. MINSA/CIES. Enfoque de riesgo y estado nutricional de los ninos menores de 5 años en la region 3. Managua, CIES, 1988.

39. Tefel, RA, Mendoza, H, and Flores, J. Social welfare. In Walker, T, ed. Nicaragua: The First Five Years. New York, Praeger, 1985.

40. See Navarro, V. Social class, political power, and the state: Their implications in medicine. In Navarro, V, ed. Medicine under Capitalism. New York, Prodist, 1977.

41. Trowbridge, FL and Newton, LH. Seasonal changes in malnutrition and diarrheal disease among preschool children in El Salvador. Am J Trop Med Hyg 28(1):136–41, 1979.

42. Teller, C, Sibrian, R, Talavera, C, Bent, V, Del Canto, J, and Saenz, L. Population and nutrition: Implications of sociodemographic trends and differentials for food and nutrition policy in Central America and Panama. Ecol Food Nutr 8:95–109, 1979.

43. Teller, CH. Demografia de la desnutricion en America Central. Intercom 6–9, 1981.

44. May, JM and McLellan, DL. The republic of Nicaragua. In May, JM and McLellan, DL, eds. The Ecology of Malnutrition in Mexico and Central America. New York, Hafner, 1972.

45. Delgado, HL, Valverde, V, Belizan, JM, and Klein, RE. Diarrheal diseases, nutritional status and health care: Analysis of their interrelationships. Ecol Food Nutr 12:229–34, 1983.

46. Aburto, A. Primer censo nacional de talla en escolares de primer grado de primaria de la Republica de Nicaragua. PAN, Managua, 1986.

47. Palacios, MA and Romero, A. Situacion y perspectiva de la nutricion en Nicaragua. Boletin Nicaraguense de Higiene y Epidemiologia 1(1):55–58, 1984.

48. CARE. Children's survival assistance program. Needs assessment team field report: Nicaragua. New York, CARE, 1988.

49. INEC. Efectos socio-economicos de la guerra de agresion. Managua, INEC, 1988.

50. Sandiford, P, Morales, P, Gorter, A, Coyle, E, and Smith, GD. Why do chilld

mortality rates fall? An analysis of the Nicaraguan experience. Am J Public Health 81(1):30–37, 1991.

51. Wolfe, BL and Behrman, I. Determinants of child mortality, health, and nutrition in a developing country. J Dev Economics 11:163–93, 1982.

52. UNICEF. Datos basicos e indicadores economicos, humanos, politicos, y sociales sobre Nicaragua. Managua, UNICEF, 1988.

53. Morales, E, Oporta, R, et al. La sobrevivencia de ninos en Nicaragua: Resultados preliminares de estudios en 33 sitios sentinelas sobre la mortalidad infantil en las regiones II, III, y V. Managua, MINSA, 1988.

54. CELADE. La mortalidad en la niñez en Centroamerican, Panama y Belice: Caracteristicas principales. San Jose, CELADE, 1988.

55. Anonymous. El drama de la salud infantil. Pensamento Proprio 6:44–48, 1988.

56. Cerezo, LV, Rodriguez, A, and Duran, R. Frecuencia de factores de alto riesgo obstetrico. Managua, MINSA, 1983.

57. Hernandez, B and Jimenez, V. Enfoque de riesgo: Estrategia para la atencion primaria en Nicaragua. Salud y Ciencia en la Revolucion 1(1):19–21, 1984.

58. Anonymous. What hope for the poor? CEPAD Reports July–September 1990, pp. 1–5.

59. Behm, H. Socio-economic determinants of mortality in Latin America. Population Bulletin of the United Nations 13:1–15, 1980.

60. Carvajal, M and Burgess, P. Socioeconomic determinants of fetal and child deaths in Latin America. Soc Sci Med 12c:89–98, 1978.

61. Scrimshaw, SCM and Hurtado, E. Anthropological involvement in the Central American diarrheal disease control project. Soc Sci Med 27(1):97–105, 1988.

62. Mata, L. Diarrhoeal disease—how Costa Rica won. World Health Forum 1:141–45, 1981.

63. Mata, L. The evolution of diarrhoeal disease and malnutrition in Costa Rica. Assignment Children 61/62:195–224, 1983.

CHAPTER 9

1. Danielson, R. Cuban Medicine. New Brunswick, Transaction Books, 1979.

2. Belmar, R and Sidel, VW. An international perspective on strikes and threatened strikes by physicians. Int J Health Services 5(27):53, 1975.

3. Medina, E and Cruz-Coke, R. Chilean medicine under social revolution. N Engl J Med 295(4):193–97, 1976.

4. Navarro, V. What does Chile mean? Milbank Memorial Fund Quarterly 52:93–103, 1974.

5. APHA Task Force on Chile. History of the health care system of Chile. Am J Public Health 67(1):31–36, 1977.

6. Belmar. R. Evaluation of Chile's health care system 1973–1976. Int J Health Services 7(3):531–40, 1977.

7. See Schmalz, J. Immigrants seek to be doctors again. *New York Times* (31 May 1989), p. A16.

8. As many as fifty leftist Nicaraguans trained as physicians in the Soviet Union during the seventies. While most of them returned to Nicaragua following the Sandinista revolution, they seem to have followed no particular political trend. Like other Nicaraguan physicians, few are FSLN members, most have private practices, and many have emigrated.

9. Anonymous. Proyecto regulador preocupa a medicos. *La Prensa* (18 August 1980), p. 5.

10. Anonymous. La medicina como comercio. *El Nuevo Diario* (12 December 1984), p. 2.

11. The precise number of emigrated physicians is not known. This estimate was made by the professional's association, CONAPRO, based on information from MINSA and the Ministry of the Interior.

12. Cahil, KM. A Bridge to Peace. New York, Maymarket-Doyma, 1988, p. 11.

13. Anonymous. Politica de estimulos a la profesion medica. *El Nuevo Diario* (10 June 1985), p. 2.

14. Vigil, C. The earthquake in Managua. Lancet 1:146, 1973.

15. Garfield, RM and Taboada, E. Health service reforms in revolutionary Nicaragua. Am J Public Health 74:1138–44, 1984.

16. Anonymous. Por que se van los doctores. *La Prensa* (12 June 1985), p. 2.

17. Anonymous. Medicos con multiples quejas. *El Nuevo Diario* (23 June 1985), p. 1.

18. Anonymous. Competitor or partner? private practice in Nicaragua. Nicaragua Health Fund Newsletter 8:8–9, 1989.

19. Anonymous. Normaran la actividad de la medicina privada. *Barricada* (24 December 1988), p. 1.

20. Alvarez, E. Medicina privada: Eficiente y economica. *La Prensa* (5 January 1989), p. 3.

21. Braveman, PA and Roemer, MI. Health personnel training in the Nicaraguan health system. Int J Health Services 15(4):699–705, 1985.

22. Haddad, J. Estado actual de la ensenanza de la salud publica en Centroamerica y Panama. Educacion Medica y Salud 16(11):69–76, 1982.

23. Morley, D. Medical education in the developing world—new approaches needed. Med Teacher 1(5):258–61, 1979.

24. Facultad de Ciencias Medicas. La educacion medica en Nicaragua: Situacion actual, logros y perspectivas. Managua, UNAN, 1981.

25. Anonymous. 25 estudiantes de medicina hacia las zonas combate. *Barricada* (1 June 1984), p. 10.

26. See Slater, RG. New family practice residency programs in Nicaragua and Costa Rica. J Family Practice 28(4):468–72, 1989.

27. Perez, R. La formacion de personal especializado en salud publica: Experiencia de Nicaragua. Managua, MINSA, 1984.

28. Galiano, S. Brief history of nursing in Nicaragua. Int J Nursing Studies 12:223–29, 1975.

29. de Borg, Z, Malespin, C, Herrera de Tercero, N, and Pineda, A. Perfil profesional de la enfermera y su responsibilidad ante la sociedad actual. Managua, Colegio de Enfermeras Nicaraguenses, 1980.

30. Garfield, RM. Health in Nicaragua today: Interview with Concepcion Huerte Ramirez. Catalyst 2(4):45–54, 1980.

31. Molina, G. Situacion actual y perspectiva de desarrollo en la carrera de enfermeria a nivel tecnico y superior. Managua, MINSA, 1985.

32. Garfield, RM. The evolution of nursing in Nicaragua. Nursing Outlook 36(1):25–29, 1988.

33. Lewis, C and Squires, A. Where every plaster counts: The reality of nursing in Nicaragua. Nicaragua Health Fund Newsletter 6:1–2, 1988.

34. Anonymous. Descentralizar la formacion de especialists medicos, tecnicos, y las enfermeras. *Barricada* (15 February 1984), p. 7.

35. Scholl, EA. An assessment of community health workers in Nicaragua. Soc Sci Med 20:207–14, 1985.

36. See Ugalde, A. Where there is a doctor: Strategies to increase productivity at lower costs. Soc Sci Med 19(4):441–50, 1984.

CHAPTER 10

1. Houtart, F and Lemercinier, G. Creencias y practicas que conciernen a la salud, en los grupos populares rurales y urbanos Nicaraguense. Louvain-la-Neuve, Universite Catholique de Louvain, 1984.

2. Anonymous. Como acabar con anarquia y explotacion con medicinas. *El Nuevo Diario* (21 August 1981), p. 1.

3. For a discussion of the tuberculosis situation see: Anonymous. Taking on T.B. Nicaragua Health Fund Newsletter 4:1–3, 1987.

4. MINSA. Informe sobre la situacion de la tuberculosis en Nicaragua. Managua, MINSA, 1980.

5. MINSA. Plan de salud 1988–1990. Managua, MINSA, 1987.

6. Cortes, G. A parar la guerra de las hormigas. *Barricada* (21 April 1982), p. 4.

7. Hernandez, L. Al "reventar" inventarios de medicamentos. *Barricada* (25 August 1988), p. 1.

8. Matheson, C. Advice from Bangladesh. Nicaragua Health Fund Newsletter 5:3–4, 1987.

9. Ruiz, M and Sanchez, R. Medicamentos como insumos criticos. Master's thesis. Managua, CIES, 1984.

10. CAM. La producion e importacion de medicamentos y la problematica de la Central de Abastecimientos Medicos. Managua, MINSA, 1981.

11. PAHO. Essential drugs revolving fund for Central America and Panama. PAHO Bull 22(3):313–16, 1988.

12. Laporte, J and Tognoni, G. Drug policy in Nicaragua. Dev Dialogue 2:121–28, 1985.

13. MINSA. Formulario nacional de medicamentos. Managua, MINSA, 1985.

14. Almasi, MS. Desarrollo del sector farmaeutico de Nicaragua. Geneva, United National Industrial Development Organization, 1985.

15. Anonymous. A survival economy. *Envio* 4:52, 1985.

16. Green, D. Rescuing their roots: Herbal medicine. Nicaragua Health Fund Newsletter 3:5–6, 1987.

17. Sotomayor, U, Cardoza, J, and Brussel, J. Rescate de la medicina popular en el uso, aplicacion y cultivo de plantas medicinales en Region I. 1(1):40–43, Salud 1987.

18. But it is a profoundly complex issue. See for example: Bonair, A, Rosenfield, P, and Tengyald, K. Medical technologies in developing countries: Issues of technology development, transfer, diffusion, and use. Soc Sci Med 28(8):769–81, 1989.

19. Joseph, SC. Iron axe, magic lamp, or Trojan horse: Issues in cross-cultural transfer of health technology. In James, G and Sax Jacoles, B, eds. The Technology Explosion in Medical Science: Implications for the Health Care Industry and the Public. New York, SP Medical and Scientific Books, 1983.

20. Mitchell, EL, Martinez-Silva, R, Vardham, H, and Vazques, IA. Administracion, mantenimiento y reparacion de equipos para laboratorios en los paises en desarrollo. Boletin de la Organizacion Sanitaria Panamericana 95(5):393–408, 1983.

21. Simon, R. Nicaragua's health system in crisis. *Miami Herald* (25 November 1990), p. 1.

22. Quoted in Lefton, D. Nicaragua: Health care under the Sandinistas. Can Med Assoc J 130:781–84, 1984.

CHAPTER 11

1. Zschock, DK. Health care financing in developing countries. Washington, DC, APHA, 1979.

2. Gish, O and Feller, LL. Planning pharmaceuticals for primary health care. Washington, DC, APHA, 1979.

3. Braveman, P. Primary health care takes root in Nicaragua. World Health Forum 6:368–72, 1985.

4. PAHO. National and international financial and budgeting implications of regional strategies and the plan of action for health for all by the year 2000. Washington, DC, PAHO, WHO, 1984.

5. OMS/OPS/UNICEF. Documentos basicos de coordinacion de la cooperacion interagencial en Nicaragua. Managua, OPS/UNICEF, 1985.

6. OPS/OMS/UNICEF. Documento de programacion de la coordinacion interagencial. Managua: OPS/UNICEF, 1986.

7. MINSA. Health plan 1988–1990. MINSA, Managua, 1987.

8. Donahue, JM. International organizations, health services, and national building in Nicaragua. Med Anthropol Q 3(3):258–69, 1989.

9. Linsenmeyer, WS. Foreign nations, international organizations, and their impact on health conditions in Nicaragua since 1979. Int J Health Services 19(3):500–29, 1989.

10. INEC. Efectos socio-economicos de la guerra de agresion. Managua, INEC, 1988.

CHAPTER 12

1. ECLA. Nicaragua: Economic Repercussions of Recent Political Events. Santiago de Chile: United Nations, 1979.

2. Fagen, R, Deere, CD, and Coraggio, JL, eds. Transition and Development: Problems of Third World Socialism. New York, Monthly Review Press, 1986.

3. JGN. The philosophies and policies of the government of Nicaragua. In Rosset, P and Vandermeer, J, eds. The Nicaragua Reader. New York, Grove Press, 1983.

4. Vilas, CM. Perfiles de la revolucion Sandinista. Buenos Aires, Editorial Legasa, 1984.

5. Walker, TW, ed. Reagan Versus the Sandinistas. Boulder, Westview Press, 1987.

6. Miller, V. Between Struggle and Hope: The Nicaraguan Literacy Crusade. Boulder, Westview Press, 1985.

7. Le Boterf, G. The challenge of mass education in Nicaragua. Assignment Children 65/68:247–66, 1984.

8. Tefel, RA, Mendoza, H, and Flores, J. Social welfare. In Walker, T, ed. Nicaragua: The First Five Years. New York, Praeger, 1985.

9. UNICEF. Datos basicos e indicadores economicos, humanos, politicos, y sociales sobre Nicaragua. Managua, UNICEF, 1988.

10. Gariazzo, A, Acosta, M, and Bermudez, A. Analisis de la situacion economico-social de Nicaragua. Managua, UNICEF, 1984.

11. CIERA/ATC/UNAG. Produccion y organizacion en el agro Nicaraguense. Managua, CIERA, 1982.

12. Solon, L, Barraclough, T, and Scott MF. The Rich Have Already Eaten. London, Transnational Institute, 1987.

13. Ministerio de Salud. Diagnostico del sector salud de Nicaragua. Managua, Ministerio de Salud, 1975.

14. Collins, J. Nicaragua: What Difference Could a Revolution Make? New York, Grove Press, 1986.

15. Austin, J, Fox, J, and Kruger, W. The role of the revolutinoary state in the Nicaraguan food system. World Development 13(1):15–40, 1985.

16. Reinhardt, N. Agro-exports and the peasantry in the agrarian reforms of El Salvador and Nicaragua. World Development 15(7):941–59, 1987.

17. Zalkin, M. Food policy and class transformation in revolutionary Nicaragua, 1979–1986. World Development 15(7):961–84, 1987.

18. Fitzgerald, V. Agrarian reform as a model of accumulation: The case of Nicaragua since 1979. J Dev Studies 22(1), 1985.

19. MIDINRA. Sector agropecuario: Resultados 1983, plan de trabajo 1984. Managua, MIDINRA, 1984.

20. CEPAL. Istmo Centroamericano: Crisis economica y planificacion del desarrollo. LC/MEX/R.2. CEPAL, Mexico, 1985.

21. Musgrove, P. The economic crisis and its impact on health and health care in Latin America and the Caribbean. Int J Health Services 17(3):411, 1987.

22. Musgrove, P. Impact of the economic crisis on health and health care in Latin America and the Caribbean. WHO Chronicles 40(4):152–57, 1986.

23. Barraclough, S. Aid that Counts: The western Contribution to Development and Survival in Nicaragua. Amsterdam, Transnational Institute/Birmingham: Third World Publications, 1988.

24. Anonymous. A survival economy. *Envio* 4:52, 1985.

25. *Barricada Internacional* 34(261):p. 10, 1988.

26. Uhlig, MA. Nicaraguan study depicts economy in drastic decline. *New York Times* (26 January 1989), p. 1.

27. MINSA. Health plan 1987. MINSA, Managua, 1986.

28. Anonymous. Devaluations in Nicaragua. *New York Times* (16 August 1989), p. D14.

29. Anonymous. How will Nicaragua survive hurricane Joan? Nicaragua Health Fund Newsletter 9:1–4, 1989.

30. ECLAC. Report on damage caused to Nicaragua by hurricane Joan. New York, United Nations, 1988.

31. Grant, J. State of the World's Children Report, 1989. London, Oxford University Press, 1988.

32. Atlimir, O. Poverty, income distribution and child welfare in Latin America: A comparison of pre- and post-recession data. World Development 3:261–82, 1984.

CHAPTER 13

1. Both quotations from Rother, L. Message for Nicaragua's victors: Things must get better, and fast. *New York Times* (4 March 1990), p. 1.

2. See also Nelson, H and Nelson, G. Health and medicine in Nicaragua. Hospital Practice 25(2):109–119, 1990.

3. Hopkinson, A and Chalmers, F. Nicaragua, the first 100 days. Lancet 300–301, 1990.

4. FSLN. Plataforma electoral: La salud y el bienestar social, pp. 22–24.

5. Anonymous. "The León Document" of UNO. Health Committee Recommendations. *Mimeo* (14 March 1990).

6. Quoted in *Barricada* (6 June 1990).

7. NCAHRN. Report of the post-election delegation to Nicaragua. New York, NCAHRN, 1990.

8. Anonymous. Debate over the agency for international development. Links 7(2): 22, 1990.

8a. N.A. Problemas en vacunacion. *La Prensa* (27 May 1991), p. 2.

9. Lomba, M. Privatizar la salud seria asestar estocada al pueblo. *Barricada* (4 July 1990).

9a. MINSA, Plan trienal de salud, 1991–1993. Managua: MINSA, 1991.

9b. MINSA, Impacto del P.C.O. en fuerza de trabajo fisico. 1991.

10. Government of Nicaragua. Document to the Donors Conference in Rome, June 1990.

11. MINSA. Plan de salud 1988–1991. Managua, 1988.

12. World Bank. Nicaragua: Country Economic Memorandum Issues Paper. 1990.

CHAPTER 14

1. See also Bommer, J. The politics of disaster—Nicaragua. Disasters 9(4):270–78, 1985.

2. Office of US Foreign Disaster Assistance. Assessment of floods in Nicaragua's north atlantic region, July 23–27. 1990.

3. Anonymous. Atlantic coast plagued by heavy rains, political squabbles. CEPAD Reports, July–August 1990, pp. 5–6.

4. Coraggio, JL and Deere, CD, eds. La transicion dificil: La autodeterminacion de los pequeños paises perifericos. Managua, Vanguardia, 1987.

5. Fagen, R, Deere, CD, and Coraggio, JL, eds. Transition and Development: Problems of Third World Socialism. New York, Monthly Review Press, 1986.

6. See for example: Manga, P. The transformation of Zimbabwe's health care system: A review of the white paper on health. Soc Sci Med 27(11):1131–38, 1988.

7. Sanders, D and Davies, R. The economy, the health sector and child health in Zimbabwe since independence. Soc Sci Med 27(7):723–31, 1988.

8. Published in JGN. The philosophies and policies of the government of Nicaragua. In Rosset, P and Vandermeer, J, eds. The Nicaragua Reader. New York, Grove Press, 1983. See also the following texts on international health.

9. Bryant, J. Health and the Developing World. Ithaca, Cornell University Press, 1969.

10. Bryant, JH. Health for all: The dream and the reality. World Health Forum 9:291–309, 1988.

11. Roemer, MI. National Strategies for Health Care Organization. Ann Arbor, Health Administration Press, 1985.

12. Roemer, MI. The changeability of health care systems. Med Care 24(1):24–29, 1986.

13. Roemer, MI. Medical care in Latin America. Washington, DC, OAS, 1963.

14. Sidel, VW and Sidel, R. A Healthy State: An International Perspective on the Crisis in United States Medical Care. New York, Pantheon Books, 1977.

15. Navarro, V. Medicine under Capitalism. New York, Prodist, 1976.

16. Basch, PF. Textbook of International Health. New York, Oxford University Press, 1989.

17. Direccion Nacional de Atencion Medica. Atencion primaria de salud en Nicaragua: Evolucion historica, logros, y dificultades. Managua, MINSA, 1984.

18. Habicht, J and Berman, PA. Strategies in primary health care. Am J Public Health 77(1):1396–97, 1987.

19. Navarro, V. Social Security and Medicine in the USSR: A Marxist Critique. Lexington, Lexington Books, 1977.

20. Harrison, P. Cuba and Costa Rica: Lessons for the third world. People 7(2): 2–4, 1980.

21. Nakajima, H. Health for all: The way ahead. World Health Forum 9:287–89, 1988.

22. Strelnick, H. Health care under fire: An interview with Dr. Myrna Cunningham. Health/PAC Bull 17(1):15-17, 1986.

23. Anonymous. Editorial. Boletin Cientifico Contingente Medico-Cuban 9(2):1, 1987.

24. See Halstead, SB, Walsh, JA, and Warren, KS, eds. Good health at low cost. New York, The Rockefeller Foundation, 1985.

25. Kendall, C. The implementation of a diarrheal disease control program in Honduras: Is it "selective primary health care" or "integrated primary health care"? Soc Sci Med 27(1):17–23, 1988.

26. Walsh, JA and Warren, KS, eds. Strategies for Primary Health Care: Technologies Appropriate for the Control of Disease in the Developing World. Chicago, University of Chicago Press, 1986.

27. See also Chen, L. Primary health care in developing countries: overcoming operational, technical, and social barriers. Lancet 2:1260–64, 1986.

28. See also Ugalde, A. The role of the medical profession in public health policy making: The case of Colombia. Soc Sci Med 13(C):109–19, 1979.

29. See also: Zukin, P. Health and economic development: How significant is the relationship? Int Dev Rev 2:17–21, 1975.

30. Chen, LC. Coping with economic crisis: Policy development in China and India. Health Policy and Planning 2(2):138–49, 1987.

31. Bell, D and Reich, M, eds. Health, Nutrition, and Economic Crises. Dover, MA, Auburn House, 1986.

32. Grant, J, ed. The impact of world recession on children. In The State of the World's Children 1984. New York, Oxford University Press, 1984.

33. See also the tables in Grant, J. State of the World's Children Report, 1989. London, Oxford University Press, 1988.

34. Smith, DL and Bryant, JH. Building the infrastructure for primary health care: An overview of vertical and integrated approaches. Soc Sci Med 26(9):909–17, 1988.

35. Smith, B. Health situation analysis, Nicaragua, 1990. Managua, Mimeo, 1990, p. 39.

APPENDICES

1, 2. Official population estimates for Nicaragua are provided by INEC via demographic projections based on the 1971 national census. This was supplemented by a household interview survey carried out in 1985 to provide the demographic assumptions needed for projections. The data presented here represent slightly higher population estimates, based in part on the following sources:

Republica de Nicaragua. Censos nacionales 1971. Managua, Gobierno de Nicaragua, 1974.

BCN. Compendio estadistico 1965–1974. Managua, BCN, 1975.

CEPAL. Anuario estadistico de America Latina. Chile, CEPAL, 1984.

IADB. Report on demographic trends and projections for Central America. Washington, DC, IADB, 1977.

Fox, RW and Huguet, JW. Population and urban trends in Central America and Panama. Washington, DC, IADB, 1977.

3. INEC. Derived by comparing data on registered events to demographic projections of expected number of births and deaths.

4. Derived by comparing mid-year black-market exchange rates with the U.S. dollar to average corboda salary levels. 1988 data from Uhlig, M. Nicaraguan study depicts economy in drastic decline. *New York Times* (26 January 1989), p. 1.

5. Ministerio de Finanza and World Bank, unpublished.

6. Interamerican Development Bank.

7. Direccion de Finanza, MINSA and INSSBI.

8. Ministerio de Finanza and Direccion de Finanza, MINSA.

9. Ministerio de Finanza.

10. MINSA, Division de Planificacion.

11. MINSA, Plan de salud 1988–1990. Managua, MINSA, 1987.

12–15. DINEI. Also Banco central de Nicaragua. Compendio estadistico 1965–1975.

16,17. MINSA, Docencia.

18–20. DINEI.

21,22. MINSA. Plan de salud 1988–1990. Managua, MINSA, 1987.

23. CONAPRO Heroes y Martires, and MINSA, Oficina de Defensa Civil.

24. DINEI and MINSA, Docencia.

25. DINEI. Also INSS. Memoria Anual 1974–1980.

26,27. DINEI. Also Banco central de Nicaragua. Compendio estadistico 1965–1975. INSS. Memoria Anual 1974–1980.

28. DINEI. Also Gobierno de Nicaragua. Anuario estadistico de Nicaragua, 1976.

29–36. DINEI. Also Banco central de Nicaragua. Compendio estadistico 1965–1975. INSS. Memoria Anual 1974–1980.

37. MINSA, Plan de salud 1988–1990. Managua, MINSA, 1987.

38. MINSA region 3. Plan de salud 1988. Managua, MINSA, 1988.

39–48. DINEI.

49. DECOPS and MINSA, Docencia.

50. MINSA, Docencia.

51–53. DINEI. Also INEC. Oficina ejecutiva de encuestas y censos, 1977. Anuario estadistico de Nicaragua, 1976.

54. MINSA, Oficina de Defensa Civil.

55. MINSA, Division de Planificacion.

56. MINSA: Plan de salud 1988–1990. Managua, MINSA, 1987.

57. CARE. Children's survival assistance program needs assessment team field report: Nicaragua. New York, CARE, 1988.

58. INSSBI. Diez años de revolucion en el INSSBI. Managua, INSSBI, 1989. Also Informe CIAV, No. 5.

59. MINSA, Oficina de Defensa Civil.

60. Ministry of the Presidency, from data provided by the Ejercito Popular Sandinista.

61–66. Direccion de Epidemiologia, MINSA.

67,68. DINEI.

69. DINEI. Also Banco central de Nicaragua. Compendio estadistico 1965–1975.

70. DINEI and PAHO. Health conditions in the Americas 1981–1984. Washington, DC, PAHO, 1986; and PAHO. Health conditions in the Americas 1977–1980. Washington, DC, PAHO, 1982; and MINSA, Division de Planificacion.

71. INSSBI. Diez años de revolucion en el INSSBI. Managua, INSSBI, 1989.

72. INEC surveys, unpublished data. Also World Bank. Food security, health, and nutrition programs in Nicaragua. Washington, DC, 1990, unpublished.

73. Although estimates vary widely on national infant mortality levels in Nicaragua and other Central American countries, an extensive review carried out by Dr. Hugo Behm in 1987 provides widely used estimates for some years. Data for intervening years were extrapolated from those years for which there were data points. Limitations of the data and a discussion of the primary studies included are provided in: CELADE. La mortalidad en la niñez en Centroamerica, Panama and Belice: Nicargua 1970–1986. San José, CELADE, 1988.

74. Data from *Barricada International* newspaper, (8 December 1988), p. 3; and Ministry of the Economy, Industry, and Commerce as reported in INEC. Nicaragua: 10 Años en cifras. Managua, INEC, 1989. Also: Gutierrez, R. La politica economica de la revolucion. Revolucion y Desarrollo No. 5, July 1989, pp. 37–58.

75. Fitzgerald, V. Agrarian reform as a model of accumulation: The case of Nicaragua since 1979. J Dev Studies 22:1, 1985. Also World Bank. Food security, health, and nutrition programs in Nicaragua. Washington, DC, 1990, unpublished.

76. CIERA. Informe de Nicaragua a la FAO. Managua, CIERA, 1983.
MINSA. Analisis preliminar de la situation de salud en Nicaragua. Tomo II: Unidad de analisis del sector salud, 1979.
MINSA: Plan de salud 1988–1990. Managua, MINSA, 1987. Also World Bank. Food security, health, and nutrition programs in Nicaragua. Washington, DC, 1990, unpublished.

77. Zalkin, M. Food policy and class transformation in revolutionary Nicaragua, 1979–86. World Development 15(7):961–84, 1987; and Banco Central de Nicaragua. Also World Bank. Food security, health, and nutrition programs in Nicaragua. Washington, DC, 1990, unpublished.

78. Zalkin, M. Ibid.; and CIERA, as reported in INEC, Nicaragua: 10 años en Cifras. Managua, INEC, 1989. Also World Bank. Food security, health, and nutrition programs in Nicaragua. Washington, DC, 1990, unpublished.

79. MINSA. Analisis preliminar de la situation de salud en Nicaragua. Tomo II: Unidad de analisis del sector salud, 1979. Also Gobierno de Nicaragua. Presupuesto general de ingresos y egresos de la republica, 1974.
MINSA: Plan de salud 1987. Managua, MINSA, 1986.
World Bank, Diagnostico del sector salud. Washington, DC, 1990. Unpublished.

80–82. CELADE: La mortalidad en la niñez en Centroamerica, Panama and Belice: Nicaragua 1970–1986. San José, CELADE, 1988.

83. DINEI and INEC.

84. DINEI and Bartlett, L. Nicaragua health services referral system: A preliminary report. 1976. Unpublished.

85,86. CEPAL. Anuario estadistico de America Latina. Chile, CEPAL, 1984.

87. Westinghouse Corporation. Child survival, risks, and the road to health. Columbia, MD, Institute for Research Development, 1987.

88. Gallardo, ME and Lopez, JR. Centro America: La crisis en cifras. Costa Rica, Flasco, 1986.

89. CEPAL. Informe anual sobre America Latina. Mexico, CEPAL, 1986.
IADB. Economic and social progress in Latin America. Washington, DC, IADB, 1983.

90–92. Grant, J. State of the World's Children Report, 1989. New York, Oxford University Press, 1988.

93,94. CEPAL. Anuario estadistico de America Latina. Chile, CEPAL, 1984.

95. Wilkie, I and Peokel, A, eds. Statistical Abstract of Latin America. Los Angeles, University of California Press, 1986.

96. CEPAL. Anuario estadistico de America Latina. Chile, CEPAL, 1984.

97. Consejo Monetario Centroamericano. Boletin estadistico. Costa Rica, Consejo Monetario Centroamericano, 1984.

98–101. CEPAL. Notas sobre la evolucion del desarollo social del Istmo Centroamericana hasta 1980. Mexico, CEPAL, 1980.

102,103. CEPAL. Anuario estadistico de America Latina. Chile, CEPAL, 1984.

104,105. PAHO. Health conditions in the Americas 1981–1984. Washington, DC, PAHO, 1986.

106. UNESCO. Apoyo a acciones estrategicos de escolarizacion, alfabetizacion, y mejoramiento de la calidad de la educacion en Centroamerica Y Panama. Costa Rica, UNESCO 514/RLA/11, 1988.

107. INEC.

108. Oficina Ejecutiva de Encuestas y Censos. 25 años de estadistica vital. Boletin Demografico 1978; 3. Also INEC-CELADE, Document F-NIC 1. Nicaragua: estimaciones y proyecciones de poblacion 1950-2025, 1983.

109. INEC.

110. DINEI.

Additional Reading

Beson, JL, Burges, WR, and Hull, HA. Vision care in Nicaragua. J Am Optometry Assoc 48(8):1047–51, 1977.

Kraudy, E, Liberati, A, Asiolo, F, Saraceno, B, and Tognoni, G. Organization of services and pattern of psychiatric care in Nicaragua: Result of a survey in 1986. Acta Psychiatr Scand 76:545–551, 1987.

Lefton, D. Nicaragua: Health care under the Sandinistas. Can Med Assoc J 130:781–84, 1984.

Lewis, V. Power or poverty: The riddle of disabled life in Nicaragua. The Independent Fall:8–29, 1980.

Missoni, E and Morelli, R. Survey of 259 cases of American cutaneous leishmaniasis in Nicaragua. J Trop Med Hygiene 87:159–65, 1984.

Rojas, AY. Perspectives in international neurosurgery: Neurosurgery in Nicaragua. Neurosurgery 7(3):297–99, 1980.

Rosenbaum, HD. Lessons learned from a radiologic paramedic training effort in Nicaragua. Diagnostic Imaging 51:180–82, 1982.

Sandiford, P, Gorter, AC, Davey-Smith, G, and Pauw, JPC. Determinants of drinking water quality in rural Nicaragua. Epidemiol Infect 102(2), 1989.

Saraceno, B. L'esperienza psichiatrica in Nicaragua. The Practitioner Edizione Italiana 74:139–45, 1984.

Saraceno, B, Asioli, F, Tognoni, G, Flores, M, Aguilar, R, and Sequeira, S. Manual de salud mental (guia basica para atencion primaria). Managua, MINSA, 1987.

Tognoni, G. L'esperanza sanitaria del Nicaragua. The Practitioner Edizione Italiana 74:40–54, 1984.

Index

Abortion, 120, 251
Afghanistan, 86
AIDS, 126–29
Alma Ata, 23, 236

Births, 115–16, 249
Bolanos, Alejandro, 11
Brazil, 50
Bolivia, 12
Brigadistas, 28, 37, 42, 46, 57, 69, 73, 74, 83, 85, 98, 107, 109, 225, 251

Cancer, 97, 113, 119
CEPAD, 15
Child health services, 229
China, 233, 240
Chile, 26, 158
CIES, 171
Civil defense committees, 17
CISAS, 125
Computers, 107
Contra War, xiv, 45, 67, 79, 136, 145–47, 156, 160, 163, 167, 199, 208, 211, 253
Community participation, 43, 235
Costa Rica, 16, 22, 59, 153, 178, 235, 261–63
Cuba, 20, 23, 50, 101, 158, 163, 176, 197, 224, 232, 233, 234, 240

Dengue fever, 61
Diarrhea, 83, 105, 131, 138, 251
Disability, 71, 253
Doctors, 89, 94, 165–72, 188, 223, 229, 244, 246, 247

Earthquake, 3, 10, 161, 232
El Salvador, 54, 56, 153, 206

Foreign Debt, 6
FETSALUD, 15, 16, 162, 224
FSLN, 6

Germany, 16, 102, 197
Guatemala, 54, 56, 153, 261–63

Health areas, 29
Health campaigns, 14, 19, 225
Health centers and posts, 12, 26, 30, 68, 164, 249, 253
Health councils, 39, 43
Health ministers, 17, 33, 90, 95, 103, 185, 189, 239
Health posts, 26, 30, 249, 253
Honduras, 12, 16, 54, 55, 56, 59, 83, 126, 151, 153
Hospitals, 29, 30, 32, 92, 93, 99, 164, 248, 249, 253, 264, 266

Infant mortality, xv, 130, 147, 257–59, 261
Immunization, xiv, 145, 155, 255–56

La Prensa, 59, 65, 96, 100, 104
Leishmaniasis, 17
Literacy crusade, 23, 24, 28, 36, 50, 57

Malaria, 10, 39, 57, 63, 75
Malnutrition, 76, 83, 85, 141, 156, 203, 251, 257
Maternal mortality, 119–20
Measles, 36, 54, 76, 254
Medical school, 165, 259
Mexico, 16, 50, 159
Ministry of Health, 13, 22, 245
Mozambique, 80

Nurses, 9, 21, 28, 31, 87, 92, 100, 168, 229, 246, 249–50

Oral rehydration, 134–38

Parteras, 13, 35, 37, 122–23, 185, 253
PAHO, 180
PIASS, 88–90, 237
Pharmaceuticals, 175–86, 188, 227, 247
Plasmaferesis, 4
Population, 7, 244, 265
Prenatal care, xiv, 144, 251
Primary care, xv, 24, 32, 86
Private care, 33, 165
Profamilia, 127

Red Cross, 17, 56, 68, 224, 232
Regions, 29, 108
Rosales, Oscar, 10

Sandinista defense committees, 39–40
Social Security, 10, 13, 19, 27, 33, 141, 175, 194, 245, 256

Tetanus, 104, 254
Tuberculosis, 61–63

UNICEF, 87, 167, 194
USAID, 14, 19, 30, 35, 131, 189, 219, 224, 241
USSR, 197, 234

Vaccinations, 32, 36, 146
Vietnam, 70, 233
Vital statistics, 105, 244

Work-Study Program, 166

Zimbabwe, 233